OXFORD PROFESSIONAL PRACTICE

Handbook of Patient Safety

Oxford Professional Practice

Handbook of Patient Safety

EDITED BY

Peter Lachman

ASSOCIATE EDITORS

John Brennan

John Fitzsimons

Anita Jayadev

Jane Runnacles

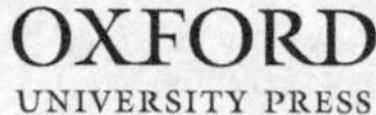

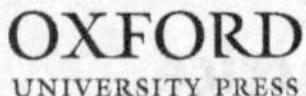

Great Clarendon Street, Oxford, OX2 6DP,
United Kingdom

Oxford University Press is a department of the University of Oxford. It furthers the University's objective of excellence in research, scholarship, and education by publishing worldwide. Oxford is a registered trade mark of Oxford University Press in the UK and in certain other countries

First Edition published in 2022

Impression: 2

Published in the United States of America by Oxford University Press
198 Madison Avenue, New York, NY 10016, United States of America

British Library Cataloguing in Publication Data
Data available

Library of Congress Control Number: 2021945574

ISBN 978–0–19–284687–7

DOI: 10.1093/med/9780192846877.001.0001

Printed in Great Britain by
Ashford Colour Press Ltd, Gosport, Hampshire

Foreword

Helen Haskell, Hussain Jafri, and Margaret Murphy
WHO Patients for Patient Safety Advisory Group

Patient safety is a field with many moving parts. It cuts across disciplines, professions, healthcare systems, business sectors, and governments. It ranges from the simple to the complex, from the intimately personal to the broadly theoretical. Perhaps more than any other area of healthcare, it embraces multiple and sometimes incompatible models of management, which have themselves evolved and changed over the years with surprising fluidity.

This sprawling combination of the philosophical and the practical is the necessary underpinning of healthcare. Without patient safety, medical treatments lose their purpose. Care flounders and can become its opposite: a source of harm. In all too many instances, in all too many parts of the world, this occurs on a regular basis. As patient leaders in patient safety, we are in a position to see the sad outcomes. For patients, safety can be everything.

In spite of the fact that patient safety is a relatively young field, there has been concern in recent years that it has ceased to be a priority of the healthcare establishment, especially in higher-income countries. Several global initiatives have aimed to reverse that trend, among them the 2014–19 Global Ministerial Summits on Patient Safety (interrupted by COVID-19 in 2020); the 2020 G20 Declaration, which names patient safety as a global priority; and the Global Patient Safety Action Plan approved by the World Health Assembly in 2021. The underlying concept is that healthcare must be made safe if the goal of universal healthcare is to have real meaning.

The goal of the present book is to address this gap by laying out the components of patient safety in a readable, yet comprehensive fashion, in a practical work of reference for anyone involved in healthcare. Its chapters include straightforward solutions that can be adopted and practised even in low-resource environments; these solutions include details of process, hygiene, medication safety, and communication. An important thread is formed by the concepts of teamwork and of flattening the hierarchy so that all can speak up for safety. Even more important is the emphasis on the role of the patient in both enabling and producing healthcare.

Why is patient engagement so important? Because, in the end, patient safety is about patients. Healthcare professionals cannot make healthcare safe without knowing what their patients experience, or without the insights and observations of patients regarding their processes and treatments. For patients, it is critical to learn to educate themselves and to advocate their own safety and that of their family members. Patients cannot, however, make themselves safe without the help of their healthcare providers. Only together can we achieve our goals.

As patient safety continues to evolve, the combined wisdom of patients and providers may yet turn out to be the major element that allows it to progress towards its goal of (dare we say it?) zero harm. This handbook, with its combination of practicality and forward thinking, is an indispensable guide along the way.

Contents

Contributors

Ahmeda Ali
General Practitioner and Assistant Director of Dublin Northeast ICGP Training Scheme
Irish College of General Practitioners
Dublin, Ireland
Chapter 2: The culture and system of patient safety

Jay Banerjee
Consultant in Geriatric Emergency Medicine
University Hospitals of Leicester NHS Trust
Leceister, England
Chapter 27: Safety in the emergency department

Rob Bethune
Consultant Surgeon
Royal Devon and Exeter NHS Foundation Trust
Exeter, England
Chapter 29: Safety in the operating theatre

Pallavi Bradshaw
Deputy Chief Medical Officer
AXA Health
London, England
Chapter 17: Open disclosure

Jeffrey Braithwaite
Professor and Founding Director
Australian Institute of Health Innovation, Macquarie University
Sydney, NSW, Australia
Chapter 11: Resilience theory, complexity science, and Safety-II

John Brennan
General Practitioner and Quality Improvement Faculty
Royal College of Physicians of Ireland
Dublin, Ireland
Chapter 4: Person-centred safety; Chapter 14 Practical approaches to safety improvement; and Chapter 26: Safety in primary care and general practice

Karen Britton
Lead Nurse Deteriorating Patient and Resuscitation
Frimley Health Foundation Trust
Frimley, England
Chapter 24: Preventing and limiting deterioration on the medical wards

Kate Churruca
Postdoctoral Research Fellow
Australian Institute of Health Innovation, Macquarie University
Sydney, NSW, Australia
Chapter 11: Resilience theory, complexity science, and Safety-II

Robyn Clay-Williams
Associate Professor
Australian Institute of Health Innovation, Macquarie University
Sydney, NSW, Australia
Chapter 11: Resilience theory, complexity science, and Safety-II

Chris Cornue
Founder & President
sláinte global partners (sgp)
Chicago, IL, USA
Chapter 19: Patient safety and information technology

David Crosby
Consultant Obstetrician and Gynaecologist, Subspecialist in Reproductive Medicine & Surgery and Perinatal & Reproductive Genetics
The National Maternity Hospital
Dublin, Ireland
Chapter 7: Communicating to be safe and Chapter 31: Safety in maternity care

Rob Cunney
Consultant Microbiologist
Children Hospital Ireland, Temple Street
Dublin, Ireland
Chapter 22: Prevention of healthcare-associated infections and Chapter 23: Sepsis and antimicrobial stewardship

Louise A. Ellis
Research Fellow
Australian Institute of Health Innovation, Macquarie University
Sydney, NSW, Australia
Chapter 11: Resilience theory, complexity science, and Safety-II

Sibylle Erdmann
Patient Carer
London, England
Chapter 4: Person-centred safety

Eoin Fitzgerald
Paediatric Registrar
Children Hospital Ireland
Dublin, Ireland
Chapter 8: Situation awareness and patient safety

John Fitzsimons
Consultant Paediatrician
Children Hospital Ireland, Temple Street
Dublin, Ireland
Chapter 2: The culture and system of patient safety and Chapter 13: Measuring patient safety on the front line

Frank Frederico
Vice President
Institute for Healthcare Improvement
Boston, MA, USA
Chapter 20: Enabling medication safety

Sean Harding
Consultant Nurse Acute Care & Trust Lead for Advanced Clinical Practice
Frimley Health NHS Foundation Trust
London, England
Chapter 28: Safety in ambulatory care

Helen Haskell
President at Mothers Against Medical Error
WHO Patients for Patient Safety
Lexington County, SC, USA
Preface

Daniel Hayes
Senior Research Fellow, Evidence Based Practice Unit
University College London and the Anna Freud National Centre for Children and Families
London, England
Chapter 32: Safety issues in mental health

Sue Hignett
Professor of Healthcare Ergonomics & Patient Safety
Loughborough Design School, Loughborough University
Loughborough, England
Chapter 9: Practical application of human factors and ergonomics to improve safety

James Hoffman
Chief Patient Safety Officer
St Judes Childrens Research Hospital
Memphis, TN, USA
Chapter 21: Safe prescribing in paediatrics

Kristen Hughes
Clinical Pharmacist, Medication Safety and Informatics
St Judes Childrens Research Hospital
Memphis, TN, USA
Chapter 21: Safe prescribing in paediatrics

Hussein Jaffrey
Patient Advocate World Patient Alliance
WHO Patients for Patient Safety
Pakistan
Preface

Kirstyn James
Consultant Geriatrician
Cork University Hospital
Cork, Ireland
Chapter 34: Safety in patients with frailty and complex long-term conditions

Anita Jayadev
Consultant Respiratory Physician
Wexham Park Foundation NHS Trust
London, England
Chapter 24: Preventing and limiting deterioration on the medical wards; Chapter 28: Safety in ambulatory care; and Chapter 37: Patient safety in a pandemic

Thomas Jun
Reader in Socio-technical System Design
Loughborough University
Loughborough, England
Chapter 9: Practical application of human factors and ergonomics to improve safety

Uma Kotagal
Emerirus Professor
Cincinnati Children Hospital Medical Centre
Cinncinati, OH, USA
Chapter 10: Reliability in healthcare

Peter Lachman
Lead Faculty Quality Improvement Programme
Royal College of Physicians of Ireland
Dublin, Ireland
Chapter 1: Introduction to patient safety; Chapter 3: Transparent leadership for safety; Chapter 7: Communicating to be safe; Chapter 8: Situation awareness and patient safety; Chapter 10: Reliability in healthcare; Chapter 14: Practical approaches to safety improvement; and Chapter 37: Patient safety in a pandemic

Thomas Lamont
Senior Lecturer and Honorary Consultant in Restorative Dentistry
University of Dundee
Dundee, Scotland
Chapter 12: Measuring patient safety at a national, organization, and system level

Michaela LaRegina
Clinical Risk Manager,
Azienda Sociosanitaria Ligure 5,
La Spezia, Italy
Chapter 37: Patient safety in a pandemic

Jason Leitch
Professor and National Clinical Director
Scottish Government
Edinburgh, Scotland
Chapter 12: Measuring patient safety at a national, organization, and system level

Janet C. Long
Senior Research Fellow
Australian Institute of Health Innovation, Macquarie University
Sydney, NSW, Australia
Chapter 11: Resilience theory, complexity science, and Safety-II

Michael Marx
Professor for International Public Health, Institute of Public Health
Universität Heidelberg
Heidelberg, Germany
Chapter 14: Practical approaches to safety improvement and Chapter 35: Safety in a multidisciplinary team

Margaret Murphy
Mother and Patient Advocate
WHO Patients for Patient Safety
Cork, Ireland
Preface and Chapter 4: Person-centred safety

Kieran Murray
Consultant Rheumatologist
University Hospital Limerick
Limerick Ireland
Chapter 35: Safety in a multidisciplinary team

Eugene Nelson
Professor
The Dartmouth Institute of Health Policy & Clinical Practice
Dartmouth, NH, USA
Chapter 4: Person-centred safety

Gail Nielsen
Consultant in Advancing Healthcare Transformation
Des Moines, Iowa, USA
Chapter 25: Preventing and limiting diagnostic error

Mark O'Brien
Associate Fellow Programme Director, Oxford Healthcare Leadership Programme
Saïd Business School, University of Oxford
Oxford, England
Chapter 17: Open disclosure

Patricia O'Connor
Honorary Professor
University of Stirling, Faculty of Healthcare Sciences and Sport
Dundee, Scotland
Chapter 6: Developing a safe clinical team

Kevin O'Hare
Consultant Histopathologist
Tallaght Hospital
Dublin, Ireland
Chapter 36: Safety in the laboratory

James F O'Mahony
Health Economist
Centre for Health Policy & Management, Trinity College
Dublin, Ireland
Chapter 5: The economics of patient safety

Susanne O'Reilly
Consultant Gastroenterologist
St Vincent's University Hospital
Dublin, Ireland
Chapter 14: Practical approaches to safety improvement

Suying Ong
Anaesthetics Registrar
Anaesthetic Department Royal Alexandra Hospital
Paisley, Scotland
Chapter 33: Patient safety in critical care

Shefal Patel
Acute Medical Consultant
Wexham Park Hospital
London, England
Chapter 24: Preventing and limiting deterioration on the medical wards

Adrian Plunkett
Consultant Paediatrician
Intensive Care
Birmingham Childrens Hospital
Birmingham, England
Chapter 15: Learning from success to become safer

Rachel Pool
Intelligence Analyst
Healthcare Safety Investigation Branch (HSIB)
Farnborough, England
Chapter 16: Investigating and learning from adverse events

Damian Roland
Professor and Consultant in Paediatric Emergency Medicine
University Hospital of Leicester NHS Trust
Leceister, England
Chapter 27: Safety in the emergency department

Kevin Rooney
Clinical Director for Critical Care, Clyde Sector
Consultant in Anaesthesia and Intensive Care Medicine
Royal Alexandra Hospital
Paisley, Scotland
Chapter 33: Patient safety in critical care

Jane Runnacles
Consultant Paediatrician
St Georges University Hospital NHS Trust
London, England
Chapter 13: Measuring patient safety on the front line and
Chapter 30: Safety in paediatrics and child health

Blair L. Sadler
Senior Fellow
Institute for Healthcare Improvement
San Diego, CA, USA
Chapter 3: Transparent leadership for safety

Kevin Stewart
Medical Director
Healthcare Safety Investigation Branch (HSIB)
Farnborough, England
Chapter 16: Investigating and learning from adverse events

Riccardo Tartaglia
Professor in Risk Management, Marconi University, Italy
Chapter 37: Patient safety in a pandemic

Kris Vanhaecht
Professor
KU Leuven Institute for Healthcare Policy
Leuven, Belgium
Chapter 18: Caring for the caregivers: The second victim

Tricia Woodhead
Associate Director for Patient Safety
West of England Academic Health Science Network (AHSN)
Bristol, England

Chapter 25: Preventing and limiting diagnostic error

Part 1

Introduction to the science and theory of patient safety

Chapter 1

Introduction to patient safety

Key points

Patient safety is a framework of organized activities that creates cultures, processes, procedures, behaviours, technologies, and environments in healthcare that consistently and sustainably lower risks, reduce the occurrence of avoidable harm, make error less likely and reduce its impact when it does occur.

World Health Organisation, *Global Patient Safety Action Plan 2021–2030*

Why patient safety is important

Every day clinicians are faced with the challenge of keeping the people they treat safe and free from harm, while, delivering the care they need. This task has become more difficult as a result of the increasing complexity of healthcare, especially in relation to chronic illness, and a continuously aging population.

Patient safety is a relatively new field of study and traditionally has not been part of the medical curriculum. The concept of patient safety, however, is not new; the maxim 'First do no harm', attributed to Hippocrates, goes back about two and a half thousand years.

Throughout the history of medicine patient safety has passed many milestones, such as Semmelweis's recommendations for handwashing in 1847 and Florence Nightingale's reports on infection rates in military hospitals in 1855.

In the 1960s, the harm caused by thalidomide led to a greater understanding of drug-related adverse events. Many consider that the modern patient safety movement started after a publication of the Harvard Medical Practice Study in 1991. This study revealed a significant and measurable problem with patient safety in US hospitals and in the following years was replicated around the world, with similar findings. This led to the development of what can now be considered as the science of patient safety.

The extent of the problem was highlighted in the Institute of Medicine's 1999 publication of *To Err Is Human*, which detailed the extent of the problem in the USA, estimating that up to 100,000 patients die each year from adverse events. Concurrently, in the UK, the NHS was responding to the emerging awareness of patient safety concerns through the development of clinical risk management and clinical governance strategies.

In 2000 an NHS review, *Organisation with a Memory*, estimated that there were over 850,000 adverse events in UK hospitals each year. Despite this awareness, serious events still occurred, and detailed enquiries revealed systematic deficits in patient safety. These deficits included the lack of a culture of safety, a blame environment, and a poor understanding of how to be safe.

The 2013 Berwick report, a response to the safety culture crisis at Mid Staffordshire NHS Foundation Trust, stated that 'mastery of quality and patient safety sciences and practices should be part of initial preparation and lifelong education of all healthcare professionals, including managers and executives'.

This handbook aims to provide frontline clinicians with an easy-to-read reference work that can address this challenge. The handbook brings the principles of patient safety to frontline health professionals such as doctors, nurses, and other health professionals. Patient safety is often seen as a complex topic. We aim to offer simple interventions to protect patients and staff from potential adverse events and harm.

Quality of care and patient safety

[illegible]

[illegible]

[illegible]

[illegible]

Quality of care and patient safety

Quality of care has always been a feature of healthcare. The modern quality in healthcare movement commenced with the publication of *Crossing the Quality Chasm* by the Institute of Medicine in the USA in 2001. Previously, standards in healthcare had been developed and services had been evaluated against the standards in the accreditation or external evaluation process. Donabedian postulated that one can achieve quality *outcomes* only if one has the *structures* or systems in place and if there are *processes* by which those outcomes are to be achieved. The past twenty years have registered the growth of improvement and implementation science, which has developed theories and methods to improve care.

One can view quality of care as being a system made up of different components or domains. If one wants to achieve good quality care, all elements of the system need to be fully operational, working together to ensure desired outcomes are achieved.

Figure 1.1 indicates how all the domains of quality are interrelated.

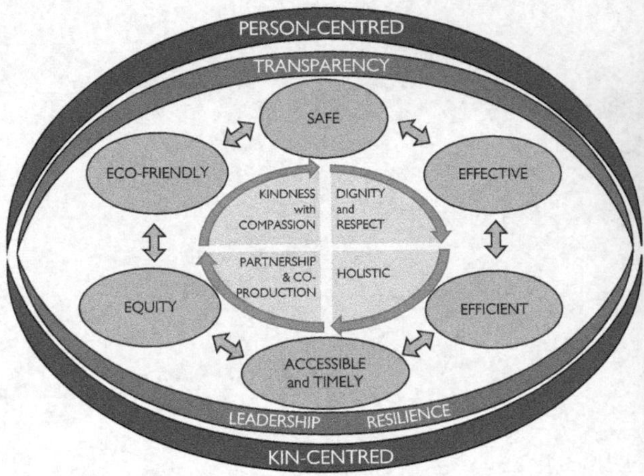

Figure 1.1 The quality system.

The quality system will function well when there is a culture that facilitates the development of the structures and processes required to produce the desired outcome. Person- or kin-centred care surrounds all the domains of quality and must be acknowledged as one develops safer care. As one explores the challenge of delivering safe care, it will become apparent that every domain of quality has a safety element. For example, one of the domains is the provision of timely care and of good access to care. Delayed diagnosis therefore is a safety and quality issue. An important quality challenge is the provision of equitable care to all, and this applies to how we design the system so that it is always safe.

This system must operate in all the domains of quality to enable the achievement of high-quality outcomes. As one learns the theories of patient safety, one will use the methods of improvement and implementation science to test and implement the changes required to achieve the care that is desired. The core values of kindness, compassion, respect, dignity, partnership, and holistic care are inherent in the quality system and central to the design of safe systems.

The WHO principles and strategy for patient safety

The WHO has guiding principles that underpin patient safety (Box 1.1). These are the principles that are applied within the theories and methods presented in the following chapters; and they are the foundation of all patient safety initiatives.

Box 1.1 World Health Organisation principles for patient safety

1. Engage patients and families as partners in safe care.
2. Achieve results through collaborative working.
3. Analyse data in order to generate learning.
4. Translate evidence into measurable improvement.
5. Base policies and action on the nature of the care setting.
6. Use both scientific expertise and patient experience to improve safety.
7. Instil a safety culture into the design and delivery of healthcare.

The WHO Action Plan has several ambitious goals, and these will require the application of the theories and methods presented in this book.

Box 1.2 Strategic objectives of the World Health Organisation Global Patient Safety Action Plan

1. Make zero avoidable harm to patients a state of mind and a rule of engagement in the planning and delivery of healthcare everywhere.
2. Build high-reliability health systems and health organizations that protect patients daily from harm.
3. Assure the safety of every clinical process.
4. Engage and empower patients and families to help and support the journey to safer healthcare.
5. Inspire, educate, skill and protect health workers to contribute to the design and delivery of safe care systems.
6. Ensure a constant flow of information and knowledge to drive the mitigation of risk, a reduction in levels of avoidable harm, and improvements in the safety of care.
7. Develop and sustain multisectoral and multinational synergy, solidarity, and partnerships to improve patient safety and quality of care.

World Health Organisation Global Patient Safety Action Plan 2021–2030

The theories of patient safety science

Patient safety science is an evolving field informed by research, debate, and real-world experience. In recent years, in what should be seen as a sign of maturity, greater space for questioning and for a critical evaluation of theories and methods has emerged. Despite achievements in the face of advancing complexity, rates of harm have remained a stubborn concern. Criticisms to the effect that patient safety has ceased to progress, has become overly bureaucratic, or has deviated from the guiding influence of safety science in general need to be addressed by examining our ability to reduce harm consistently. Many of the chapters in this book seek to address new and emerging ideas, so that they may be blended into a systematic approach to safety practice.

As the field has evolved, there is better understanding of what is needed in order for us to measure and achieve safety. The theories covered in this book are practical, so that the busy clinician can make patient safety part of day-to-day work. To be safe, we need always to manage risk proactively; and each theory aims to provide a way to do this.

- Individual responsibility and accountability are the foundation of most safety initiatives. However, given the complexity of healthcare, one needs to have a safe context within which one can deliver it safely.
- Risk/critical incident management has been the mainstay, and the original approach to patient safety was limited to risk/incident management and the review of adverse events. This included the introduction of root cause analysis and failure mode effects analysis, which aimed to understand the causation of harm. This is insufficient to ensure a safer system but is essential for highlighting where we need to improve.
- Human factors and ergonomics (HFE) is a domain that originates in engineering and aviation and provides the framework upon which most patient safety initiatives are based. Safety results from the successful interaction of related parts of a complex system of interactions between humans, the environment, and the technologies that are required to complete complex tasks.
- Reliability theory emanates from the study of 'high reliability organizations' (HROs) in other industries, which are designed to have low defect rates—for example in nuclear power, in the military, and in air traffic control, where safety is core to all operations. HFE is central to the design of highly reliable processes. Interventions such as the standardization of processes and care pathways have achieved considerable success, for example in the elimination of central line-associated bloodstream infections.
- Systems theory and the proactive management of risk combine how the system operates at different levels and introduce the concept of complex adaptive systems, in which there are no linear processes but rather a set of ever changing interactions, and therefore safety cannot be taken as a given but needs to be planned and managed. Processes are not linear, and therefore the complexity of the system implies that one cannot have a simple solution that fits all. The proactive management of risk in each clinical area requires an assessment of how the system works and how reliable can it be under varying conditions.

For example, highly predictable clinical care processes such as blood transfusion need to be highly reliable, others may aim for the ability to adapt under changing conditions. For example, routine surgery and some similar trauma need to be highly adaptable.

- Resilience theory considers safety as occurring on a day-to-day basis, with constant adaptation to changing conditions. Safety II looks at safety from the prism of what works well. It studies this process and also analyses adverse events, in order to enable a process to be safe under all conditions.

The most important component in the development of a safe system relates to a culture of safety, where safety is embedded in everything we do. Healthcare is a high-risk industry, and therefore safety must be central to all its strategies and policies. A safe organization has safety as its core business, aims to ensure that all those who work in the system make safety a priority, and does everything it can to help them achieve this goal.

There are many challenges to developing a safe culture, and the most complex of these is offering employees *psychological safety*, the foundation of developing a safe system. Individuals need to feel safe in order to challenge the status quo, report deficits, and feel empowered to improve the process. This requires a leadership that fosters safety, protecting and supporting staff in what is called a just culture. It involves the development of teams and the co-creation of safety both with the team and with the people who receive care. It involves making people feel safe, so that they may deliver safe care.

Despite our knowing why we need to be safe and what we need to do to deliver safe care, healthcare is still not safe (see Wears and Sutcliffe 2020). This may be due to changing definitions of safety and to the lack of agreement on what constitutes harm and how to measure it. We have tended to measure it retrospectively, but the latest theory calls for anticipating harm and predicting where it may occur, so that we can minimize the risk through active mitigation.

It is intended that this book will encourage the development of safer systems, in which all staff members feel psychologically safe, work together without fear, and share expectations of delivering safe care and minimizing all potential harm.

Summary box

How to use the book

This book has been designed and written as an accessible and practical guide to patient safety. Our primary aim in presenting this diverse subject through this format is to help everyone in healthcare to bridge the know–do gap by making care safer for patients.

Whether carried as hardcopy or accessed electronically, this rapid reference work is meant for everyone in healthcare, from bedside to boardroom, healthcare workers, and patients. We hope that it will be useful from day one of professional preparation until your very last day of involvement in healthcare.

Part I provides the current theories and methods that can be used in developing a safer system.

Part II applies these theories to specific challenges we face in patient safety.

Part III focuses on safety in different clinical areas.

There are cross-references throughout the book, so readers can move seamlessly from theory to practice and back again.

References and further reading

A global patient safety action plan

World Health Organisation, *Global Patient Safety Action Plan 2021–2030*. 2021. WHO, 3 August. https://www.who.int/teams/integrated-health-services/patient-safety/policy/global-patient-safety-action-plan.

The start of modern patient safety

Berwick, D. M. et al. *A Promise to Learn—a Commitment to Act*. London: Crown copyright, 2013. https://www.gov.uk/government/uploads/system/uploads/attachment_data/file/226703/Berwick_Report.pdf.

Department of Health. *An organisation with a memory: report of an expert group on learning from adverse events in the NHS*. London: The Stationery Office, 2000.

Donaldson, L. An organisation with a memory. *Clinical Medicine* 2.5 (2002): 452–7. https://www.rcpjournals.org/content/clinmedicine/2/5/452.full.pdf.

Francis, R. (chair). *Report of the Mid Staffordshire NHS Foundation Trust Public Inquiry. 2012.* London: Crown copyright, 2013. https://www.gov.uk/government/uploads/system/uploads/attachment_data/file/279124/0947.pdf.

Kohn, L. T., Corrigan, J., and Donaldson, M. (eds). *To Err Is Human: Building a Safer Health System.* Washington, DC: National Academy Press, 1999.

Leape, L. L. *Making Healthcare Safe: The Story of the Patient Safety Movement*. Springer, 2021. https://library.oapen.org/handle/20.500.12657/49509.

Leape, L. L. et al. The nature of adverse events in hospitalized patients: Results of the Harvard Medical Practice Study II. *New England Journal of Medicine* 324.6 (1991): 377–84.

Learning from Bristol: The Report of the Public Inquiry into Children's Heart Surgery at the Bristol Royal Infirmary 1984–1995. London: Crown copyright, 2002. https://www.gov.uk/government/uploads/system/uploads/attachment_data/file/273320/5363.pdf.

Reason, J. Human error: Models and management. *BMJ* 320.7237 (2000): 768–70. https://doi.org/10.1136/bmj.320.7237.768.

Scally, G. and Donaldson, L. J. Clinical governance and the drive for quality improvement in the new NHS in England. *BMJ* 317 (1998): 61–65.

Recent theories

Bates, D. W. and Singh, H. Two decades since to err is human: An assessment of progress and emerging priorities in patient safety. *Health Affairs* 37 (2018): 1736–43.

Chassin, M. R. and Loeb, J. M. High-reliability health care: Getting there from here. *Milbank Quarterly* 91 (2013): 459–90.

Edmondson, A. C. *The Fearless Organization: Creating Psychological Safety in the Workplace for Learning, Innovation, and Growth*. Hoboken, NJ: John Wiley & Sons, 2018.

Heifetz, R. and Linsky, M. *Leadership on the Line: Staying Alive through the Dangers of Leading*. Boston, MA: Harvard Business Review Press, 2017.

Vincent, C. and Amalberti, R. *Safer Healthcare: Strategies for the Real World*. London: Springer, 2016.

Wears, R. and Sutcliffe, K. *Still Not Safe: Patient Safety and the Middle-Managing of American Medicine*. Oxford: Oxford University Press, 2020.

Weick, K. E. and Sutcliffe, K. M. *Managing the Unexpected*. Hoboken, NJ: Jossey-Bass, 2007.

Quality improvement

Lachman, P., Batalden, P., and Vanhaecht, K. A multidimensional quality model: An opportunity for patients, their kin, healthcare providers and professionals to coproduce health. *F1000Research* 9 (2021):1140 (https://doi.org/10.12688/f1000research.26368.3).

Chapter 2

The culture of patient safety

Key points

Safety culture is that aspect of organizational culture that reflects and influences how safety is prioritized, resourced and practiced in a work setting.

Safety culture is the result of the interaction between individual and group beliefs, values, and attitudes.

Safety climate refers to an employee's perceptions of particular aspects of the organization's safety culture.

Introduction

Culture is the foundation of all the processes and resultant outcomes in an organization. In healthcare, patient safety is dependent on the prevailing safety culture. When one assesses either the success or the failure of the safety of an organization, both will be attributed to the prevailing culture, which determines every action that is taken by every person in the organization to achieve outcomes. This chapter introduces the concept of safety culture in healthcare.

Key components of a safe culture

The safety psychologist James Reason (1998, 2000) suggested that a strong safety culture is made up of five overlapping component cultures, as shown in Box 2.1:

Box 2.1 Safety culture components

In an *informed culture* all staff members have a level of knowledge and awareness of safety science that is appropriate to their role. Leaders and managers apply safety thinking in how work is designed and carried out. This requires the open and transparent sharing of information related to safety. In an informed culture, the *organization* collects, analyses, and shares safety information.

In a *reporting culture* people have the willingness and the confidence to report any safety concerns (such as near misses and errors) without any fear of blame or punishment. Some reporting may require confidentiality, in which the staff has much faith. In a reporting culture people know that the information they submit will be acted upon.

A *just culture* is one in which the right actions occur after an adverse event. There are two elements. The first one is *retribution*, whereby individuals are held accountable for their actions by peers who can understand the nature and context of an error. In a just culture a person who performs an unsafe act will not be punished if his or her act was well intentioned and justified. On the contrary, a person who acts recklessly or takes a deliberate and unjustified risk will be subject to disciplinary action. If someone has been injured, that person should be compensated appropriately. The second element is *restoration*, whereby any individual, be it a patient or a practitioner, who has been hurt by an incident is identified and supported towards recovery. Restoration also aims to repair the trust and the relationships damaged by an incident.

In a *flexible culture* the organization and its people are capable of adapting to changing demands.

A *learning culture* is one in which it is possible to analyse safety data, draw the right conclusions, learn from mistakes, and act upon recommendations.

How to measure safety culture and climate

An understanding of safety culture is important because the safety culture of a team or an organization impacts on crucial outcomes such as harm reduction, team performance, or learning from adverse events. Understanding is also important because safety culture can be examined, measured, and shaped so as to improve safety. There are validated tools that facilitate the measurement of safety culture, providing both summative and formative insights into how organizations perform over time and identifying where they might best focus their improvement efforts (see Box 2.2).

Box 2.2 Examples of patient safety culture instruments

Hospital surveys on patient safety culture: Agency for Healthcare Research and Quality (AHRQ) in the USA

The AHRQ Surveys on Patient Safety Culture (SOPS™) enable healthcare organizations to assess how their staff perceives various aspects of patient safety culture in multiple settings such as hospitals, nursing homes, ambulatory outpatient medical offices, community pharmacies, and ambulatory surgery centres. The hospital SOPS has, for example, forty survey items covering areas such as communication, reporting and teamwork. See www.ahrq.gov/sops/about/index.html, AHRQ Publication No. 19-0076, September 2019.

Manchester Patient Safety Assessment Framework (MapSaF)

This framework covers multiple dimensions of safety culture and five levels of safety culture development. This allows the generation of a profile of an organization's safety culture in terms of areas of relative strengths and challenges, which can be used to identify a focus for change and improvement. See https://webarchive.nationalarchives.gov.uk/ukgwa/20171030124256/http://www.nrls.npsa.nhs.uk/resources/?EntryId45=59796.

How to develop a safe culture

The means and effectiveness of interventions to change safety culture remain controversial. Some components of a safety culture require structures and processes (data systems, education, named roles) that need to be resourced and supported. These features contribute to an organization's governance for safety and are most effective in influencing safety culture when combined with good leadership practices.

Six leadership practices necessary to develop and sustain a culture of safety were identified in the report *Leading a Culture of Safety*:

- establish a compelling vision for safety;
- build trust, respect, and inclusion;
- engage and develop a board;
- prioritize safety in the selection and development of leaders;
- lead and reward a just culture; and
- establish organizational behaviour expectations.

There are many additional practices and tools that support leaders and organizations in their task of shaping a culture. Many of these have their basis in person centredness and are an extension to staff of concepts that are used to improve patient care (see Box 2.3).

Box 2.3 Practices that support a good safety culture

Patient participation (power of partnership)

Involves patients and families in the co-creation and accountability of safety governance structures (Berwick et al. 2013).

Transparency (power of openness)

Ensures open, timely, and accessible sharing of all data related to safety with patients, staff members, and the public (Berwick et al. 2013).

Psychological safety (power of respectful listening)

Uses trust to create a sense of confidence that the team will not embarrass, reject, or punish someone for speaking up (Edmondson 2018).

Appreciative inquiry (power of the positive)

Uses appreciation for what and why is working well, in order to discover organizational strengths (Cooperrider et al. 2008).

Humble inquiry (power of the curious)

Uses curiosity to build respectful relationships (Schein 2013).

Intelligent kindness (power of belonging)

Uses ideas of kinship to build supportive and nurturing teams (Ballatt and Campling 2020).

The idea of setting out to change culture on purpose is not necessarily helpful, except in extreme circumstances. Culture may be seen as flawed or poor, and changing it may be considered an essential action; however, this broad brush can be overly simplistic. An organization's culture also tends to be a source of strength and character, and recognizing this can yield results. Issues regarding safety governance, management, or leadership should be considered before addressing any concerns with culture.

Another approach is to focus on behaviour and performance as the means to building culture over time. Here shared activities (handover, huddles, debriefs) may be used to model good behaviours and to highlight their benefits on performance. Over time, through the sincere enacting of the behaviours that represent a safe culture, a virtuous cycle is created that can change deeply held attitudes and beliefs. This requires leadership, psychological safety, and patience.

It is important to recognize that any efforts to address safety culture benefit from highlighting staff safety as a goal, in addition to patient safety. In a workplace with multiple hazards for staff (lifting injuries, assault, contagion), the power of a staff safety culture has an important influence on shared values.

Finally, regulators must understand the influence that safety culture has on efforts to reduce harm. As Dr Don Berwick noted in the Berwick report, 'culture will trump rules, standards and control strategies every single time'. This means that regulators must not only pay attention to compliance and critical outcomes, but also have a role in encouraging and guiding the emergence of supportive safety cultures.

Summary box

- Safety culture refers to the way patient safety is thought about and implemented within an organization and the structures and processes in place to support it.
- Measuring safety culture or the safety climate is important because the culture of an organization and the attitudes of its teams have been found to influence patient safety outcomes, and these measures can be used to monitor change over time.
- Safety tools that are short, easily repeatable over time, and adaptable to different contexts may be the ones most practical to adopt.
- Organizations with a positive safety culture base their communication processes on mutual trust, shared perceptions of the importance of safety, confidence in the effectiveness of preventive measures, and support for the workforce.

Further reading

American College of Healthcare Executives and Institute for Healthcare Improvement/NPSF Lucian Leape Institute. *Leading a Culture of Safety: A Blueprint for Success*. Boston, MA: American College of Healthcare Executives and Institute for Healthcare Improvement, 2017. http://www.ihi.org/resources/Pages/Publications/Leading-a-Culture-of-Safety-A-Blueprint-for-Success.aspx.

John Ballatt J, Campling P, Maloney C. *Intelligent Kindness: Rehabilitating the Welfare State*. 2nd edition. RCPsych/Cambridge University Press, 2020.

Berwick, D. M. et al. *A Promise to Learn—a Commitment to Act*. London: Crown copyright, 2013. https://www.gov.uk/government/uploads/system/uploads/attachment_data/file/226703/Berwick_Report.pdf.

Cooperrider, D. L., Whitney, D., and Stavros, J. M. *Appreciative Inquiry Handbook* (2nd ed.). Brunswick, OH: Crown Custom Publishing, 2008.

Edmondson, A. *The Fearless Organization: Creating Psychological Safety in the Workplace for Learning, Innovation, and Growth*. Hoboken, NJ: John Wiley & Sons, 2018.

Health Foundation. *Measuring Safety Culture*. London: Health Foundation, 2011. https://www.health.org.uk/publications/measuring-safety-culture.

Reason, J. Human error: Models and management. *BMJ* 320.7237 (2000): 768–70. https://doi.org/10.1136/bmj.320.7237.768.

Schein, E. *Humble Inquiry: The Gentle Art of Asking Instead of Telling*. San Francisco: Berrett-Koehler Publishers, 2013.

Sorra, J. et al. *AHRQ Hospital Survey on Patient Safety Culture Version 2.0: User's Guide*. Rockville, MD: Agency for Healthcare Research and Quality, 2019. AHRQ Publication No. 19-0076. https://www.ahrq.gov/sops/surveys/hospital/index.html.

Chapter 3

Transparent leadership for safety

Key points

The safety of an organization is set by the culture that exists, as this culture will determine how people act and behave.

A safety culture requires leadership that defines the expected behaviours of all and the desired outcomes to be achieved.

A leader for safety addresses the complexity of care and does not avoid conflict. Safety will be planned and supported at every level of the organization.

Candour with patients and support for staff will be key features of leadership.

A leader for safety addresses the complexity of care and does not avoid conflict.

A leader for safety will be compassionate and reflective and will develop a learning organization that takes lessons from successes as well as failures.

Introduction to leadership for safety

A safe organization requires leadership at all levels, from the frontline clinical team to middle and executive management. This chapter discusses the key leadership attributes that are needed in order for an organization to be safe. The theme of leading for safety will be present and evident in every subsequent chapter.

Leadership for safety and quality of healthcare should be part of a quality management system in every part of the organization. Box 3.1 lists the essential elements.

Box 3.1 Leadership for safety

Promotes and enhances a culture of safety:

- Creates an environment for safety.
- Promotes psychological safety for staff.
- Asks if as a leader one is just and transparent.
- Values person centredness, intelligence, kindness, respect, and being humble.

Develops a safety management system plan for safety:

- Develops a vision for safety and makes safety the business plan.
- Promotes reliable systems to deliver services.
- Proactively manages risk within the system.
- Develops a risk management system to protect and mitigate against risk.
- Effectively responds to incidents that occur.
- Learns from incidents in real time and spreads the learning.
- Supports the people who have been harmed.
- Supports those who have caused the harm.
- Exercises a just culture.

Sets up controls for safety:

- Measures outcomes proactively and with transparency.
- Uses data in real time to assess safety.

Develops an improvement and learning organization:

- Continually improves and implements changes designed to improve safety.
- Learns from what works and what does not.
- Educates staff for safety and continually learns from experience.

How to promote and enhance a culture of safety

Achieving optimal levels of safety throughout an organization requires highly visible, consistent, and empathetic leadership. Patient safety must be a priority that is recognized, rewarded, and supported by leadership. Failure to satify this condition will be a major barrier to success.

Without an overt commitment to safety the following may occur:

- Frontline staff members will be uncertain as to whether safety really is a top priority and will not know how to proceed if they see suboptimal care.
- When harm occurs, there can be confusion and paralysis caused by fear.
- Safety will become reactive to incidents rather than proactive

Leadership provides the platform of confidence in support of patient safety and is the glue that connects individual patient safety efforts.

Effective leaders create a just culture in which team members feel safe both physically and mentally/psychologically, so that they in turn can provide safe care to the people seeking care, who in turn feel safe about the care they receive.

Genuine ownership of safety at the front line begins with a core belief that all patients deserve to be free of harm. This belief is expressed in all organizational literature, in conversations during the recruitment of new personnel, and in daily activity. Such expressions could involve doing regular presentations with staff members who work on projects about safety, thinking about how to implement their recommendations across the organization, appointing safety champions among both staff and patients, and regularly discussing the business of safety.

One way to develop a culture of safety is for leaders to do the gemba (i.e. 'real place') walks or the safety walkrounds. Leadership walkrounds show commitment to the concepts of safety. They are learning opportunities, which can be used for understanding what the front line is doing to achieve safety and to listen to patients and their families. Frontline staff has the chance to discuss its safety achievements and improvement projects.

A team can use tools such as MaPSaF to assess the current state of its culture, so that improvement in that culture may be assessed. There are tools available to do this and it is important to implement them at the beginning of the assessment, so that improvement may be measured.

Walkrounds have been shown to assist in the prevention of burnout if they are done within the wider context of a culture that supports patient safety. That will be a just culture, which encourages learning from mistakes and supports reporting both clinical incidents and excellence in care (see Box 3.2).

Box 3.2 Leader for safety characteristics

- Creates a just culture with responsibility and accountability, not a blame culture.
- Embraces transparency in internal and external communication, while protecting individual rights.
- Acts with empathy, courage, and urgency when harm occurs.
- Acts with compassion and kindness.

How leaders can develop a safety system

Safe organizations will have safety management systems at every level, from the front line to the board. This applies to executive leaders as well as to leaders of clinical teams. Juran proposed a trilogy of actions for a quality management system that can be applied to the safety system (see Figure 3.1).

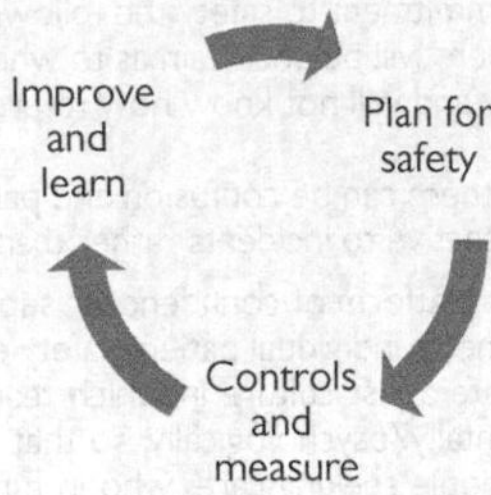

Figure 3.1 A clinical leader for safety will apply these three interventions on a daily basis, using improvement theories and methodologies to implement change.

Plan for safety

[illegible]

Box 2.3 [illegible] safety

[illegible]

Promote reliable systems

[illegible]

Plan for safety

As one assesses the complexity of healthcare, it is clear that we need to plan all aspects of care in order to ensure that we can achieve its safe delivery. It cannot be assumed that professionals will be safe. Safety needs to be the focus of the organization and of the clinical teams.

Each of the steps outlined in Box 3.3 is part of a proactive planning and continual adjustment to changing environments.

The planning for safety has three key elements:

Box 3.3 Key actions of a leader who supports patient safety

A leader in safety who has planned for safety will

- develop a common purpose of achieving patient safety for all those who work in the organization;
- set the behaviours required for safety within the values of the team and of the organization;
- create a culture of respect and belonging;
- have a clear understanding of the potential risks and harms to staff and patients that may occur;
- train the staff in the knowledge topics required for safe care, including in human factors;
- train the staff in communication skills, so as to prevent misunderstandings;
- have clear policies and standard operating procedures for developing reliable care;
- undertake regular simulation in order to ensure competence in the response to risk;
- respond to incidents in real time with support for all those affected and with a rapid investigation of the cause;
- create a learning organization ready to take lessons from what works well and have a plan as to how to spread that learning;
- work with patients and families to develop safety.

Promote reliable systems

Leaders for safety will assess how work is actually done and will promote the reliability of the process – doing what we are supposed to do. They will pay attention to detail, listen to the front line, and apply human factors assessments of the work system and processes of care, so that reliability can be achieved. A leader will look at reliability. An example is antibiotic stewardship, where daily assessment of adherence to protocols will improve safety. Improving reliability may involve redesigning processes (e.g. with LEAN), standardizing processes, redesigning tasks around the expertise of staff members, and introducing simulation training.

Proactively manage risk

Healthcare is complex and has inherent risks. The leader for safety will accept these inherent risks. This will allow for a proactive management whereby the clinical and support teams are able to mitigate risks and prevent harms. An example is having daily safety huddles, in which current risks are identified and action is taken before the safety event occurs. Also, rapid response teams are to manage proactively people who are at risk of deterioration.

Respond to clinical incidents

Despite the best efforts, errors will occur in all healthcare organizations, and harm may result. The litmus test is what an organization or a clinical team does to minimize harm and how it responds when harm occurs.

When harm occurs, an immediate and appropriate response should occur, and it is tailored to the level of severity involved. Depending on the level and scope of the harm, results should be shared with the organization's leadership and, where appropriate, with external monitoring and review bodies. The aim of the response is to support those involved and to learn by studying what happened, so that processes may be improved.

As discussed in Chapters 17 and 18, a transformational leader will actively promote and support candour, so as to enable staff members to have an open disclosure and at the same time feel supported by their leadership.

Box 3.4 A leader for safety's response to incidents

A safe organization and clinical team will

- have duty of candour, that is, a policy of apology and disclosure when harm occurs;
- support those directly harmed and their immediate relatives;
- support those who work at the organization, including volunteers and board members;
- be able to investigate, learn, and make changes (See Chapter 18 (second victim)).

Controls and measures for safety

A leader for safety will ensure that there are standards of care and measures by which one can assess whether these standards are met. The real-time measurement of safety at each system level allows for immediate reactions and makes safety more likely. The measures need to be regularly reviewed and widely understood by frontline staff, as described in Chapters 12 and 13

Metrics need to be reviewed at various levels of the organization, including by the board and by each department and clinical team. Organizations should participate in relevant quality review systems, where their results can be compared with others. An annual outside review of the overall safety and quality programme could be conducted, and results should be shared widely.

An example is medication harm. To prevent erroneous prescriptions and possible adverse events from them, one should follow a standard operating procedure (SOP) that needs to be adhered to. A leader for safety will make this a priority at both executive and clinical team level. This will entail making accuracy in prescribing a daily measure, with the help of an associated improvement programme. (See ch. 13)

Development of a transparent and learning organization

Underpinning all safety efforts is how an organization or a clinical team learns. A safety leader at any level of the organization will constantly ask:

- Are we safe now?
- Will we be safe in the future?
- Does our staff feel safe (psychological safety)?
- Do the patients feel safe?
- What do I/we need to do to ensure safety?
- How can we learn so as to be able to improve safety?

A transparent leader will use tools such as failure mode and effects analysis (FMEA) to discover potential failures within an organization and clinical teams.

A transparent organization or team is one that is willing to share what happens openly, with duty of candour, and one that will learn from these experiences. The safety leader will actively seek out comparator teams or organizations in order to see whether the standard of care is as safe as it could be.

A progressive safety leader recognizes that leadership in patient safety is important at all levels, not just at the top, and will place safety at the centre of all decisions.

Summary box

Safety management system

Further reading

Summary box

Culture

- Achieving optimal levels of safety in an organization and in clinical teams requires visible, consistent, and empathetic leadership.
- Genuine ownership of safety begins with a core belief that all patients, however long their stay, deserve to be free of harm.
- Effective leaders for safety are those who create a just culture, enthusiastically support safety in their own work, and embrace transparency in communication.

Safety management system

Plan

- A leader for safety will proactively plan for safety.
- A key test of an organization's commitment to safety is what it does to proactively minimize harm and how it responds when harm occurs.

Controls and measures

- Standards for safe care and metrics of safety will be set at all the organizational levels that are regularly reviewed; they are essential to success.

A learning and improving organization

- Leaders for safety will remove barriers to transparency, such as fears of blame and punishment, litigation, and reputational harm.
- Leaders for safety will enable an education for safety and will facilitate learning from incidents and from what works well as part of everyone's daily work.
- Leaders for safety will include patients and their families in safety planning.

Further reading

Baker, R. and Axler, R. Creating a high performing healthcare system for Ontario: Evidence supporting strategic changes in Ontario. University of Ontario, October 2015. http://ihpme.utoronto.ca/wp-content/uploads/2016/03/Baker-OHA_HSR-Creating-High-Performing-Healthcare-System_policy_paper_oct...Final_.pdf.

Barson, S. et al. What initiatives do healthcare leaders agree are needed for healthcare system improvement? Results of a modified Delphi study. *Journal of Health Organization* and Management 32.8 (2018): 1002–12. https://doi.org/10.1108/jhom-08-2017-0216.

Clay-Williams, R. et al. Medical leadership, a systematic narrative review: Do hospitals and healthcare organisations perform better when led by doctors? *BMJ Open* 7.9 (2017): e014474. https://doi.org/10.1136/bmjopen-2016-014474.

Drew, J. R. and Pandit, M. Why healthcare leadership should embrace quality improvement *BMJ* 368 (2020): m872. https://doi.org/10.1136/bmj.m872.

Martin, G. P. and Dixon-Woods, M. After Mid Staffordshire: From acknowledgement, through learning, to improvement. *BMJ Quality and Safety* 23 (2014): 706–8.

Rosenbaum, L. Cursed by knowledge: Building a culture of psychological safety. *New England Journal of Medicine* 380.8 (2019, 21 Feb.): 786–90. https://doi.org/10.1056/nejmms1813429.

Regulation 20: Duty of candour. London: Quality of Care Commission, 2015. https://app.croneri.co.uk/care-standards/cqc-fundamental-standards-england/regulation-20-duty-candour.

Sadler, B. and Stewart, K. *Leadership in a Crisis: The Power of Transparency*. London: The Health Foundation, 2015. https://www.health.org.uk/sites/default/files/LeadingInACrisisThePowerOfTransparency.pdf.

Savage, M. et al. Effective physician leaders: An appreciative inquiry into their qualities, capabilities and learning approaches. *BMJ Leader* 2 (2018): 95–102. https://bmjleader.bmj.com/content/leader/2/3/95.full.pdf.

Vincent, C., Burnett, S., and Carthey, J. *The Measuring and Monitoring of Safety*. London: The Health Foundation, 2013.

Chapter 4

Person-centred safety

Key points

- Patients, as people, are central to improving patient safety.
- There are many practical approaches to creating person-centered safety.
- These include patient-held records, co-production and co-design of services, and sharing in the decision-making process.
- Tools such as teach back and peer-to-peer support can lead to improved safety.
- Partnership with patients can improve safety at all levels of care.

What is person-centred safety?

> Are patients and their families ... someone to whom we provide care? Or are they active partners in managing and redesigning their care?
>
> Don Berwick, MD

As the ultimate recipient and victim of unsafe care, the patient *as a person* has the greatest interest in improving safety. Traditionally, patients have been largely excluded from efforts to improve care. It is increasingly recognised that patients, caregivers, and family members have a critical role to play in making healthcare safer and often notice safety issues that busy healthcare workers may miss. Positive patient experience is associated with increased clinical effectiveness and fewer adverse events. Everyone shares a responsibility for safe care.

Partnering with people to achieve safer care occurs across a continuum, *from remote involvement and feedback* to basic care delivery to co-leadership in care redesign (see Figure 4.1).

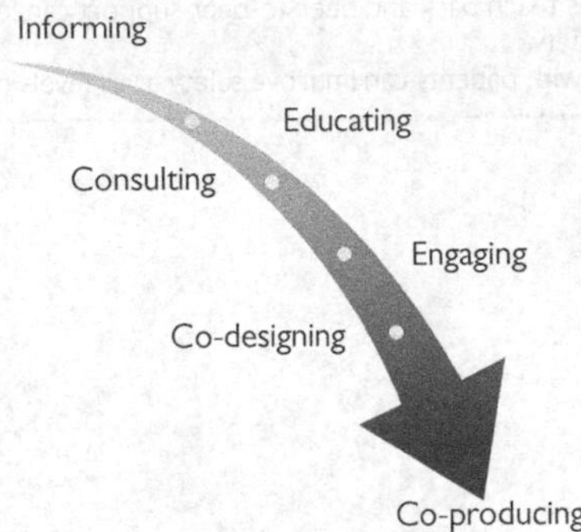

Figure 4.1 Continuum of patient partnership for safety

Person-centred care has been defined as care that is coordinated, personalized, enabling, and delivered with dignity, compassion, and respect. While aspiring to improve in these four areas is laudable, true enablement of effective patient involvement in care delivery through the facilitation of patient agency is core to co-producing safer care. Agency is the power and courage to make change. It seems reasonable to state that patient-centred care and patient-centred safety exist only when perceived as such by the patient.

Why is person-centred safety a challenge?

> Nothing about me without me.
>
> Valerie Billingham, patient

The greatest challenge to unlocking person-centred safety lies in disrupting the traditional hierarchy of healthcare so as to create space for patients to feel comfortable to ask questions and to get adequately involved in their own care. This requires every effort to establish an equal relationship between the clinician and the patient as a person, in order to generate a respectful exchange on an equal footing. The first step is for the clinician to listen and to allow patients and members of their families to speak up and be part of the care process. By realizing a true and equal partnership and by fostering a sense of psychological safety between the clinician and the patient as a person, one can generate a culture of safety in all aspects of health and care.

> Paying attention to the quality of language is the foundation for successful dialogue and everyday collaboration. Many patients and carers can describe the pain caused by a single word they encountered while being treated. (Sibylle Erdmann, parent carer)

There are many practical approaches to enhancing this kind of relationship and ensuring that the voice of patients can be heard; such approaches are listed in Box 4.1.

Box 4.1 Approaches to developing person centred care

My favourite aunt

By imagining a cherished family member such as a 'favourite auntie' in the role of the patient, we can begin to recognize where care can be more personalized and communication improved.

Hello, my name is...

This is a worldwide movement started by Kate Granger, a practising clinician turned patient who recognized that redistributing power in the therapeutic relationship starts with a name and an introduction.

What matters to you?

This question summarizes an initiative aimed at creating space for patients to discuss the elements and goals of care that are most important to them, as well as any fears or concerns about their condition or treatment alternatives, in addition to what may be prioritized by their treating clinician on the basis of biomedical knowledge

Take 5/patient/personal stories

Clinicians are encouraged to take the opportunity to sit with a patient and listen to his or her story in an unstructured or semi-structured conversation, outside a normal clinical encounter and relationship.

Patient/personal experience surveys

This is a structured quantitative or qualitative approach to gathering data on the patient experience. Qualitative surveys offer an opportunity to collect a rich account of how care either served or failed the patient.

Patient-reported outcome measures

These are standardized measures designed to capture patient-reported information on symptoms and functional aspects of specific illnesses.

Patient champions/representatives

These are patients, caregivers, and family members recruited to offer a representative view, on behalf of themselves and other patients, at micro, meso and macro levels of the healthcare system. Patient representatives wish to have a sense that their efforts add value to the healthcare process. Achieving this often requires mentorship, familiarization, and training in navigating the healthcare system.

Patient leadership

Patients, carers, and family members can lead healthcare system change and redesign this system so as to introduce innovation and improvement. One example is the WHO Patients for Patient Safety network and its cohort of international patient safety champions, who provide leadership for safety at all levels in their respective countries: policymaking, standard setting, regulation, research, and education.

How can person-centred approaches achieve safer care?

Partnership with patients and the incorporation of the patient voice facilitates patient-centred improvements in safety at all levels of the healthcare system. In general, informed patients who build meaningful therapeutic relationships with clinicians, relationships underpinned by psychological safety, have a greater opportunity to take an active part in making their own care and the care of their loved ones safer. This stems from their greater situational awareness of all parties involved and their ability to focus on the goal of safe care, shared with their clinician and the wider health system (see ch. 8, p. 00 (situation awareness)). For many clinicians, adopting this approach may require some radical change to current practice and to the healthcare system design. Achieving safer care in partnerships with patients as persons who receive care requires a change in the power relationship. NHS England has produced a framework designed to facilitate the co-production of services together with patients and their families (Box 4.2).

Box 4.2 Methods to improve person-centred safety

- patient-held medical record
- co-design and co-production
- shared decision making
- structured tools for enhancing interactions
- teach-back
- peer-to-peer or group support
- shared medical review

Addressing hierarchy and power differentials is a logical place to start. A *patient-held medical record* addresses transparency and encourages the sharing of information about how to be safe. While robust data about improved overall safety are lacking, anecdotal evidence suggests that, when patients have open access to healthcare information about themselves, many of them feel empowered to take a more active role in partnering with their clinician in order to achieve safer care. When both the patient and the clinician view the medical record, it is more likely to have correct information on critical facts such as prescribed medications and medical history. This also offers patients the opportunity to track their health progress and to highlight potential safety concerns of their own.

Safer care can be *co-created and co-produced* at the individual level of patient and clinician; at group level, for patients who share a common illness or healthcare resource; and across the wider healthcare system.

Co-production allows patients, as persons, to design how care could be delivered and what safety measures could be included in the design from the perspective of the service user as well as from that of the service provider (see Box 4.3).

A change in the way we interact with patients as persons can lead to safer clinical encounters and safer experiences. Shared decision-making is a two-way relational process of helping people to reflect on, and express, their preferences on the basis of their unique circumstances, expectations, beliefs, and values (see Box 4.4)

Box 4.3 Coproduction with a single patient

Case example: Matt, forty-two years old

Matt is a healthy and active engineer who rarely interacts with healthcare professionals and is not on any regular medication. He enjoys hillwalking. Last weekend he stumbled and fell on his right knee, which became bruised, swollen, and sore. He was concerned that he may need an x-ray or an MRI scan to rule out a serious injury due to the pain. He visited his GP for further assessment. After carefully examining Matt's knee, the GP suggested that the most likely diagnosis was soft tissue bruising and a bad sprain. What happened next?

Scenario 1 The traditional approach

While the GP was reasonably certain that an MRI scan was not indicated for Matt's injury, he was afraid that Matt would feel let down without an MRI. The GP arranged an MRI and prescribed a course of anti-inflammatories.

Matt worried about his knee, feeling that it was better to rest completely and refrain from walking until after the scan. He took sick leave from work. During the MRI scan, he felt uncomfortable in the confined space. The result revealed minor soft tissue bruising, as the GP had suspected; however, the knee now felt *stiffer because of* not being used and Matt required the pain relief *daily* for three weeks. This medication caused him heartburn and nausea, for which the GP then prescribed an antacid and further follow up.

Scenario 2 Shared decision-making

The GP used a structured approach, to share with Matt the decision about how to proceed. The two agreed that medical imaging was unlikely to add significant further diagnostic value, unless pain and function in the knee did not improve as expected. Matt's concerns about the need for further investigation were allayed. They agreed a treatment plan that involved rest, ice packs, a lightly compressive knee support bandage, elevation when possible, and anti-inflammatory painkilling medication as required.

The GP then used a teach-back technique, to make sure that Matt was aware of the common risks and side effects associated with taking these medications and knew what to do if he had any further concerns or questions. After the consultation, Matt had a better understanding of the underlying cause of his knee discomfort, felt confident about using the knee again, and did not need to take painkilling medication regularly.

To encourage active participation, clinicians need to address the power imbalances that may be present in the clinician–patient dynamic. There are several tools that can assist the clinician; and *structured question tools* can be used to encourage patients to ask questions of their clinician at every healthcare interaction. These questions can relate to diagnosis, treatment options, medications, and other aspects of care. Examples include programmes such as Ask Me 3 (IHI), 5 Moments for Medication Safety (WHO), Know Check Ask (HSE Ireland), and Take 2 (CEC, NSW).

Box 4.4 Shared decision-making

Why
- increased patient knowledge
- more accurate perception of risk
- increased congruence between the patient's values and informed care choices
- decreased passivity in decision-making
- improved patient–clinician communication
- the patient's preference for less invasive interventions
- improved situational awareness

How
Step 1 – Choice talk
- ➢ step back
- ➢ offer choice
- ➢ justify choice
- ➢ check reaction
- ➢ defer closure

Step 2 – Option talk
- ➢ check knowledge
- ➢ list options
- ➢ describe options
- ➢ provide patient decision support
- ➢ summarize

Step 3 – Decision talk
- ➢ focus on patient preferences
- ➢ elicit a preference
- ➢ move towards a decision
- ➢ offer a review

Often patients do not understand what is said to them; and a useful method to improve comprehension in a non-hierarchical manner is *teach back*. This is an evidence-based health literacy intervention where patients explain back to their provider, *in their own words*, what they must know and do about their condition (see Box 4.5).

Peer-to-peer support, either individual or in a group, can be used to give patients opportunities to raise, share, and solve individual and group concerns from others, who have similar experiences and fears.

Structures like the one presented in Box 4.6 can facilitate a *shared medical review* for a group of people with a common condition or treatment need. For example, a shared medical appointment is arranged for a group of people newly diagnosed with asthma. They meet with the doctor and the specialist nurse simultaneously, to learn about optimal management of asthma. Concerns can be shared among the group, and patients may learn from each other's questions and experiences. Direct links between this model of care delivery and improved safety have yet to be made; nevertheless, associated improvements in treatment effectiveness and lower rates of hospitalization may lead to safer care for patients overall.

Possible ways to take a systems approaches to patient safety are listed in Box 4.7.

Box 4.5 Teach Back

Why: Improved patient comprehension of medication, self-care, and follow-up instructions

How:
1. Use an empathetic tone of voice.
2. Make eye contact and use open, relaxed body language.
3. Use simple words and plain language.
4. Ask the patients to explain in their own words what they have heard.
5. Ask non-judgemental, open-ended questions.
6. Avoid asking closed ('yes'–'no') questions.
7. Make it clear that the responsibility is on you, the clinician, to explain things clearly.
8. If the patient is unable to teach back correctly the first time round, explain again and retry.
9. Use print materials in plain language to support the process.
10. Document that teach back has been used and describe the patient's response.

Box 4.6 Peer to peer support

Case example: Anne, 66 years old

Ann is a recently retired teacher married to Paul. She has two children and four grandchildren. She enjoys reading and has a passion for gardening. Three years ago, after several respiratory infections and a particularly severe bout of pneumonia requiring hospital treatment, Anne was diagnosed with chronic obstructive pulmonary disorder.

After speaking with her doctor, she was advised that her condition was probably caused by years of smoking cigarettes. She felt ashamed. She immediately quit smoking, but was very reluctant to speak even with her closest friends and family about her diagnosis and its impact on her life. She stopped participating in her book club and in her gardening group, as she worried about what others would think of her breathlessness and cough.

Over the following months she left the house less and less, and her family noticed how withdrawn she had become. On a routine visit to the respiratory clinic, a respiratory physiotherapist met with Anne and assessed her. She shared a leaflet with Anne that had been designed and written by other patients attending the clinic. While Anne had read some details about her condition previously, this was the first time that the information really made sense to her; it answered many of the questions that she had but was too embarrassed to ask.

The physiotherapist recommended that Anne join the local COPD support group. Anne attended the group meetings and met many people who suffered from similar symptoms and had similar worries. They shared solutions, stories, and connections. Through the group, Anne gained confidence in managing her chronic condition optimally. She was also enabled to recognize her own COPD and act early to manage it safely during an exacerbation.

Box 4.7 Systems approaches to person-centred safety

- patient-focused registries;
- co-designed health information;
- community coordination support networks;
- choosing diagnostics and treatment wisely;
- experience-based co-design.

Co-produced, *condition-specific registries* can prompt patients to monitor and continually assess their health in partnership with their clinician. This allows early detection and shared awareness of deterioration. For example, the use of the Swedish Rheumatology Quality Register has led to improved rates of disease remission for patients with rheumatoid arthritis.

Co-designing health information resources (e.g. information leaflets, consent forms, websites, etc.) with the patients can make these resources more relevant to other patients, more approachable, more understandable, and easier to read.

Groups of people with specific needs that are based on geographic location or minority group are enabled to build, around existing care services, *support networks* that are based on social and cultural values rather than on traditional healthcare structures. This can facilitate safer care through community support.

Population-based health literacy initiatives aimed at achieving safer healthcare can involve the voices of patients. One example of such an initiative is the Choosing Wisely campaign, an international health information movement aimed at building a shared understanding of current scientific evidence for patients and clinicians, as it applies to common medical concerns.

In this book there are many examples of how systems understanding is essential for safe care. When developing a process map of how the system works, one should include people who receive care, because their experiences will provide a much deeper understanding. As people, patients may have skills that enhance the potential for effective system redesign and thus contribute to realizing safer care. The experience-based co-design toolkit is a structured partnership approach that involves patients and clinicians and aims to co-design improvements in safety driven by experiences of care and by evoked emotions (see Box 4.8).

Finally, the most important way to achieve safety is to listen and hear and to treat the patient as a person. This includes involving him or her in investigations.

> 'You ignore at your peril the concerns of a mother', as Mother and Patient Representative Margaret Murphy once said.

Box 4.8 Experience-based design

Why

- Design principles and techniques are used to improve an experience from the perspective of the service user.
- Through partnership, patients and clinicians are empowered to make changes.
- The approach provides rich qualitative insights and can be tailored to a variety of care settings.

How

1. Use observation to appreciate how care happens on a daily basis.
2. Interview and record the experiences of patients, carers, families, and clinicians.
3. Edit the interviews to create a film.
4. Meet with clinicians and agree on the elements that they are happy to share with patients.
5. Show the film to patients.
6. Identify improvement areas together with patients.
7. Hold a joint meeting of patients and clinicians to share experiences and agree on improvement priorities.
8. Organize structured design groups comprised of patients and clinicians in order to drive improvement.
9. Celebrate improvements in safety together.

Summary box

Top tips

- Treat a patient as a person rather than as someone with a disease.
- Appreciate patients' ideas, expectations and contributions in creating safer care.
- Co-design solutions and co-produce safer care in partnership with patients (regarded as persons) and with those closest to them.
- Use available tools to assist you in the way care is delivered.
- Never disregard the concerns of a patient or family member.

Additional resources

Vincent, C. and Amalberti, R. *Safer Healthcare; Strategies for the Real World*. Ebook, Springer Open, 2016.

Further reading

de Iongh, Anya and Erdmann, Sibylle. Better healthcare must mean better for patients and carers. *BMJ* 361 (2018): k1877. doi: https://doi.org/10.1136/bmj.k1877.

Doyle, C., Lennox, L., and Bell, D. A systematic review of evidence on the links between patient experience and clinical safety and effectiveness. *BMJ Open* 3 (2013): e001570. doi: 10.1136/bmjopen-2012-001570.

Elwyn, G. et al. Shared decision making: A model for clinical practice. *Journal of General Internal Medicine* 27.10 (2012), 1361–7. doi:10.1007/s11606-012-2077-6.

Griffey, R. T. et al. The impact of teach-back on comprehension of discharge instructions and satisfaction among emergency patients with limited health literacy: A randomized, controlled study. *Journal of Community Healthcare* 8.1 (2015): 10–21. https://doi.org/10.1179/1753807615y.0000000001.

Health Foundation. Person-centred care made simple (Version 1). 2014. London. https://www.health.org.uk/publications/person-centred-care-made-simple.

NHS England. *Framework for Involving Patients in Patient Safety*. 2021. NHS, June. https://www.england.nhs.uk/wp-content/uploads/2021/06/B0435-framework-for-involving-patients-in-patient-safety.pdf.

The Point of Care Foundation. Experience-based co-design. n.d. London. .https://www.pointofcarefoundation.org.uk/resource/using-patient-experience-for-improvement/improving-care/experience-based-co-design.

Teach Back Training Kit. Website. n.d. http://teachbacktraining.org/home.

Chapter 5

The economics of patient safety

Key points

- An understanding of health economics is essential when making clinical decisions as well as when improving the safety of care.
- Harm to patients accounts for up to 15% of the budget of a hospital, and there is a broader impact in terms of litigation and loss of earnings for the individual affected.
- It is far more cost-effective to deliver safe care.
- The measurement of the cost effectiveness of patient safety initiatives can be calculated.

Abbreviations used

CEA	cost-effectiveness analysis
QALY	quality-adjusted life years
ICER	incremental cost-effectiveness ratio
LYG	life year gained

Overview

This chapter considers the health economics framework and its application to patient safety in healthcare. It begins with a brief outline of cost-effectiveness analysis (CEA), then goes on to examine some illustrative examples of published health economic analyses of safety initiatives. The discussion section explores how the health economic perspective can be both aligned and in conflict with the objective of patient safety.

The objective of this chapter is to equip you with an understanding of the basics of health economics and its application to patient safety, so as to enable you to identify cost-effective patient safety initiatives.

What is health economics?

Health economics is a branch area of study that applies the concepts of economic analysis to the production, maintenance, and consequences of health at both individual and population level. Health economics contains many subspecialties, but, in the context of palliative care, the most relevant one is cost-effectiveness analysis (CEA).

CEA is the study of the costs of providing health interventions and their resulting health benefits. Its objective is to maximize overall population health. CEA is motivated by the scarcity of resources. This means that the health gains generated by healthcare interventions need to inform difficult choices about which healthcare interventions to provide and which to withhold. CEA combines both technical and ethical judgements in order to decide which interventions should be funded and implemented. While the technical judgements are matters of fact, the ethical or normative issues are matters of values and are not always characterized by consensus. Accordingly, different approaches to CEA have emerged, depending on the extent to which government has a role in providing healthcare and on the trade-offs [illegible] between equity and individual liberty.

CEA aims to appraise the total cost of an intervention, including the opportunity costs of providing the intervention and any downstream savings that may occur, irrespective of where in the health system. CEA could also include costs and savings that accrue to other government departments, private businesses, and the broader economy, depending on the prevailing norms in each country or jurisdiction.

CEA also attempts to estimate the total health benefits that follow from an intervention, from now until the patient's death. These include the positive therapeutic outcomes, but also any harms that may result as a consequence of the intervention such as side effects, mistakes, or adverse events.

Definitions

CEA

A cost-effectiveness analysis is the study of the costs of providing health interventions and their resulting health gains. Its objective is to maximize overall population health.

QALY

The quality-adjusted life year (QALY) is a multidimensional metric of health gain that combines reductions in both morbidity and mortality.

Cost-effectiveness ratios

Cost-effectiveness ratios are obtained by dividing the expected cost of an intervention by its total QALY gains.

ICER

The incremental cost-effectiveness ratio estimates how many additional costs are incurred in order to achieve one more unit of additional health when comparing alternative intervention strategies.

Cost-effectiveness threshold

The cost-effectiveness threshold represents an upper bound on ICERs and corresponds to a judgement about what represents good value for money.

What is health economics?

Health economics is a broad area of study that applies the concepts of economic analysis to the production, maintenance, and consequences of health at both individual and population level. Health economics contains many subdisciplines and, in the context of patient safety, the most relevant one is cost-effectiveness analysis (CEA).

CEA is the study of the costs of providing health interventions and their resulting health benefits; its objective is to maximize overall population health. CEA is motivated by the scarcity of resources. To maximize the health generated by healthcare budgets, we need to make difficult choices about which healthcare interventions to provide and which to withhold.

CEA combines both technical and ethical judgements in order to decide which interventions ought to be funded and which not. While the technical or positive judgements are matters of fact, the ethical or normative issues depend on matters of value and are not always supported by consensus. Accordingly, different approaches to CEA have emerged, depending on the extent to which central government has a role in providing healthcare and on the preferences within society for trade-offs between equity and individual liberty.

CEA aims to appraise the total cost of an intervention, including the up-front costs of providing the intervention and any downstream savings that may occur later and in other areas of the health system. Whether or not CEA should also include costs and savings that accrue to other government departments, private businesses, and the broader society depends on the prevailing norms in each country or national setting.

CEA also attempts to appraise the total health benefits that follow from an intervention, both now and in the future. These include the positive therapeutic outcomes, but also any harms that may result as consequence of unavoidable side effects, misdiagnosis or adverse events.

Definitions

CEA

Cost-effectiveness analysis is the study of the costs of providing health interventions and their resulting health benefits; its objective is to maximize overall population health.

QALY

The quality-adjusted life years (QALY) is a unidimensional metric of health gain that combines reductions in both morbidity and mortality.

Cost-effectiveness ratios

Cost-effectiveness ratios are obtained by dividing the total net cost of an intervention by the total net QALYs gained.

ICER

The incremental cost-effectiveness ratio estimates how many additional costs are incurred in order to achieve this or that additional health gain, when comparing alternative intervention strategies.

Cost-effectiveness threshold

The cost-effectiveness threshold represents an upper bound on ICERs that corresponds to a limit on what represents good value for money.

Quantification of health gains

Health gains are typically quantified in CEA using QALYs.

- The QALY is a unidimensional metric that combines reductions in both morbidity and mortality.
- A unidimensional metric is used deliberately to provide a measure of health gain that can be employed to compare many different types of interventions that work on different aspects of health improvement across different illnesses in different patients.
- This compromises the resolution with which we appraise the multifaceted improvement in health from diverse interventions, but such a simplification is required if we want to achieve comparability across multiple candidate interventions.

CEA employs a simple decision rule to determine which interventions represent sufficiently good value to merit funding.

- This decision is based on cost-effectiveness ratios and on what is known as the cost-effectiveness threshold.
- Cost-effectiveness ratios are obtained by dividing the total net cost of an intervention by the total net QALYs gained with its help.
- Importantly, the costs and effects within the ratio are not necessarily formed by comparison to no intervention, but are relative to the costs and effects of the next best alternative intervention strategy. This is in order to estimate what is known as the ICER, which tells us how many additional costs are incurred in order to achieve this or that additional health gain when comparing alternative intervention strategies.
- The cost-effectiveness threshold represents an upper bound on ICERs that corresponds to a limit on what represents good value for money.
- Health economists would recommend that all interventions with ICERs below the threshold be accepted and all those above the threshold be rejected.
- In principle, allocation according to this decision rule yields the largest health gain possible for the corresponding number and magnitude of healthcare resources available.
- The earlier description of the ICER-threshold decision rule assumes that new interventions are both more costly and more effective than existing interventions. In some cases, new interventions are both more effective and less costly than the previous standard of care. In such cases, new interventions demonstrate what is known as dominance and can be recommended without reference to a threshold.
- CEA is most useful when there are clearly identifiable net total costs and QALYs that can be appraised for a specific intervention, such as a drug. Conversely, the appraisal of the cost-effectiveness of nursing care is a less meaningful proposition, as clearly nurses carry out a range of tasks, some of which might be highly cost-effective while others might not. Accordingly, CEA must be applied carefully to produce meaningful recommendations for resource allocation.

Cost-effectiveness analyses of safety

Typically, the hierarchy for the adoption of a new intervention is to demonstrate that

- it is safe and does not harm patients;
- it has greater efficacy than existing interventions; and
- it is cost-effective.

Improved safety is, typically, an ongoing and explicit objective of all health services. Furthermore, it will often be the case that what is safer will also demonstrate dominance in terms of cost effectiveness. For example, the reduction in adverse events within a service may lead to better health outcomes and lower additional care costs. In such cases, the objectives of safety and cost effectiveness are aligned.

There are three scenarios to consider:

1. If it can be demonstrated that safer care is likely to be more effective and to cost less (which demonstrates dominance), then there is little need for a comprehensive CEA. A decision maker does not need to know how much more effective and how much less costly a safer service improvement will be to endorse that improvement. Indeed, research that carefully quantifies the size of the increase in effectiveness and cost savings would itself be a waste of research effort, and therefore should be avoided.
2. Where a safety improvement leads to an increase in effectiveness, but also to an increase in costs, the objectives of safety and cost effectiveness are potentially in tension. While ideally we would like all services to be as safe as possible, the fact that some safety initiatives can be net costly requires us to consider the trade-off of increased cost for increased safety. Many safety initiatives may be good value, but others may not be worth paying for. In other words, we choose, naturally, safer healthcare services, but not at all costs.
3. Where there is a trade-off of increased cost for additional safety, we must carefully quantify the improved effectiveness in terms of QALYs and the increased costs of the new intervention or service improvement. If the ICER of the safety improvement is within the cost-effectiveness threshold, then the objectives of safety and cost effectiveness remain aligned. Conversely, if the ICER of the safety improvement exceeds that threshold, then the objective of improved safety conflicts with the objective of achieving cost-effective care. Accordingly, we may reject a safety initiative that is not within our threshold.

There are studies that attempt to estimate the overall costs to health systems of medical errors, both in terms of damaged health and additional healthcare costs and in terms of lost employment and wider economic damage.

- For example, in the USA, estimates from 2008 appreciated medical errors to have costed £19.5bn (from 1.5 million avoidable medical injuries).
- While such estimates can be useful in demonstrating the urgency of attending to the issue of healthcare safety and in creating an overall motivation to promote related policies, they do not provide a useful guide to policymakers or service planners as to what specific service improvements are worth adopting (or not). CEAs of particular service changes or innovations are more specific.

Box 5.1 Case 1: Computer-ordered entry systems

Forrester et al. (2014) provide a good example of where an initiative to improve safety is estimated to be cost-effective. An analysis used a model to estimate the costs and consequences of implementing a computerized order entry form instead of the conventional paper prescription. The researchers found that the computerized system cost less and resulted in fewer medication errors and adverse drug events. While the analysis did not estimate the health consequences in terms of QALYs, it still clearly indicates a case of dominance. This is because the reduction in medication errors and adverse events is highly likely to result in improved QALY outcomes. The fact that the computerized prescribing system demonstrates dominance in terms of reduced costs and fewer negative outcomes obviates the need for quantifying the health benefits in QALYs. Accordingly, in the case of such an intervention, the safety and cost-effectiveness perspectives are in alignment.

Box 5.2 Case 2: Blood transfusions

An example of a CEA of an intervention designed to improve the safety of blood transfusion services is offered by Teljeur et al.'s (2012) analysis of prion filtration in Ireland. That analysis noted that Ireland had suffered a history of blood scandals, and consideration was given to a filtration service that would reduce the risk of the variant Creutzfeldt–Jakob disease (vCJD) being passed from asymptomatic donors to recipients.

A cost-effectiveness model showed that, although the risk of vCJD transmission could be reduced, this would be achieved at a cost of €3.7 million per life year gained (LYG). A LYG can be considered commensurate with a QALY.

The reason for the very high ICER in this case is that, although the intervention would improve blood safety, it was estimated that, over ten years of implementing the service, only two cases of vCJD would be spared through prion screening.

The estimated ICER far exceeds the cost-effectiveness threshold of €45,000/QALY conventionally applied in Ireland. Accordingly, in this context prion filtration would be considered very poor value for money and has not been adopted by the Irish Blood Transfusion Service.

Box 5.3 Case 3: Nurse-to-patient ratios

An example of the difficulty of finding clear evidence of interventions that improve safety in a cost-effective way can be encountered in the literature on nurse to patient ratios. While it seems intuitively highly plausible that there would be a positive relationship between staffing and patient safety, the literature does not appear to offer clear evidence to support this assumption.

A recent review of the cost-effectiveness evidence on changing nurse to patient ratios found no studies that give estimates on the cost per QALY of changing staff intensity and only two studies on the cost per LYG of such service changes (Twigg et al. 2015). While both studies reported favourable cost-effectiveness ratios for the staff intensifications they assessed, the overall conclusion is that there is a very slim body of evidence reporting beneficial changes in the metrics required for comparability with other healthcare interventions. Moreover, the current literature certainly does not seem to provide sufficient information to judge at what point the increased staff-to-patient ratio ceases to be cost-effective in improving safety and other beneficial outcomes.

The example of an absence of clear evidence showing that improved staff-to-patient ratios are a cost-effective way of improving safety probably simply reflects the fact that it is difficult to gather evidence on such relationships between staffing and safety; it is not necessarily an indication that improved staffing is not effective or cost-effective at improving care. Indeed, it is important to remember that the absence of evidence of cost effectiveness is not evidence of an absence of cost effectiveness.

Box 5.4 Case 4: Antibiotics effectiveness

Robotham et al. (2016) conducted a CEA to estimate the effectiveness of alternative methods for screening for meticillin-resistant Staphylococcus aureus (MRSA) on admission to English hospitals. While it is expected that the screening methods considered in their analysis would improve the safety of hospital care by reducing the anticipated number of clinical infections and deaths, the costs of the screening strategies were such that the estimated cost per QALY estimates exceeded UK cost-effectiveness thresholds. Accordingly, although hospital-acquired infections impose a known and heavy healthcare burden, it appears that screening for such infections on admission is not a good value means of improving the safety of care.

How health economics can align and conflict with patient safety

[illegible]

How health economics can align and conflict with patient safety

It is tempting to assume that all initiatives that improve patient safety will necessarily enhance the cost effectiveness of healthcare services. Indeed, in many cases they will do. Unfortunately, reassuring statements that safer care is more efficient care are simplistic, as they are not always true.

- Safety is a desirable feature of healthcare systems and should be enhanced, but not if the costs of doing so exceed the benefits of better uses of resources required elsewhere in the health system.
- CEA provides decision makers with a clear, consistent analytical tool for appraising the benefits and costs of improved safety initiatives.
- Moreover, CEA offers a very clear decision-making framework within which one can judge which safety initiatives represent value for money.
- In cases in which the cost-effectiveness perspective conflicts with the drive to improve safety, decision makers must act with conviction to avoid the temptation to enhance safety at all costs.
- Insisting on prioritizing safety without regard to cost will lead to an overall reduction in the health gains achieved by the healthcare system.
- Resisting the temptation to increase safety at all costs is difficult, as the forgone additional safety will belong in the part of the health system that the decision maker has responsibility for, while the resources saved may purchase health benefits that are purchased elsewhere. Accordingly, it is understandably difficult for a decision maker to knowingly prioritise the health of patients outside of their area of management at the detriment of those within their area of control.
- Achieving cost-effective improvements in safety is, arguably, as much about the discipline of decision makers and their resolve to make efficient choices as it is about the clinical, technical, and cultural processes required to enhance care.

This chapter presented some examples of health-economic evaluations of safety drawn from the existing literature. Nevertheless, the literature on the cost effectiveness of safety improvements remains relatively thin and immature. Accordingly, those wishing to understand the health-economic consequences of safety initiatives within their area of practice may need to generate the cost-effectiveness evidence themselves, as there is little published evidence at present.

Summary box

Health economics provides a well-developed framework for the appraisal of safety initiatives. In many cases there will be a happy alliance between improving safety and enhancing the efficiency of care.

Where safety and cost effectiveness conflict, decision makers need to remember that cost-ineffective services reduce population health.

The shortage of published evidence to date means that decision makers may need to conduct their own analyses of safety improvements in order to make evidence-based decisions regarding the efficient use of resources at their disposal.

References

Forrester, S. H. et al. Cost-effectiveness of a computerized provider order entry system in improving medication safety ambulatory care. *Value in Health* 17.4 (2014): 340–9.

Robotham, J. V. et al. Cost-effectiveness of national mandatory screening of all admissions to English National Health Service hospitals for meticillin-resistant Staphylococcus aureus: A mathematical modelling study. *Lancet Infectious Diseases* 16.3 (2016): 348–56.

Teljeur, C. et al. Cost-effectiveness of prion filtration of red blood cells to reduce the risk of transfusion-transmitted variant Creutzfeldt–Jakob disease in the Republic of Ireland. *Transfusion* 52.11 (2012): 2285–93.

Twigg, D. E. et al. Is there an economic case for investing in nursing care—what does the literature tell us? *Journal of Advanced Nursing* 71.5 (2015): 975–90.

Further reading

Andel, C. et al. The economics of health care quality and medical errors. *Journal of Health Care Finance* 39.1 (2012): 39–50

Bouvy, C. et al. The cost-effectiveness of periodic safety update reports for biologicals in Europe. *Clinical Pharmacology & Therapeutics* 93.5 (2013): 433–42.

Cook, A. et al. The effect of a hospital nurse staffing mandate on patient health outcomes: Evidence from California's minimum staffing regulation. *Journal of Health Economics* 31.2 (2012): 340–8.

Etchells, E. et al. Comparative economic analyses of patient safety improvement strategies in acute care: A systematic review. *BMJ Quality & Safety* 21.6 (2012): 448–56.

Pauker, S. G., Zane, E. M., and Salem, D. N. Creating a safer health care system: Finding the constraint. *JAMA* 294.22 (2005): 2906–8.

OECD papers

Auraaen, A., Slawomirski, L., and Klazinga, N. The economics of patient safety in primary and ambulatory care: Flying blind. OECD Health Working Papers, No. 106, OECD Publishing, Paris 2018, https://doi.org/10.1787/baf425ad-en.

de Bienassis, K., Llena-Nozal, A., and Klazinga, N. The economics of patient safety, Part III: Long-term care: Valuing safety for the long haul. OECD Health Working Papers, No. 121, OECD Publishing, Paris 2020, https://doi.org/10.1787/be07475c-en.

de Bienassis, K., Slawomirski, L., and Klazinga N. The economics of patient safety Part IV: Safety in the workplace: Occupational safety as the bedrock of resilient health systems. OECD Health Working Papers, No. 130. OECD Publishing, Paris 2021, https://doi.org/10.1787/b25b8c39-en.

Slawomirski, L., Auraaen, A., and Klazinga, N. The economics of patient safety: Strengthening a value-based approach to reducing patient harm at national level. OECD Health Working Papers, No. 96. OECD Publishing, Paris 2017, https://doi.org/10.1787/5a9858cd-en.

Chapter 6

Developing a safe clinical team

Key points

- The achievement of patient safety requires teamwork.
- The degree of teamwork reflects the culture of the system.
- Safe clinical teams exhibit psychological safety, where every team member feels safe to raise concerns and always feels supported.
- In a safe clinical team there is meaning to work and a sense of belonging.
- Respect, compassion, and kindness are core values of a safe clinical team.

What is the safety issue?

- Harm occurs in all healthcare settings and is a concern for all healthcare staff.
- Most multidisciplinary professional training offers little regarding the practical application of how to assess risk and continuously improve safety in clinical practice.
- As patients, we all assume that healthcare is safe.
- Team training is not routine in healthcare, yet it is the operational norm in all healthcare settings.
- All healthcare environments are currently experiencing a deficit in staff availability.

Why is it a challenge?

- Many processes in healthcare are not standardized. Healthcare is complex and not considered a highly reliable industry.
- Many clinical leaders are focused on day-to-day operations and outputs rather than on a systems approach and patient outcomes.
- Clinical discussions carried out every day as a team, specifically on safety matters that occur throughout the day, are not routinely practised.
- The culture of the clinical context needs to be receptive to open and honest discussions.
- Person- and family-centred approaches are not always paramount.
- The technology for standardizing care can be unaffordable and poorly designed.

What is the theoretical basis?

- Team learning enables outcome improvement, task mastery, and adaptive and responsive practices.
- Adopt systems thinking: understanding the interactions and interdependencies of the whole healthcare system is crucial for the local impact of behaviours and practices and for the patient's outcomes.
- Practise open disclosure: the open, honest, and timely disclosure of medical errors to patients develops a culture based on transparency (see Chapter 17, open disclosure).

What do you need to do to be safe?

- Speak up when you are aware of harmful and potentially harmful practices or situations and create the conditions for others to do the same.
- Embed and practise clear communications tools, to be used daily.
- Listen to patients and carers, aiming to understand care from their perspective.

How can the hierarchy affect the team's professional autonomy?

- Historically, all healthcare systems are hierarchical.
- Seniority in organizational team structures does not necessarily amount to skill.
- Defer clinical responsibility to individuals who have the highest expertise, be that the most junior member of the team, or perhaps even the patient, if that person has the skills best suited for undertaking the tasks at hand in a manner that improves safety and reliability.
- Develop leaders who can practice open communication.
- Provide mentorship to suport clincal leaders.

Training in non-technical skills, focused on teamwork knowledge and attitudes

- Non-technical skills (NTS) are the cognitive (decision-making, situation awareness) and interpersonal (communication, teamwork, leadership) skills that underpin technical proficiency. They are considered particularly important for preventing errors.
- NTS are interpersonal skills such as communication skills, leadership skills, teamwork skills, decision-making skills, and situation awareness skills.
- Technical skills are the abilities and knowledge needed to perform specific tasks. They are practical and often relate to mechanical, information technology, mathematical, or scientific tasks. Examples include knowledge of programming languages and the capacity to use mechanical equipment or tools.

What is known to work to build safe teams?

- Train the clinical team together, to improve care.
- Support staff training, to enable the teams to understand the critical conditions required for patient safety.
- In context, agree to a set of rules and behaviours that are upheld by all team members, to sustain and improve safety.
- Make the right thing easy to do. Consider areas of care that can be standardized.
- Hold daily safety briefing sessions, to discuss the elements of risk that could require optimum clinical care.
- Create safe opportunities for people to speak up in the clinical area, and create the conditions for everyone to speak freely, expressing concerns and sharing opportunities to prevent harm.
- Implement Schwartz rounds, that is, evidence-based group discussions where staff members from all backgrounds come together to discuss the emotional and social challenges of caring for patients, to support each other, and to share stories.
- Seek opportunities for care to be co-designed with patients and carers, so that you deliver improved outcomes.
- Practise, practise, practise. As a team, use simulation to identify, mitigate, and reduce harm,
- Build confidence in team members by celebrating success and focus learning on the elements of care that go well, in order to understand the critical behaviours and practices. Then replicate these elements.

How do you measure your team's safety?

- Use standard measures to determine outcomes, measuring what matters to patients and staff members.
- Make measuring the system's performance and outcomes easy tasks to do.
- Understand the difference between work imagined and work done.
- Analyse safety across the patient's journey by defining individual processes and timelines from the patient's perspective, using process mapping (see ch. 13, measurement of safety).

Practising team safety: Tips

- Encourage and create opportunities to discuss risk openly in your conversations.
- Use a standard template to guide conversations, for example:
  - Are we all clear about the care planning today?
  - Are there any concerns?
  - Where do we anticipate that there may be problems?
  - What can we do to mitigate any issues identified?
  - Who will be responsible for each aspect?

Summary box

- Seek to build a whole system of care where the potential harms are openly discussed and active plans are made to avoid harm.
- Embed and practise clear communications tools, to be used on a daily basis.
- Build training opportunities to use tools and techniques that improve and maintain safe practice.
- Measure staff compliance alongside patient outcomes.
- Practise using simulation techniques for both simple and complex tasks and use key communication tools within the scenarios.
- Hierarchy does not necessarily correspond to knowledge. Defer to the expert, be that the patient or a junior member of the team, if that person can deliver the tasks at hand when safety is paramount.
- Seek to understand and create joy at work.
- Encourage your team to be the best that it can be.

Further reading

Aggarwal, R. et al. Training and simulation for patient safety. *BMJ Quality & Safety* 19 (2010): i34–i43.

Edmonson, A. C. (1999). Psychological safety and learning behavior in work teams. *Administrative Science Quarterly* 44: 350–83.

Gandhi, T. K. et al. Transforming concepts in patient safety: A progress report. *BMJ Quality & Safety* 27 (2018): 1019–26.

Gordon, M., Darbyshire, D. and Baker, P. Non-technical skills training to enhance patient safety: A systematic review. *Medical Education* 46 (2012): 1042–54.

McDowell, D. S. and McComb, S. A. Safety checklist briefings: A systematic review of the literature. *AORN Journal* 99.1 (2014): 125–37, e13.

Nabhan, M. et al. What is preventable harm in healthcare? A systematic review of definitions. *BMC Health Services Research* 12 (2012), https://bmchealthservres.biomedcentral.com/articles/10.1186/1472-6963-12-128.

Perlo, J. et al. *IHI Framework for Improving Joy in Work* (IHI White Paper). Cambridge, MA: Institute for Healthcare Improvement, 2017.

Robert, G. et al. Exploring the adoption of Schwartz Center Rounds as an organisational innovation to improve staff well-being in England, 2009–2015. *BMJ Open* 7 (2017): e014326.

Studdert, D. M., Piper, D., and Iedema, R. Legal aspects of open disclosure, II: Attitudes of health professionals: Findings from a national survey. *Medical Journal of Australia* 193 (2010): 351–5.

Chapter 7

Communicating to be safe

Key points

- Communication reflects the culture of a system at every level in healthcare.
- In the course of one day there are multiple transfers of information that can lead to a communication error.
- Most patient safety incidents and adverse events have a communication component.
- Communication methods can be implemented so as to improve communication between people, either with the patient and his or her family or within the clinical teams.

What is the safety issue?

Effective communication among team members and between team members and patients is of paramount importance in the provision of safe and reliable person-centred care. Effective clinical communication is clear, explicit, respectful, collaborative, and attentive. It can lead to an improved flow of information, effective interventions, the patient's and the healthcare professional's satisfaction, and patient safety.

Ineffective communication among healthcare professionals can have serious repercussions and may even result in harm for the patient.

Why is it a challenge?

Ineffective communication puts patient safety at risk for various reasons. These include the lack of exchange of critical information, the misinterpretation of information, and the overlooking of changes in the patient's status. The sources of ineffective communication are often multifactorial and can span the entire multidisciplinary team. Patients need an open communication system instead of experiencing adverse events stemming from communication failures. Ineffective communication is a common problem and may be caused by barriers to effective communication or by human factors (see Table 7.1).

Table 7.1. Barriers to communication

Barriers	Human factors
Lack of confidence	Cognitive overload
Saving face	Stress and fatigue
Preserving relationships	Distractions and interruptions
Deference to hierarchy	Poor interpersonal skills
Fear of repercussions	Imperfect information processing
Conflict avoidance	Flawed decision-making

Data from (Lyndon et al. 2011)

How can one be safe?

As a precaution, to develop a safe and effective framework for handovers one should involve collaboration, open communication, clear identification of all parties, shared decision making, and shared responsibilities.

The components of a safe work culture include:

- implementing safe handovers
- using a common language (e.g. SBAR, I-PASS)
- critical interventions to stop unsafe behaviour.

Implementing safe handovers

Patient handovers are prone to communication errors owing to the presence of barriers to effective communication. Large amounts of complex information may be sludged and frequently can result in misinterpretations and omissions. On the other hand, the use of a structured format, such as the framework of SBAR (situation, background, assessment, and recommendation) or I-PASS (illness severity, patient summary, action list, situation awareness and contingency planning, and synthesis by receiver) are crucial to the development of safe, effective handovers.

Using a common language

Structured communication support tools such as SBAR and I-PASS have been used successfully in clinical practice to improve patient safety (see Table 7.3).

Table 7.3 [illegible] of structured communication to support safety

They provide a common language across [illegible]
They [illegible] expected [illegible]
They [illegible] a common [illegible]
They improve efficiency, safety, and accuracy
They [illegible]

SBAR (situation, background, assessment, and recommendation) [illegible] 2002 [illegible] to reduce communication errors at the time of [illegible]. It was adopted by the [illegible] and is now commonly used for handover in healthcare (see Table 7.3).

I-PASS was developed from best evidence, expert practices in the literature, feedback from a pilot study, and observations made by the handover [illegible] and has been shown to be highly reliable [illegible] (see Table 7.4).

Documentation to be safe

Documentation is a vital component of safe and effective patient care. It provides a mechanism to record and communicate the data, information, and knowledge about a patient that the care provider [illegible]. The fundamental principles of documentation to be safe are [illegible].

How can one be safe?

An intervention to develop a communication framework in healthcare should involve collaboration, open communication, coordination of all parties, shared decision-making, and shared responsibilities.

This communication framework can include

- implementing safe handovers;
- using a common language (e.g. SBAR, I-PASS)
- critical interventions to stop unsafe behaviour.

Implementing safe handovers

Patient handovers are prone to communication errors, owing to the presence of barriers to effective communication. Large amounts of complex information may be included and frequently can result in informational gaps and omissions in the handover report. Use of a structured communication framework such as SBAR (situation, background, assessment, and recommendation) or I-PASS (illness severity, patient summary, action list, situation awareness and contingency planning, and synthesis by receiver) are critical to the development of safe, effective handovers.

Using a common language

Structured communication support tools such as SBAR and I-PASS have been used successfully in clinical practice to improve patient safety (see Table 7.2).

Table 7.2. Benefits of structured communication support tools

They create a common language for communication.
They flatten the perceived healthcare hierarchy.
They guarantee regularity and predictability in handover communication.
They improve efficiency, efficacy, and accuracy.
They promote a culture of patient safety in healthcare settings.

SBAR was successfully adapted in 2002 from the US Army; the goal was to reduce communication errors at the time of clinical handover. It was adopted by the Kaiser Permanente organization in Colorado, USA, and is now commonly used worldwide in healthcare (see Table 7.3).

I-PASS was developed from best cited handover practices in the literature, user feedback from a pilot study, and observations made by the handover team; and it has been shown to be highly reliable (Clements 2007; see Table 7.4).

Documentation to be safe

Documentation is a vital component of safe and effective patient care. It provides a mechanism to record and communicate data, information, and knowledge about a patient and the care provided. It can be written or electronic. The fundamental principles of documentation to be safe are found in Box 7.1.

Table 7.3. Example of user of Kaiser Permanente SBAR tool, 2002

Situation What is going on with the patient?	'I am calling about Mrs. Joseph in room 251. Chief complaint is shortness of breath of new onset.'
Background What is the clinical background or context?	'Patient is a 62-year-old female post-op day one from abdominal surgery. No prior history of cardiac or lung disease.'
Assessment What do I think the problem is?	'Breath sounds are decreased on the right side with acknowledgment of pain. Would like to rule out pneumothorax.'
Recommendation What would I do to correct it?	'I feel strongly the patient should be assessed now. Are you available to come in?'

Source: Institute for Healthcare Improvement, n.d.

Table 7.4. Example of user of I-PASS handover tool

Illness severity Stable, 'watcher', unstable	'This is our sickest patient.'
Patient summary • summary statement • events leading up to admission • hospital course • ongoing assessment • plan	'AJ is a 4-year-old boy with a history of ex 26 week gestation admitted with hypoxia and respiratory distress secondary to a left lower lobe pneumonia. He presented with cough and high fevers for two days before admission, and on the day that he presented to the emergency department he had worsening respiratory distress. In the emergency department, he was found to have a Na of 130, likely secondary to volume depletion versus syndrome of inappropriate secretion of antidiuretic hormone. He received a fluid bolus and was started on O2 at 2.5L. He is on ceftriaxone.'
Action list • to do list • time line and ownership	'Please look in on him at approximately midnight and make sure his vitals are unchanged and his oxygen saturation is stable. Check to determine if his blood culture is positive tonight.'
Situation awareness and contingency planning • know what's going on • plan for what might happen	'If his respiratory status worsens, please get another chest radiograph to determine if he is developing an effusion.'
Synthesis by receiver • receiver summarizes what was heard • asks questions • restates key action/to do items	'OK, so AJ is a 4 year old ex premie admitted with hypoxia and respiratory distress secondary to a lower lobe pneumonia on ceftriaxone, O2 and fluids. You want me to check on him at midnight to make sure he's stable and check his blood culture. If his respiratory status worsens, I will repeat a radiograph to look for an effusion'

Data from Starmer et al. 2011

Box 7.1 Fundamental properties of documentation to be safe

Documentation to be safe should be:

- clear, concise, and comprehensive;
- accurate, true, and honest;
- relevant;
- reflective of observations that have been made;
- timely and completed during or immediately after giving care;
- chronological order;
- a complete record of the care provided;
- permanent;
- retrievable;
- confidential; and
- patient-focused.

Using technology to improve patient safety

In recent times there has been an increase in the development and implementation of healthcare technologies. The application of technology to enhance patient safety is of paramount importance. The World Health Organization (WHO) has developed four working groups for the use of technology to improve patient safety, giving particular consideration to the needs and challenges of settings in Lower and Middle Income countries. (see Table 7.5).

Table 7.5. WHO Themes for the safe introduction of technology

Introducing new technology safely	• regulation • health technology assessment • clinical engineering • training and surveillance
Making existing technologies safer	• reporting systems • human factors • home care • hospital care • primary care • quality assurance
Information technology	• electronic records • computerized physician order entry • decision support • bar coding
Simulation and training	• improvement of patient safety through education and training, moving the learning curve from patient to simulator • use of low- and high-tech simulation • use of research, design, and testing

Source: Adapted from Aggarwal et al. 2010

Critical interventions to stop unsafe behaviour

Healthcare organizations need to encourage providers to report unsafe behaviour. Reporting mechanisms should be made easy and must be supported by the presence of a non-punitive environment. Mechanisms of reporting unsafe behaviours include reporting to a senior, filing an incident report, using a suggestion box, or reporting directly to a task force with assigned responsibilities for addressing these issues.

Educational programmes can teach the basic skills necessary to promote effective communication and safe behaviour. However, for individuals who consistently exhibit unsafe behaviour, educational programmes may need to be supported by more focused sessions and targeted counselling.

Summary box

- Effective communication is of critical importance to the provision of safe and reliable person-centred care.
- Ineffective communication can have serious repercussions and may even result in harm to the patient.
- The development of a communication framework should involve collaboration and open communication.
- The development of effective handovers and of a common language with structured communication support tools is necessary for the provision of safe patient care.
- Documentation is a vital component of safe and effective patient care, and fundamental principles should be followed.
- The application of technology to enhance patient care should be considered.
- Educational programs can teach the skills necessary to promote safe behaviour, more targeted counselling being applied to those who consistently exhibit unsafe behaviour.

References

Aggarwal, R. et al. Technology as applied to patient safety: An overview. *BMJ Quality & Safety* 19 (2010): i3–i8.

Clements, K. High-reliability and the I-PASS communication tool. *Nursing Management* 48,3 (2017): 12–13.

Institute for Healthcare Improvement. Guidelines for communicating with physicians using the SBAR process. n.d. Cambridge, MA. http://www.ihi.org/resources/Pages/Tools/SBARToolkit.aspx.

Lyndon, A., Zlatnik, M. G., and Wachter, R. M. Effective physician–nurse communication: A patient safety essential for labor and delivery. *American Journal of Obstetrix and Gynecology* 205,2 (2011): 91–96. doi:10.1016/j.ajog.2011.04.021.

Starmer, A. J. et al. I-PASS, a mnemonic to standarize verbal handoffs. *Pediatrics* 129 (2012): 201–4.

Further reading

Berwick, D. M. Seeking systemness. *Healthcare Forum Journal* 35 (1992): 22–8.

Building the Nurse–Physician Partnership: Restoring Mutual Trust, Establishing Clinical Collaboration. Washington, DC: Health Care Advisory Board, 2005.

Joint Commission on Accreditation of Healthcare Organizations. *The Joint Commission Guide to Improving Staff Communication.* Oakbrook Terrace, IL: Joint Commission Resources, 2005.

Leonard, M., Graham, S., and Bonucom, D. The human factor: The critical importance of effective teamwork and communication in providing safe care. *Quality and Safety in Health Care* 13 (2004) (Suppl. 1): 185–90.

O'Daniel, M. and Rosenstein, A. H. Professional communication and team collaboration. In R. G. Hughes (ed.), *Patient Safety and Quality: An Evidence-Based Handbook for Nurses*. Rockville, MD: Agency for Healthcare Research and Quality, 2008, ch. 33.

Shahid, S. and Thomas, S. Situation, background, assessment, recommendation (SBAR) communication tool for handoff in health care: A narrative review. *Safety in Health* 4 (2018). https://safetyinhealth.biomedcentral.com/articles/10.1186/s40886-018-0073-1.

Chapter 8

Situation awareness and patient safety

Key points

- Situation awareness implies that all team members have the same level of understanding of the real-time safety challenges.
- This requires constant collection of information, comprehension and sharing of the information, and then making decisions to mitigate risk.
- Methods to improve situation awareness include safety huddles and crew resource management.

What is situation awareness?

- In its simplest sense, situation awareness means being aware of what is going on around you.
- In the healthcare context, effective situation awareness begins with the collation of relevant patient information in a systematic fashion, followed by the analyses and sharing of this information, which allows for a unified understanding among the members of the clinical team. This in turn allows for the early identification of potential risks, enabling appropriate mitigating actions to be taken in a timely fashion.
- Situation awareness is widely used in other high-risk industries such as aviation, nuclear energy, construction and the military.
- Interesting fact: situation awareness was recognized as an essential tool for military aircraft crews already during the First World War.

What is the safety issue?

- All organizations in which people work have latent weaknesses, which are multifactorial in nature and increase the likelihood of errors. This is particularly true of complex adaptive systems such as healthcare organizations.
- Even the most experienced professionals can be lacking in situation awareness, particularly when performing tasks that are routine to them.
- A study analysing the causative factors in airline accidents identified problems related to situational awareness in 88% of the accidents that involved human error.
- Indeed, medical error was estimated as the third leading cause of death in the USA.
- Failure to recognize and treat patients whose condition is deteriorating is a cause of significant unintended harm in healthcare environments.

Why is it a challenge?

- The way in which we read situations can be influenced by a number of factors such as our level of experience, the numbers of distractions, the amount of relevant information at our disposal, and tiredness—to name only a few.
- The science that examines the relationships between humans and the systems they interact with is known as human factors or ergonomics.
- The early detection of deteriorating patients is key to improving patient outcomes, and this is facilitated through better situation awareness.
- Improving situation awareness in the healthcare setting is a complex task, which requires significant efforts to embed it as part of the culture.
- Clinicians may initially view it as an additional pressure on top of an already busy workload, given that the benefits are not immediately apparent.

How can one be safe?

What is known to work?

What is the theoretical basis?

It has been proposed that situation awareness includes three levels (see Figure 8.1):

- the perception of what is happening (level 1);
- the understanding of what has been perceived (level 2);
- the use of what is understood to think ahead (level 3).

What we need to do to be safe

How can one be safe?

What is known to work?

- Effective teamwork and communication are essential components in the delivery of high-quality, safe patient care.
- It has been recognized that effective communication can depend on the personnel involved or may vary according to circumstances.
- The implementation of standardized tools and behaviours has proven to be very effective at reducing this variation in other high-reliability organizations such as aviation, therefore improving performance in a consistent fashion and reducing risk.

What is the theoretical basis?

It has been proposed that situation awareness includes three processes (see Figure 8.1):

- the perception of what is happening (level 1);
- the understanding of what has been perceived (level 2);
- the use of what is understood to think ahead (level 3).

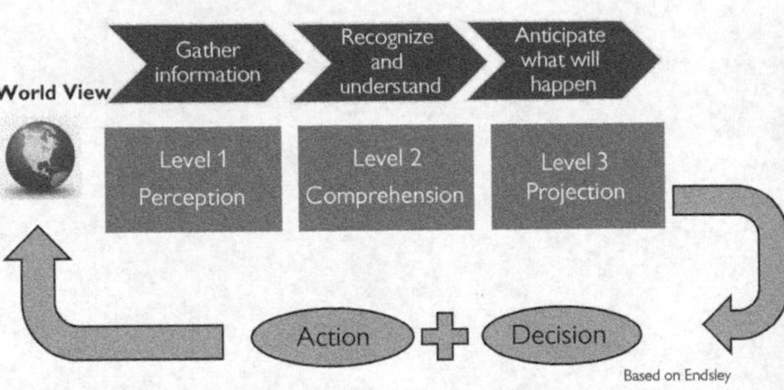

Figure 8.1 Processes designed to develop situation awareness.

The theory of change proposes that short meetings such as safety huddles (discussed later) facilitate the development of situation awareness and allow for a more collaborative teamwork, with a more efficient sharing of information. This further expedites a common understanding of the clinical condition of patients, which in turn enables actions to be taken to mitigate any potential harm and to respond in a timely fashion to any deterioration in these patients' condition.

What you need to do to be safe?

- Given the complexity of healthcare organizations, no single intervention taken in isolation, can solve a problem. What is required instead is a combination of interventions targeting the various contributory factors involved in the clinical deterioration of patients.
- Central to this process is the need to adopt a systems approach, which will assess the various interacting components of the healthcare machine as a whole rather than as a series of distinct silos. Indeed, it is often at the interface between these components that information is lost and errors can occur.

- One of the key benefits of improving situation awareness is that it facilitates the shift from a reactive to a more proactive approach to patient care. This allows for mitigating actions to be taken to avoid preventable harm.
- Given that a significant number of potential interventions exist and that the effectiveness of each one can vary between institutions, any intervention should be tailored, before implementation, to meet the specific needs of the institution.

Use of huddles to facilitate situation awareness

- Huddles are among the key tools for improving situation awareness in healthcare settings. They have been borrowed from other high-reliability industries with the aim of minimizing harm and errors.
- Huddles in the healthcare setting consist in bringing together multidisciplinary team members involved in patient care to share relevant information.
- They should be brief and structured, should focus on essential information only, and should optimize staff engagement in an inclusive fashion. Also, they should occur frequently, given the dynamic nature of healthcare.
- The primary objectives of huddles are to identify patients who are at risk of deterioration along with any other relevant safety issues; to develop among all team members a shared understanding of these patients and of their risks; and to implement interventions aimed at mitigating against any of the risks identified.

Box 8.1 Clinical example: The WHO surgical safety checklist

The WHO Safe Surgery Checklist provides an excellent clinical example of situation awareness in action.

It was developed after extensive consultation with key stakeholders, an essential step for any new initiative if it is to be successful.

The checklist is split into three components that reflect the process steps taken with a patient who is due to undergo a surgical procedure:

- before induction of anaesthesia ("sign in");
- before incision of the skin ("time out");
- before the patient leaves the operating room ("sign out").

The aim of the checklist is to minimize errors and adverse events, as well as to increase teamwork and communication in the surgical setting.

A significant reduction in both morbidity and mortality as a result of using the checklist has been demonstrated, and the checklist is now adopted by a majority of surgical providers around the world.

Crew resource management

- Another tool that can be used to improve communication and teamwork is the tool known as 'crew resource management' (CRM). The concept was originally developed in the aviation sector, in response to assessments of the causative factors in plane crashes.
- While a variety of different CRM programmes exist, all of them focus on the role that human factors play when operating in stressful and high-risk environments. Individual CRM programmes should be tailored to meet the specific needs of the organization.
- The benefits of CRM in aviation have been well demonstrated and CRM has become a standard component of aviation training. In healthcare, while studies have shown that CRM can have a positive impact on team performance, more robust evidence is required to clearly demonstrate its effect on clinical care outcomes.

Summary box

- Situation awareness means being aware of what is going on around you. This concept is widely used in other high-risk industries, and with proven benefits.
- Medical error was estimated as the third leading cause of death in the USA, and therefore its mitigation requires a conscious effort.
- The early detection of deteriorating patients is key to improving patient outcomes and is facilitated by better situational awareness.
- One of the key benefits of improving situation awareness is facilitation of a shift from a reactive to a proactive approach to patient care.
- Huddles and CRM are very useful tools for improving situation awareness in healthcare settings.
- The WHO Safe Surgery Checklist is an excellent clinical example of situation awareness in action.

Further reading

Brady, P. W. et al. Improving situation awareness to reduce unrecognized clinical deterioration and serious safety events. *Pediatrics* 131 (2013): 298–308.

Edbrooke-Childs, J. et al. Development of the huddle observation tool for structured case management: Discussions to improve situation awareness on inpatient clinical wards. *BMJ Quality & Safety* 27 (2018): 365–72.

Endsley, M. R. A taxonomy of situation awareness errors. In R. Fuller, N. Johnston, and N. McDonald (eds), *Human Factors in Aviation Operations*. Aldershot: Ashgate, 1995, 287–92.

Endsley, M. R. Toward a theory of situation awareness in dynamic systems. *Human Factors Journal* 37(1) (1995): 32–64.

Goldenhar, L. M. et al. Huddling for high reliability and situational awareness. *BMJ Quality & Safety* 22(11) (2013): 899–906.

Hayes J., et al. Assessing risks to paediatric patients: Conversation analysis of situation awareness in huddle meetings in England. *BMJ Open* 9 (2019): e023437. doi:10.1136/ bmjopen-2018-023437

Kohn, L. T., Corrigan, J. M., and Donaldson, M. S. (eds). *To Err Is Human: Building a Safer Health System*. Washington, DC: Committee on Quality of Health Care in America, Institute of Medicine, National Academy Press, 1999.

Lachman, P., et al. Perspectives of paediatric hospital staff on factors influencing the sustainability and spread of a safety quality improvement programme. *BMJ Open* 11(3) 202: e042163. doi:10.1136/ bmjopen-2020-042163

Leonard, M., Graham, S., and Bonacum, D. The human factor: The critical importance of effective teamwork and communication in providing safe care. *BMJ Quality & Safety* 13 (2004): i85–i90.

Makary, M. A. and Daniel, M. Medical error: The third leading cause of death in the US. *BMJ* 353 (2016): i2139. https://doi.org/10.1136/bmj.i2139.

O'Dea, A., O'Connor, P., and Keogh, I. A meta-analysis of the effectiveness of crew resource management training in acute care domains. *Postgraduate Medical Journal* 90 (2014): 699–708.

Stapley, E., et al. Factors to consider in the introduction of huddles on clinical wards: perceptions of staff on the SAFE programme. *International Journal for Quality in Health care*.30,1 (2018): 44–49. doi:10.1093/intqhc/mzx162

Chapter 9

Practical application of human factors and ergonomics to improve safety

Key points

- Human factors and ergonomics (HFE) aims to understand the complexity of the interaction between humans and the other elements of an increasingly complex system.
- HFE integrates and applies theories from psychology, anatomy and physiology as well as organization management to design safe clinical systems.
- The design of all healthcare systems and processes should apply HFE theory and methods.

Introduction

Healthcare has developed, borrowed and applied various tools and approaches from other industrial sectors in order to improve safety. It has often done so dogmatically, without understanding how different tools and approaches would address different types of risk in healthcare.

Despite efforts over the past two decades to improve patient safety in various areas of healthcare, it is very hard to find clear evidence of widespread and sustained improvement.

Calls to integrate HFE into healthcare and patient safety have been growing, but there is a risk of misunderstanding what HFE is and how it should be applied. This chapter aims to present the definition, core principles, models and methods of HFE and their applications to healthcare.

Human factors and ergonomics

HFE is a unique academic transdisciplinary subject that brings together knowledge from disciplines such as psychology (attention, motivation, memory, cognition, perception, decision-making, and situation awareness), anatomy and physiology (vision, hearing, strength, posture, reach, and fit) and organization management (teamwork and organizational culture).

This multi-, inter- and cross-disciplinary subject aims to better understand the nature of interactions at multiple levels (= social science) and seeks to create a system or to change the existing one (= design and engineering) so as to suit people's needs rather than expecting people to adapt to designed interactions.

At the same time, HFE understands that complexity, uncertainty, and ambiguity from continuously changing work situations and conditions inevitably create the need for a flexible adaptation of people as they interact with a system. The 'system' here can be a technology, a software, a medical device, a team, a procedure, a policy, or a guideline and has the physical, cognitive, and organizational dimensions with which people interact.

Domains of HFE

HFE has the following three domains of specialization, as defined by the International Ergonomics Association:

Physical

Physical HFE focuses primarily on the physical characteristics and activities of a person. Relevant topics in healthcare include design of workplace layout (e.g. intensive care environments and emergency room), work-related musculoskeletal disorder (e.g. patient-handling activities and surgeons performing minimally invasive surgery) and impact of environmental factors (e.g. noise, alarm, temperature, humidity, airflow, and lighting).

Cognitive

Cognitive HFE focuses primarily on the cognitive characteristics and activities of a person (perception, memory, decision-making and human error). Relevant topics in healthcare include usability analysis and design of medical devices (e.g. inhalers), medical equipment (e.g. anaesthesia machines) and information technologies (e.g. electronic patient records). Human error is a cognitive ergonomic issue that has been studied in order to better understand underlying causal factors and reduce patient safety incidents.

Organizational HFE

Organizational HFE, which is also called macro ergonomics, focuses primarily on psychosocial characteristics of people and on organization-level structures, policies, and processes. Relevant topics in healthcare include work schedule, job stress and burnout of healthcare workers, teamwork, work system, and organizational culture.

As used in this chapter, the acronym HFE combines two distinct terms, 'human factors' and 'ergonomics', in a kind of shorthand designed to indicate that they can be used interchangeably, to designate the same thing. Human factors specialists (also known as ergonomists) are professionals who applies theory, principles, data and methods to optimize human well-being holistically and to improve overall system performance. Human factors professionals usually avoid focusing on short-term or local outcomes and aim to understand trade-offs between system performance and human well-being.

HFE is the relevant purposive human behaviour in 'designed' human technology organizational systems. People in healthcare integrate their physical, cognitive and social skills while having multiple goals and the means to carry out a vast variety of tasks through interactions with a wide range of devices and systems. Besides, the individuals' increasing ability to customize, adapt, and design their own work tasks and workplace setup means that we are unable to predict the way in which people complete their work tasks.

Therefore HFE applies methods in order to consider the variety of ways in which work tasks might be completed and ensures that systems are designed for use in a range of contexts.

In simple terms, the core question that HFE aims to address is: *Can this person, with this training and information, using these tools and technologies, perform these tasks to these standards, under these conditions?*

Applications of HFE

Box 9.1 Applications of HFE

HFE has a wide range of applications:

(i) design for people (human-centred design);
(ii) design by or with people (participatory design); and
(iii) incident analysis.

The HFE applications to design (both 'design for people' and 'design by or with people') are relevant at all stages in the lifecycle of equipment, environment and services: planning, prototyping, implementing, operating, training, evaluating, maintaining and recycling.

Design for people

HFE helps designers to understand better the physical, cognitive, and social capabilities and limitations of critical characteristics across their huge diversity and variability. It establishes exactly which critical characteristics must be designed for at the early stage of a design process, then it takes a pragmatic, real-world approach in order to suit best, or at least to include, around 95% of the population by providing adjustability or fitting to the average in certain circumstances.

Design by or with people

HFE recognizes the importance of the active involvement of healthcare workers, patients and their families in co-designing and improving systems and processes. HFE empirical knowledge about human capabilities is important, but insufficient for implementing successfully HFE-based interventions; hence a participatory way of applying HFE knowledge is important. Various traditional HFE methods (e.g. system maps, persona, risk analysis, etc.) can be applied for participatory design with very busy healthcare staff and vulnerable patients; one example is designing a safer integrated medicine management pathway.

Incident analysis

HFE has been applied to improve learning from healthcare safety incidents and near misses as well as successes. It provides tools such as the Human Factors Analysis and Classification System (HFACS), which is based on the Swiss cheese model (Box 9.2).

Box 9.2 The HFACS framework

The HFACS framework consists of four main categories

1. organizational influences;
2. unsafe supervision;
3. precondition for unsafe acts and twenty-one subcategories;
4. HFE also provides various accident analysis methods that help to identify patient safety incidents and to understand the underlying causal factors systematically (rather than attributing blame to individuals). HFE-based incident analysis encourages both systems thinking and resilience thinking.

Systems thinking highlights that incidents are not usually caused by a single catastrophic decision or maladaptive action, but by dynamic interactions between people, tasks, technology, and working conditions—including management, regulation, and policy. Resilience thinking acknowledges that human adaptations are essential, yet no particular adaptation is 'right' or 'wrong' in itself but depends on its own context, which is always slightly different from any other.

HFE principles

Box 9.3 HFE principles

All the HFE applications are based on the following three core principles:

1. systems orientation;
2. person centredness;
3. design-driven improvements, which are very relevant to healthcare.

Systems orientation

Performance results from the interactions of a sociotechnical system in which the person is but one embedded component. This principle has motivated healthcare to replace a 'blame the person' culture with a more holistic, system-based approach.

Person centredness

The person or the group of people is central in a healthcare work system. This means that efforts must be made to support people by designing work systems that fit their capabilities, limitations, performance needs, and other characteristics—and not the other way around.

Design-driven improvements

A person-centred design of work structures and processes, when grounded in robust HFE science and practice, can improve myriads of important patient, provider, and organization outcomes.

One of the most widely used healthcare HFE system models depicting the three HFE principles is the Systems Engineering Initiative for Patient Safety (SEIPS). This model was initially introduced in 2006 and an extended version, SEIPS 2.0, was introduced in 2013 (see Figure 9.1).

SEIPS models are based on Donbedian's structure–process–outcome model of healthcare quality and on the feedback loop concept of systems theory.

The general composition of this model is that the sociotechnical work system produces work processes, which shape outcomes. The left side of the model (Figure 9.1) depicts a sociotechnical work system with six interacting components: person(s), tasks, tools and technologies, organization, internal environment and external environment. The middle part of the model depicts work processes; these can be broken down into physical, cognitive, and social performance processes of work by both professionals and patients. The right side of the model depicts work outcomes (states or conditions resulting from the work processes) at three levels: patients, professionals, and organizations. Table 9.1 describes all the elements of SEIPS 2.0 model.

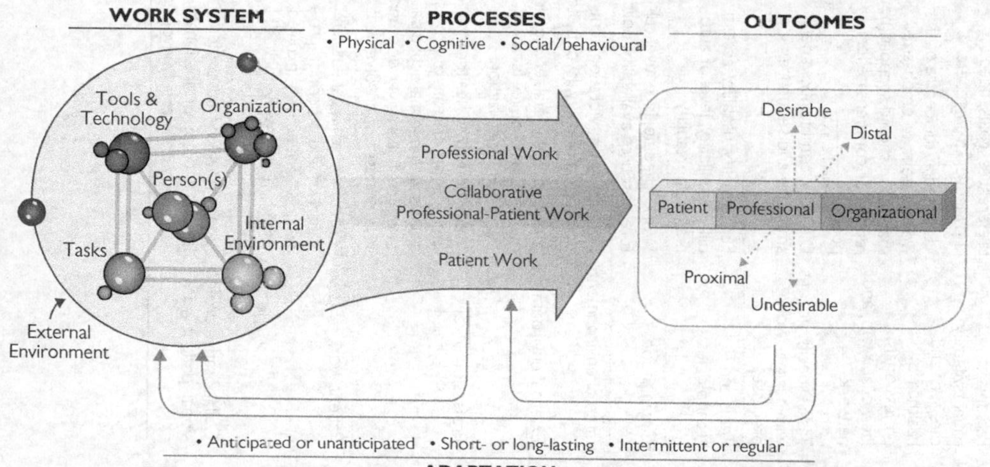

Figure 9.1 Systems Engineering Initiative for Patient Safety 2.0.

Reproduced with permission from Holden et al. (2013).

Table 9.1. SEIPS components

Components	Sub-components	Characteristics
WORK SYSTEM	Person(s): patients/family caregiver and healthcare professionals; individual, team, and network	Preferences, goals, needs, knowledge, strength, etc. * Located at the centre of the work system, to emphasize that design should support (not replace or compensate for) people
	Tasks: specific actions within larger work processes	Difficulty, complexity, variety, ambiguity and sequence
	Tools and technologies	Functionality, usability, accessibility, familiarity, level of automation, portability
	Organization	Work schedule, incentive, culture, resource availability, policy
	Internal environment	Lighting, noise, vibration, temperature, air quality, layout, etc.
	External environment	Macro-level societal, economic, ecological and policy factors outside an organization
PROCESSES	Professional work	Work done by a healthcare professional or team of professionals with minimal active patient, family caregiver or other non-professional involvement
	Patient work	Work in which a patient, family caregiver and other non-professional are actively involved with minimal involvement of healthcare professionals
	Collaborative professional–patient work	Work in which both professionals and non-professionals are jointly and actively involved

OUTCOMES	Patients	Proximal	Distal
		Stress, satisfaction, quality of care, adherence, etc.	Health, survival, engagement, happiness, finance, etc,
	Professionals	Stress, fatigue, discomfort, trust, mood, etc.	Health, burnout, job satisfaction, legal consequence, etc.
	Organizations	Short-term earning, compliance with regulations, press, staffing difficulties, etc.	Long-term financial performance, market share, staff turnover and shortage, culture change, etc.
ADAPTATION	Anticipated or unanticipated, short or long-lasting, intermittent or regular *Adaptations are made to reduce the gap between actual and ideal performance. *Not all adaptations are easily predictable or beneficial.		

The SEIPS 2.0 model has been used in many areas, including

- quality and safety improvement research and practice;
- health technology evaluation;
- patient safety education.

The SEIPS 2.0 model facilitates systems thinking and resilience thinking in order to deal with the complexity of designing, evaluating, monitoring and auditing systems, services, and processes as well as of investigating incidents.

In Chapters 29 and 35 the model will be used to demonstrate how one can design safe work systems and processes of care.

There are systems frameworks and a variety of HFE approaches and methods that can help us to understand complex interacting systems and subsystems involving people. HFE aims to take the right approach, and this almost always involves collaboration with other specialities and disciplines. There are advantages to integrating HFE with quality improvement science and with implementation science, as discussed in Chapter 14.

HFE approaches can have greater impact when HFE expertise is embedded in the healthcare system and HFE awareness is extended to a wider range of healthcare professionals by instilling HFE education into the medical and healthcare curriculum.

Summary box

- HFE provides a scientific approach to how systems work.
- There are three main strands in HFE—physical, cognitive and organizational—and all of them are important to understanding how systems work.
- Key principles include a focus on systems, person cenredness and design-driven improvements.
- The SEIPS 2.0 model brings these aspects together, so as to allow an analysis of how systems work, processes are undertaken and outcomes are achieved.
- The SEIPS 2.0 model can be used by clinical teams in their day-to-day analysis of their own work and safety.

Reference

Holden, R. J. et al. SEIPS 2.0: A human factors framework for studying and improving the work of healthcare professionals and patients. *Ergonomics* 56.11 (2013): 1669–86. https://doi.org/10.1080/00140139.2013.838643.

Further reading

Carayon, P. et al. Work system design for patient safety: The SEIPS model. *Quality & Safety in Health Care* 15 (Suppl 1) ((2006): i50–8. http://dx.doi.org/10.1136/qshc.2005.015842.

Chartered Institute of Ergonomics and Human Factors. *Human Factors for Health & Social Care* (White Paper). Birmingham: CIEHF, 2018. https://www.ergonomics.org.uk/Healthcare.

Cohen, T. N. et al. Using HFACS–Healthcare to identify systemic vulnerabilities during surgery. *American Journal of Medical Quality* 33.6 (2018); 614–22. https://doi.org/10.1177%2F1062860618764316.

Dul, J. et al. A strategy for human factors/ergonomics: Developing the discipline and profession. *Ergonomics* 55.4 (2012): 377–95. doi: 10.1080/00140139.2012.661087.

Hignett, S. et al. Human factors and ergonomics and quality improvement science: Integrating approaches for safety in healthcare. BMJ Quality & Safety 24.4 (2015): 250–4. http://dx.doi.org/10.1136/bmjqs-2014-003623.

International Ergonomics Association. Definition and Domains of Ergonomics. 2019. https://www.iea.cc/whats/index.html.

International Journal Quality in Healthcare Supplement on Human Factors 33.1 (2021). https://academic.oup.com/intqhc/issue.

Holden RJ, Carayon P. SEIPS 101 and seven simple SEIPS tools. *BMJ Quality & Safety* 2021;**30**:901-910. http://dx.doi.org/10.1136/bmjqs-2020-012538

Jun, G. T. et al. A participatory systems approach to design for safer integrated medicine management. *Ergonomics* 61.1 (2018): 48–68. https://doi.org/10.1080/00140139.2017.1329939.

Jun, G. T. and Waterson, P. Systems thinking: A new direction in healthcare incident investigation (4 min-long animation). 2017. https://youtu.be/5oYV3Dqe0A8.

Wilson, J. and Sharples, S. Methods in the understanding of human factors. In J. Wilson and S. Sharples (eds), *Evaluation of Human Work* (4th edn). Boca Raton, FL: CRC Press, 2015, pp. 1–32.

Chapter 10

Reliability in healthcare

Key points

- Healthcare is unreliable in many of its operations. This is unsafe and inefficient.
- High reliability aims to produce error-free operations under various conditions.
- Reliability in healthcare implies that the patient receives the right care and that the processes deliver care in a standardized way.
- Reliability theory offers interventions such as care bundles standardization and process redesign, which can improve the reliability of care and its outcomes.
- The key features of a reliable team are a capacity for anticipation, frontline ownership of the process, and learning.

What is reliability in healthcare?

Reliability theory is a scientific approach designed to achieve the elimination of error rates in a process. High-reliability organizations (HROs) are characterized by the high potential to eliminate error through processes that are organized in a systematic and scientific way, and thereby to reduce risk and deliver unprecedented outcomes. Examples of HROs are firefighters, rescue services and the nuclear industry.

Reliability is a concept that derives from everyday life. We normally expect a process to produce the same result every time we use it. These processes can vary between being relatively simple—for example opening a carton of milk, or washing one's clothes in the washing machine—and being extremely complex—for example launching a rocket. If the outcome of a process is inconsistent or unpredictable, the process will be recognized as unfit for purpose. What use would a car be that does not start when the key is turned in the ignition, or a lamp that fails to light when one turns the switch on?

Why is it important?

Much of what we do in healthcare achieves the desired outcome most of the time. However, there are many processes that are not reliable. For example:

- the time when the operating list or outpatient clinic will start;
- whether the correct medication is prescribed, and whether it will be given on time;
- whether a clinical protocol is adhered to all the time.

To achieve the best possible outcomes for patients and to enhance the overall healthcare provider experience, it is essential to aim for high reliability in healthcare systems and processes.

Definitions of reliability

Reliability is defined as the capability of an object or process to perform its intended function over time, under specified conditions. It can be measured as the amount of failure-free operations over time.

The translation of this definition into healthcare is as follows: *reliability is a situation in which every single time the correct patient receives the correct treatment, in the correct place, at the correct time, from the correct person.* The aim is to decrease potential error, that is to enhance the number of failure-free operations.

If one measures human behaviour, there are nominal errors that occur, and these increase with stress. In healthcare the chances of error increase with the complexity of a task and the levels of stress under which the corresponding action is taken. Stressful clinical processes in the emergency department (ED), in the operating room, or in the intensive care unit (ICU) are prone to error.

Nominal human error rates

error of commission, e.g. misreading a label: 0.003%
error of omission without reminders: 0.01%
simple arithmetical errors with self-checking: 0.03%
error rate under very high levels of stress: 0.25%

What is the theory?

A study of high reliability organizations undertaken by Weick and Sutcliffe (2011) has identified five key characteristics of HROs (see Figure 10.1).

High Reliability (Weick and Sutcliffe)

The application of the theory is demonstrated in Table 10.1. The first three steps consist in anticipating possible safety events and proactively mitigating against them; the second two consist in containing an event and learning in real time.

Table 10.1. Characteristics of HRO applied to healthcare

	Characteristic	Example
Anticipation	Preoccupation with failure	Making sure that every prescription is 100% correct every time
	Sensitivity to operations	Using the SEIPS M model to assess the work system in real time
	Reluctance to simplify	Understanding the complexity of clinical processes and that good and poor outcomes are not due to linear action
Containment	Commitment to resilience	Applying learning to any event and working within a just culture
	Deference to expertise	Asking the patient, house officer, or nurse what the solution could be rather than coming up with solutions

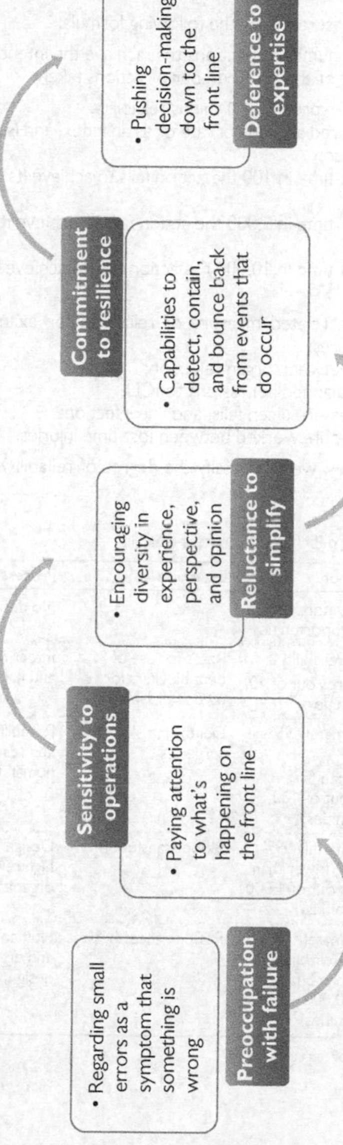
Preoccupation with failure
• Regarding small errors as a symptom that something is wrong
Sensitivity to operations
• Paying attention to what's happening on the front line
Reluctance to simplify
• Encouraging diversity in experience, perspective, and opinion
Commitment to resilience
• Capabilities to detect, contain, and bounce back from events that do occur
Deference to expertise
• Pushing decision-making down to the front line

Figure 10.1 Characteristics of HROs.

Measures of reliability

Reliability can be measured using the following formula:

reliability = the number of actions that achieve the intended result, out of the total number of actions taken

The defect rate of a process is 1 minus reliability.

Reliability is measured as a defect rate or as an index, and is expressed as an order of magnitude:

- 10-2 means that 1 time in 100 the action fails to achieve its intended result;
- 10-3 means that 1 time in 1,000 the action fails to achieve its intended result;
- 10-4 means that 1 time in 10,000 the action fails to achieve its intended result.

One can also use a related measure of reliability, for example time or counts between failures:

- transplant cases between organ rejection;
- days between unplanned admissions to ICU;
- days between pressure ulcer, falls, and line infections;
- employee work hours worked between lost-time injuries.

Using these measures, we can classify the degree of reliability, as indicated in Table 10.2.

Table 10.2. Starting definitions of process reliability

Level	Description	Examples	Process design
Chaotic process	Failure in more than 20% of opportunities		No design
Level 1 (10-1)	80–90% reliability (1-2 failures out of 10 opportunities)	Rates for use of beta blockers for myocardial infarction	Intent, vigilance, and hard work
Level 2: (10-2)	Approximately 95% reliability (fewer than 5 failures out of 100 opportunities)	Deaths in risky surgeries	Reliability science and research in human factors
Level 3: (10-3)	Approximately 99% reliability (fewer than 5 failures out of 1,000 opportunities)	Blood transfusion	Design of high reliability organizations
Level 4: (10-4)	Approximately 99.99%rReliability (fewer than 5 failures out of 10,000 opportunities)	Routine anaesthesia	Human factors and ergonomics design, resilience

10^{-5} = Deaths from major radiation

Translating theory into practice

[illegible]

Translating theory into practice

For a clinician, there are many ways to approach the task of improving reliability.

- It is important to recognize that one can have difficulty with this task as an individual, because many healthcare processes are complex and involve multiple providers with different kinds of knowledge, types of attitude and varieties of behaviour.
- A useful starting point can be to concentrate on processes that one can control (e.g. one could draw a personal checklist to ensure that tasks are completed). Unfortunately, given human nature, this approach is often insufficient for developing constant reliability. If these lists fail to yield reliability, the default attitude is often simply to 'try harder'. However, if the system of which the individual is a part is not reliable, it will not be possible to achieve perfect reliability, no matter how hard one tries.
- Many processes in healthcare delivery involve common equipment, standard order forms, protocols and written policies or procedures. These elements of care can be helpful for providers but do not guarantee adherence and reliable care.

Recognizing the human element in care provision is essential if we want to move towards a more reliable system-based care. Practical ways to improve reliability include the use of human factors theory (see Chapter 9) and simple tools designed to act as enforcers of reliable processes. With these we can achieve a high degree of reliability. Examples are:

- The introduction of decision aids and reminders that are built into systems. These need to be reviewed and revised regularly, as the brain learns to ignore them in time.
- The development of evidence-based processes that ensure that the desired action is the default action. This guarantees that there is no other way to complete a certain task or process.
- The implementation of redundant processes that ensure that a given action is reliable. A good example is the double-checking of a prescription by another person, independent of the prescriber, to ensure that the prescription is correct.
- The careful examination of the process flow and the subsequent redesign around the habits of providers.

This implies that we need to design the processes of care to achieve reliability. In Figure 10.2 the conceptual approach is shown and in Table 10.3 examples of actions to take at each level are indicated.

Table 10.3. Concepts of reliability

Level of reliability	Concepts
Level 1 Designing basic failure prevention Intent vigilance and hard work	Standardized order sets, pathways Feedback of information on compliance Awareness and training
Level 2 Human factors, reliability science Designing sophisticated failure prevention, basic failure identification and mitigation	Decision aids and reminders built into the system Desired action the default function Redundancy—extra steps Real-time identification of failures Checklists Examples: Patients receive standard asthma education at Discharge Standard Scheduling rules
Level 3 Tackling reliability in healthcare level 3 concepts on the basis of sophisticated behavioural patterns	Mindfulness Taking advantage of habits and patterns Making the system visible
Level 4 A 3-tier design strategy to embed reliability into the system, as in Figure 10.2	Prevent initial failure using intent and standardization Create a redundancy function (identify failure and mitigate) Critical failure mode function (identify critical failures and then redesign)

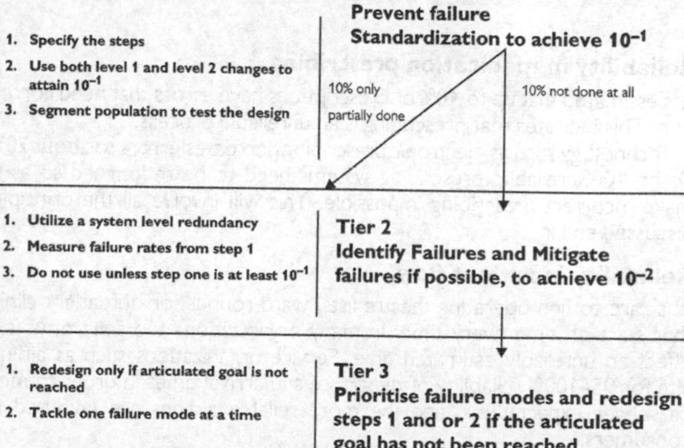
Generic Three Tier Design for Reliability
Tier 1
Prevent failure
Standardization to achieve 10^{-1}
1. Specify the steps
2. Use both level 1 and level 2 changes to attain 10^{-1}
3. Segment population to test the design
10% only partially done
10% not done at all
1. Utilize a system level redundancy
2. Measure failure rates from step 1
3. Do not use unless step one is at least 10^{-1}
Tier 2
Identify Failures and Mitigate failures if possible, to achieve 10^{-2}
1. Redesign only if articulated goal is not reached
2. Tackle one failure mode at a time
Tier 3
Prioritise failure modes and redesign steps 1 and or 2 if the articulated goal has not been reached

Figure 10.2 Design for reliability.

Practical actions to adopt to achieve reliability

Standardization

The most important way to improve the reliability of a facet of care is to standardize the care process. Standardization:

- is based on the clear specification and articulation of the desired process;
- should be agreed by all those who will use the process; and
- must be subject to scrutiny and study to be assessed for variability.

Care bundles are an example of a standardized process.

Care bundles

Box 10.1 Care bundles

A bundle is an all-or-nothing collection process, in other words all elements are required for the effective care of patients under treatment.

Each element is scientifically grounded and is essential to the improvement of clinical outcomes. When these elements are bundled together and combined, there is significant improvement of patient care.

For a care bundle to be effective, it must be adhered to exactly and in its entirety.

Examples are care bundles used to prevent

- surgical site infection
- central line infection
- pressure ulcers
- falls
- venous thromboembolism
- acute myocardial infarction

Reliability in medication prescribing

It is estimated that up to 40% of prescriptions have errors that need correction. This indicates that prescribing is an unreliable process.

Technology such as electronic prescribing decreases errors to about 20%. To be 100% reliable, prescribing systems need to be redesigned so as to make incorrect prescribing impossible. This will involve all the principles discussed so far.

Reliability in patient flow

It is rare to find operating theatre lists, ward rounds, or outpatient clinics that start on time every time. In many organizations the start time is in effect an unreliably estimated time. Service organizations such as airlines aim for 95–100% reliability of departure and arrival times in order to meet passenger expectations, and the more reliable airlines are favoured by consumers.

In healthcare the start time of most procedures is approximate, and this results in a significant waste of time. Many reasons are often cited for this unreliability, but it is possible to design a process that starts and ends on time.

Reliability in effective practice

A strong scientific evidence base, provided through randomized controlled trials and meta-analytical data, guides the practice of modern medicine. However, the implementation and use of evidence-based medicine is not reliable. It is estimated that doctors follow clinical guidelines approximately 30–40% of the time, often because of personal preference and professional autonomy. To improve the overall quality of care, it is necessary to find ways to implement evidence-based care reliably.

Top tips

Practical steps to improve reliability:

- Study the process carefully.
- Draw a detailed process map of what happens.
- Compare it to what is supposed to happen.
- Measure whether the steps in the process deliver the desired outcome (e.g. medications on time every time).
- If something is not reliable, ask why.
- Redesign and test a new process with one patient at a time.
- Measure against the old process.
- Spread the new process gradually, as reliability is achieved.

Summary box

Characteristics of a highly reliable clinical team:

A: anticipation of what may happen:

- **preoccupation with small elements** of process that do not function well, in addition to more serious systems failures;
- recognition that **small failures** are as important as large failures (e.g. delayed cardiotocograph reading, delays in giving antibiotics);
- awareness that **deviation from what is supposed to happen** can become the new normal over time: ask whether the wrong way becomes the status quo;
- **guarding against complacency:** healthcare providers may be involved in an adverse event any time, even if they have never been involved in one before; therefore it is not enough to be reliable less than all the time;
- **being reluctant to simplify** interpretations of the processes followed, and showing willingness to examine comprehensively the root causes in real time;
- encouraging **sensitivity to operations** and supervising how things are working on the front line in the context of complex daily work: this gives frontline staff the authority to improve and make processes safer; staff members can make continuous adjustments that prevent errors from accumulating and enlarging;
- basing actions on reports from those who see patients.

B: learning all the time:

- commitment to **learn** continually **from what works and what does not**: this grants authority to study the process and improve;
- developing capabilities to detect, contain, and bounce back from errors that are part of day-to-day activities;
- **deference to the expertise** of staff working on the front line;
- **making decisions on the front line**, authority being delegated to those with the greater expertise, regardless of rank.

Reference

Weick, K. E. and Sutcliffe, K. M. *Managing the Unexpected: Assuring High Performance in an Age of Complexity*. San Francisco, CA: Jossey-Bass, 2001.

Further reading

Chassin, M. R. and Loeb, J. M. High-reliability health care: Getting there from here. *Milbank Quarterly* 91.3 (2013): 459–90.

Health Foundation. *Evidence Scan: High Reliability Organisations*. 2011, November. https://www.health.org.uk/sites/default/files/HighReliabilityOrganisations.pdf.

Pronovost, P. et al. Creating high reliability in health care organizations. *Health Services Research*, 41 (2006): 1599–617.

Chapter 11

Resilience theory, complexity science, and Safety-II

Key points

- Traditionally, safety in healthcare relied on linear assumptions and solutions—such as restructuring processes to minimize human error, constraining behaviours, or standardizing procedures.
- The approach is challenged by the recognition that healthcare behaves as a complex adaptive system.
- In line with this, resilience engineering suggests that humans, with their ability to adapt their own behaviour to changing conditions, are an important resource for maintaining safety in the system.
- The application of resilience ideas to healthcare includes the disjuncture between work-as-imagined and work-as-done and Safety-II, an approach that focuses on how and why things go right, rather than paying attention exclusively to the occasions where things go wrong (Safety-I).
- Two methods for examining resilience in healthcare are considered here, namely the resilient assessment grid and the functional resonance analysis method.

Safety in healthcare

Safety, as approached by most healthcare systems worldwide, has traditionally relied on beliefs that adverse outcomes can be explained by linear cause–effect chains, as originally proposed by the domino effect and later, by Reason's Swiss cheese model.

This approach is underpinned by the assumption that adverse outcomes, whether mild or serious, have causes that can be found and fixed, and that these differ from the causes of ordinary, successful care. This assumption has had consequences for how adverse events have been investigated. The focus has been on identifying specific components that failed, for instance via root cause analysis (RCA); and a consequent regime of reactive safety management procedures followed—such as enforcing compliance with policies and processes. From this perspective, humans, acting alone or collectively, appear predominantly as a liability or hazard. However, healthcare is much more complex than this approach to safety suggests and few ultimate sources of problems are amenable to simplistic fixes.

More recently, there has been a shift towards complexity-based safety thinking, where safety is no longer viewed as a static product or service but as an emergent property in a complex adaptive system (CAS). Healthcare is increasingly being recognized as a CAS, which functions in a non-linear fashion and is composed of interdependent and interacting parts (e.g. clinicians, patients, equipment). This means that cause and effect are not always linked in a predictable manner; they are mediated through all the complexities.

The challenge: ensuring safety in complex systems

There are many challenges to maintaining safety within a complex system. Traditional responses to safety focus retrospectively, addressing adverse events or restructuring systems or processes so as to minimize human error, or by attempting to constrain behaviours and standardize procedures.

But this traditional approach does not align with what actually happens in clinical practice, which represents the dynamic, ever-changing nature of health settings; nor does it take into account the inherent interdependencies and connections between various parts of the system. Health professionals constantly adjust their practices to changing conditions; they do not realize safer care by slavishly following guidelines or policies. For example, many areas in health are chronically understaffed and people must work within the constraints imposed by this situation, which sometimes means fluctuating numbers of staff with differing skill sets.

Changing service demands also introduce unanticipated challenges: for example, multiple trauma patients arriving *en masse* at an emergency department, or increased demand for isolation beds during a difficult *Clostridium difficile* outbreak can seriously stretch the resources. The intricacies of the context add so many variables to the equation that simple directives or procedures (e.g. standard operating procedures) with instructions to follow them faithfully are not sufficient for managing safety effectively.

A related challenge is how the work of safety is conceptualized. The complexity of the health system means that the way in which the work of keeping patients safe is imagined to occur rarely comes close to the reality of its occurring. The concepts of work-as-imagined (WAI) and work-as-done (WAD) seek to highlight this discrepancy and provide a useful framework for addressing it. WAI refers to how work is planned and thought through before acting, while WAD refers to the actual carrying out of that work. Those who develop policies and directives distant from the clinical "coal face" are sometimes derogatively thought of as producing WAI, but even work planned by those at the bedside may not adequately account for the unpredictable variables and for the web of interactions within a complex health system. And it is a truism that no one doing WAI can predict all the things that can happen on the front lines of care. No one could write a policy manual to cover so many contingencies—and no clinician would have the time to consult it, anyway.

Safety-II and resilience

To look at WAD is to gain a deeper understanding of everyday clinical work. When we step back to observe the practices of nurses, doctors, and allied health staff in a setting like a hospital, what is noticeable is the extraordinary capacity they have, both individually and collectively, to adjust their behaviour to the changing circumstances of healthcare delivery (e.g. a complex patient, a piece of broken equipment, weather conditions, a riot or major accident that puts pressure on emergency services and reverberates across the hospital). This ability to maintain performance in the face of variable conditions is known as resilience. It may overlap with individual psychological resilience—both often involve coping with crises—but we think of it as a potential of systems rather than of individuals.

The concept of systems resilience comes from resilience engineering. It views people as a positive force for coping with disturbances in complex organizations. It involves the capacity, shared among people within a system to anticipate, monitor, learn, and adapt, making trade-offs between diverse and often conflicting demands. Hollnagel (2009) invented the efficiency thoroughness trade-off (ETTO) principle, bringing to attention the fact that efficiency and thoroughness are not readily achievable at the same time. Being thorough can mean that you are not necessarily being efficient, and being efficient means that you might skimp on thoroughness. The capacity to balance and adjust between these two contrasting goals expresses both a resilient system and self-organization among healthcare professionals. ETTO is near-ubiquitous in healthcare. For example, staff members in intensive care spend energy redistributing tasks, risks, and care between different patients on the basis of their assessments of morbidity and need.

Recognition of both the complexity of healthcare and the potential for humans to respond productively to this complexity leads resilience to a somewhat radical reconceptualization of safety in healthcare. The traditional 'find-and-fix' approach, which has been termed Safety-I, assumes that systems are tractable and focuses on eliminating things that go wrong. On the other hand, the resilience-inspired Safety-II approaches safety proactively, by enabling things to go right.

In this regard, Safety-II shares some broad themes with the concept of positive deviance, where one looks for the best performing individual and for learning from excellence (Chapter 15). Yet Safety-II focuses on the spectrum of everyday clinical work rather than just on the strongly good or bad. Both Safety-I and Safety-II give useful perspectives, and indeed are complementary (see Figure 11.1). The point is that looking at the ordinary (Safety-II)—most cases when things go right—rather than just at the extraordinary (Safety-I)—the small number of times when things go wrong—provides us with information about the way the system operates safely and affords us opportunities to engineer greater levels of resilience.

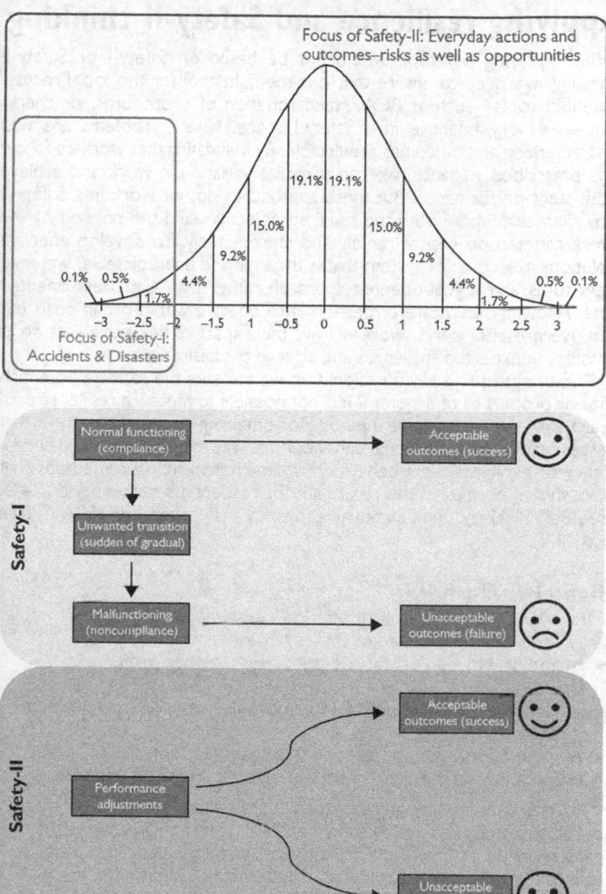

Figure 11.1 Comparison of Safety-I and Safety-II perspectives on safety.
Adapted from Hollnagel, Braithwaite, and Wears (2013).

Applying resilience and Safety-II thinking

When applying any tool, whether it be based on Safety-I or Safety-II thinking, we need to ensure that it is the right tool for the job. Process-oriented tools—such as RCA, standardization of procedures, or check-lists—are very effective in a Safety-I space, where problems are well characterized and outcomes predictable. By mandating that workers follow the prescribed guidance, we can minimize variation in work and achieve consistent performance. But these approaches do not work in a Safety-II environment, where both the required objectives and the context of the work can and do change rapidly and unexpectedly. To develop effective solutions in a complex system that is dynamic and unpredictable, we need new tools and a goal-oriented approach rather than a process-oriented one. Allowing healthcare professionals to operate within broad goals but not overprescribing their work will give them space to flex and adjust, so as to meet unexpected challenges and achieve the desired aims.

This brings us to a key question. Can we measure the resilient potentialities or properties of a system? It is not possible to measure resilience prospectively, but we do have methods for obtaining proximal measures that assess team or organizational behaviour in a way that will predict their tendency to exhibit resilient behaviours when challenged. Two methods that have shown promise in this regard are the resilient assessment grid (RAG) (see Box 11.1) and the functional resonance analysis method (FRAM) (see Box 11.2).

Box 11.1 The RAG

The RAG consists of four 'abilities' of organizations in relation to how they cope with unexpected or challenging events:

- **monitor**: How do organizations monitor their performance? (critical);
- **anticipate**: How do they anticipate a crisis or an adverse event? (potential);
- **respond**: How do they respond to a crisis? (actual);
- **learn**: How do they learn from experiencing a crisis? (factual).

Within the four abilities and subvariables are nested a series of probing or diagnostic questions, which should be developed specifically for the organization to be studied, and are answered on a six-point Likert scale ('excellent', 'satisfactory', 'acceptable', 'unacceptable', 'deficient', 'missing').

The answers to the probing questions can be quantified, and the results aggregated to derive an overall resilience rating. The answers can also be used to construct a resilience profile (usually presented as a web chart), in which a high aggregated score and a balanced web chart (i.e. scores for all elements towards the perimeter of the chart) indicate that the organization is likely to be resilient if challenged.

Example, taken from the work of Damen et al. (2021), shows how the FRAM can be used to understand the differences between WAI and WAD in a clinical department. This understanding can then be used to better align procedures so as to enable clinicians to flex and adjust to changing circumstances in ways that are safe for patients.

Box 11.2 The FRAM

The FRAM is a process-mapping tool that maps a series of interconnected activities that make up the task under consideration. In addition to activity inputs and outputs, the FRAM allows for activity preconditions, controls, timing, and resources to be considered.

This tool can also pay heed to variations in the timing of each subcomponent of a task and enables the user to see how that variability may affect subsequent or dependent activities and the progress of the task overall.

The study was conducted at two cardiothoracic surgery departments, one in Australia and one in Europe, around patient anticoagulation procedures associated with surgery. The WAI FRAM was developed from international guidelines. The FRAM was modified to show pathways for WAD using data derived from semi-structured interviews with eighteen healthcare professionals who were involved in anticoagulation processes.

The analysis provided a clinical view of preoperative anticoagulation management overlaid on the institutional view, and highlighted some of the everyday practical considerations that led to variability in relation to the guidelines. While the implementation of the modelling tool revealed a number of places where clinicians did not follow processes that aligned with international guidelines, it provided insights into why this might be the case and offered some suggestions as to what to do about it.

Summary box

- Healthcare is a complex adaptive system; this makes the control, prediction, and understanding of cause and effect difficult.
- Resilience is a system's capacity to maintain performance in response to variable conditions. Humans are an important resource for system resilience.
- Traditional safety management (Safety-I) focuses on the few occasions where things go wrong. This leads to an increasing disconnect between WAI (by managers, policymakers) and WAD (by frontline staff).
- Safety-II, on the other hand, encourages us to gain a deep understanding of everyday clinical work and system resilience by focusing on the cases, usually taken for granted, where things go right.
- The FRAM and the RAG are two tools that assist in the study of resilience.

In the real world on the front lines of care, clinicians have always flexed and adjusted their practices, accommodating to the demands placed upon them, whether they are stimulated by patient needs, resource constraints, technological limitations, test delays, deficits in the team, poor cultures, or systems that are not completely fit for purpose.

Concepts drawn from resilience engineering and complexity theory help us to understand better how healthcare works and what keeps patients safe. Policies, guidelines, standard operating procedures and regulations have a place, but are not ultimately definitive in describing how clinical work is done.

The Safety-I paradigm has helped us to think how care can be delivered if everything goes to plan and has supported efforts to reduce harm whenever it occurs in a stable, predictable environment. The Safety-II paradigm has drawn our attention instead to the actual work that keeps patients safe and has encouraged us to focus on what makes things go right when care is delivered under pressures and demands.

References

Damen, N. L. et al. Preoperative anticoagulation management in everyday clinical practice: An international comparative analysis of work-as-done using the functional resonance analysis method. *Journal of Patient Safety* 17.3 (2021): 157–65.

Hollnagel, E. *The ETTO Principle: Efficiency–Thoroughness Trade-Off: Why Things That Go Right Sometimes Go Wrong*. Surrey: Ashgate, 2009.

Hollnagel, E. Epilogue: RAG: The resilience analysis grid. In E. Hollnagel et al. (eds), *Resilience Engineering in Practice: A Guidebook*. Surrey: Ashgate, 2011, pp. 275–96.

Hollnagel, E. *FRAM: The Functional Resonance Analysis Method*. Surrey: Ashgate, 2012.

Hollnagel E., Braithwaite, J., and Wears, R. L. (eds). *Resilient Health Care*. Surrey: Ashgate, 2013.

Further reading

Braithwaite, J., Wears, R. L., and Hollnagel, E. (eds). *Resilient Health Care: Reconciling Work-as-Imagined and Work-as-Done*. Boca Raton, FL: CRC Press, 2016.

Braithwaite, J., Wears, R. L., and Hollnagel, E. Resilient health care: Turning patient safety on its head. *International Journal for Quality in Health Care* 27.5 (2015): 418–20.

Heinrich, H. W. *Industrial Accident Prevention: A Scientific Approach*. New York: McGraw Hill, 1941

Hollnagel, E., Braithwaite, J., and Wears, R. L. (eds). *Delivering Resilient Health Care*. London: Routledge, 2018.

Hollnagel, E, Wears, R. L., and Braithwaite, J. *From Safety-I to Safety-II: A White Paper*. The Resilient Health Care Net/University of Southern Denmark, University of Florida, USA, and Macquarie University, Australia, 2015. https://www.england.nhs.uk/signuptosafety/wp-content/uploads/sites/16/2015/10/safety-1-safety-2-whte-papr.pdf.

Hollnagel, E. and Woods, D. D. Epilogue: Resilience engineering precepts. In E. Hollnagel, D. D. Woods, and N. Leveson (eds), *Resilience Engineering: Concepts and Precepts*. Aldershot: Ashgate, 2006, pp. 347–58.

Iflaifel, M. et al. Resilient health care: A systematic review of conceptualisations, study methods and factors that develop resilience. *BMC Health Services Research* 20 (2020): 1—21.

Johnson, A., Clay-Williams, R., and Lane, P. Framework for better care: Reconciling approaches to patient safety and quality. *Australian Health Review* 43 (2019): 653–5.

Nyssen, A. and Bérastégui, P. Is system resilience maintained at the expense of individual resilience? In J. Braithwaite, R. L. Wears, and E. Hollnagel (eds), *Reconciling Work-as-Imagined and Work-as-Done*, Boca Raton, FL: Taylor & Francis, 2017, pp. 37–46.

Sujan, M., Spurgeon, P., and Cooke, M. The role of dynamic trade-offs in creating safety: A qualitative study of handover across care boundaries in emergency care. *Reliability Engineering & System Safety* 141 (2015): pp. 54–62.

Wears, R. L., Hollnagel, E., and Braithwaite, J. (eds). *Resilient Health Care: The Resilience of Everyday Clinical Work*. Surrey: Ashgate, 2015.

Part 2

Practical application and methodologies of patient safety

Chapter 12

Measuring patient safety at a national, organization, and system level

Key points

- Measurement is the foundation of improving the safety of the clinical process.
- Measurement is done at national, regional, local, and team levels.
- Data can be collected routinely or for a specific programme.
- Clinical teams will benefit from measures that are relevant to them and to the patients.
- All measurements should tell a story and should lead to improvement in care.

Measuring patient safety

This chapter presents an overview of measuring patient safety at national, organization, and system level. The measurement of safety varies according to the level one works at. These definitions are fluid, depending on one's specific context, but the key is always to measure for learning.

Why should we measure patient safety?

- To improve patient care and safety, we need to understand the harm, both actual and potential, that we cause our patients.
- Measuring patient safety and harm allows patients, relatives, health and care staff, policymakers, funders—in short, everyone interested in patient care—an opportunity to understand the causes and the impact of harm and to start to identify possible interventions designed to prevent its recurrence in the future.
- Measurement is therefore an important first step towards improving patient care, but should also be used continually, to ensure monitoring and ongoing improvement over the long term.
- Through assessment, measurement yields a method that can facilitate learning and improvement throughout the patient's journey and throughout healthcare systems.
- Measuring safety is valuable in all health and care settings in the developed and developing world.

How to measure patient safety?

Given the complexity of modern care, it is recommended to use a range of data from multiple measurement strategies in order to capture information about any patient safety risks and harm(s) caused. Using multiple measurement methods can produce greater understanding of care delivery, of the areas for possible improvement, and of the systems that work well.

Adverse event reporting

- Adverse events are untoward consequences of care that cause unnecessary harm to patients.
- Reporting adverse events allows analysis and learning from the incidents, so as to reduce the likelihood of their recurrence.
- The system relies upon acknowledgement of harm coming from the professionals involved in the patient's care.
- All relevant data should be recorded in the report in order to allow for event analysis and for the identification of opportunities to improve care.
- Learning and corrective measures should be shared with those involved and with wider teams, so as to prevent future harm of a similar kind.
- Adverse events are underreported in healthcare, as many professionals worry about punitive consequences and a 'blame culture'.
- This underreporting leads to missed opportunities to improve health systems and to prevent future harm.
- Adverse event systems can be voluntary or mandatory for defined patient harm incidents; examples are 'never events' in the UK and USA (Box 12.1) and 'sentinel events' in Australia.

Box 12.1 Examples of 'never events'

Surgical	• wrong site surgery • wrong implant/prosthesis • retained foreign object, post procedure
Medication	• mis-selection of a strong potassium solution • administration of medication by the wrong route
Mental Health	• failure to install functional collapsible shower or curtain rails
General	• falls from poorly restricted windows • misplaced nasopharyngeal or orogastric tubes • scalding of patients

Retrospective medical records review

- Reviewing medical records can identify patient safety events.
- The IHI Global Trigger Tool is a two-stage process of reviewing medical records.
- At the first stage, medical records are selected randomly and screened by health professional staff with a view to identifying predetermined triggers or events.
- The second stage involves a nurse and a physician reviewing the identified records of sources of patient harm.
- The data can be much richer and broader than those obtained by other measurement methods, but this method is resource-intensive.

Routinely collected data

- Data collected for administrative or funding management can be used to identify harm at different levels of care. These data could be clinical information from electronic health records, health administrative data, or data furnished by disease registries and epidemiologic surveillance systems.
- Healthcare services, organizations, and national systems routinely collect data that can be used to assess patient safety and to identify potential areas of improvement.
- The ability to capture reliable and comparable data depends on the quality of the underlying infrastructure and systems.
- Routine data require sustained resource investment over time.
- National databases with unique patient identifiers can link patient experiences across several settings.

Patient-reported measures

- Patient feedback and input are invaluable for the identification of harm; moreover, the involvement of patients encourages person-centred care (Box 12.2).
- Patient feedback can identify good practice, contribute to the sharing of learning, and encourage improvement.
- Patient-reported measures focus on event-predisposing factors, on circumstances of harm, and on the management of the harm incident.

Everyone can see the services response and the implemented changes.

Box 12.2 Real-time patient feedback system: Care Opinion

- Care Opinion is an online platform that allows patients to share their experiences of health and care services.
- Patients can share honest feedback that is anonymized for all involved.
- The Care Opinion team shares feedback directly with the teams most likely to make a difference.

What should be measured?

Challenges of measuring patient safety

What should be measured?

Box 12.3 Top tips for patient safety measurement

- Measure patient safety for improvement, not for punishment.
- Measure patient safety over time, to be able to see trends.
- Measure as closely to the front lines as possible.
- Make measurement a part of the daily process.
- Look at data in real time.
- Maintain a broad definition of safety.
- Prioritize the resources that tackle harms in your system.
- Measure near misses as well as harm or adverse events.
- Measure what works well.

- To understand the level of avoidable harm and to identify areas for improvement requires more than one single measurement.
- Before choosing patient measures, it is important to understand the system in which improvement will be delivered.
- Measurements should be relevant to the user, and the choice of measurement will vary depending on setting, locality, and country.
- When selecting what to measure, involving key stakeholders is vital for ensuring continuous engagement and for creating a positive safety culture.
- Measurement selection can involve patients, healthcare professionals, management teams, and policy makers.
- Co-production of measurement with patients and frontline staff is beneficial.
- Each system can learn from other systems, but each system should purposively select the measures of patient safety that are most relevant and useful to its context.

Challenges of measuring patient safety

Establishing the true level of patient harm is very challenging, for several reasons:

- Adverse event reporting relies on professionals to be aware that they have caused harm (or a near miss) in the first place.
- Blame cultures and punitive measures (including litigation) taken after harm reporting have led to a tendency to underreport adverse events.
- Routinely collected data rely upon the accuracy of coding and reporting.
- Measuring patient safety requires resource allocation. System, organizational, and national monitoring needs financial and workforce resources.

Metrics of patient safety

National-level data

There are several metrics that are routinely used at a national level for monitoring [illegible] improvements.

Hospital standardized mortality ratio

The hospital standardized mortality ratio or rate (HSMR) is a measure [illegible] and a tool that can be used to reduce the incidence of avoidable deaths in acute [illegible], several [illegible] England, [illegible], Scotland, and United States use the HSMR [illegible] and to identify areas in which patient care should be improved.

[illegible]

- [illegible]
- [illegible]
- [illegible]
- [illegible]
- number and severity of [illegible]
- number of [illegible]
- [illegible]

There is continuing debate about the use of HSMR and the results should be considered with caution but the primary role of HSMR is to identify areas that warrant further investigation.

- The results should be investigated carefully, with the focus on supplementary data, [illegible] may exist [illegible] in the data
- Mortality [illegible] may or may not be related to the quality of patient care; [illegible] such as data quality can also contribute to changes in the HSMR
- HSMRs can help [illegible] to areas that require improvement [illegible]
- However, over time, HSMRs can help [illegible] national bodies [illegible] their improvement work resulted in reduced number of [illegible]
- HSMR should not be [illegible]

Metrics of patient safety

National-level data

There are several metrics that are commonly used at a national level for monitoring, learning, and improvement.

Hospital standardized mortality ratio

The hospital standardized mortality ratio or rate (HSMR) is a measurement or screening tool that can be used to reduce the incidence of avoidable death in acute settings. Several countries (Australia, Canada, England, Netherlands, Scotland and United States) use the HSMR to monitor mortality and to identify areas in which patient care should be improved.

Box 12.4 Hospital standardized mortality rate

HSMR is calculated by comparing the actual number of deaths with the predicted number of deaths.

HSMR = observed deaths/predicted deaths.

HSMR > 1 is interpreted as indicating more deaths than predicted.

HSRM < 1 is interpreted as indicating fewer deaths than predicted.

Normal variation over time is to be expected; hence the HSMR score is rarely 1.

HSMR considers mortality data and adjusts for some of the factors that are known to affect the underlying risk of death.

Scottish hospitals adjust for:

- primary diagnosis
- age and gender
- place where the patient was admitted
- type of admission (elective/non-elective)
- number and severity of prior admissions to hospital in the past year or five years
- number of emergency admissions to hospital
- admission as day patient or inpatient

- There is continuing debate about the use of HSMR and the results should be considered with caution. But the primary role of HSMR is to identify areas that warrant further investigation.
- The results should be investigated locally, with the help of supplemental data, in order to establish what other factors may cause variation in the data.
- The variation may or may not be related to the quality of patient care; issues such as data quality can also contribute to changing the HSMR.
- HSMR can help teams to focus on areas that require improvement or, conversely, on areas to learn from.
- Reviewed over time, HSMR can help systems, organizations, and national bodies to find out whether their improvement work results in a reduced number of preventable deaths.
- HSMR should not be used to rank hospitals or health systems but can be used to learn from one another and to aid improvement.

Emergency hospitals readmissions

- Emergency hospital readmissions have been correlated to the quality of the care that patients receive along the clinical pathway.
- There are quality improvement frameworks in many countries, for instance in Denmark, England, Germany, and the United States.
- Recognized limitations to this type of measure include the following:
    - it is difficult to separate avoidable readmissions from readmissions due to patient complexity;
    - they have links with factors outside hospital control (e.g. primary or social care);
    - they have unclear links with other measures of safety (e.g. mortality).

Emergency department twelve-hour waits

- This is a measure of the number of patients who remain in emergency departments for more than twelve hours after the decision to admit them has been made and recorded.
- It can serve as an indicator of hospital bed occupancy, healthcare performance, and safety.

Hospital-associated infections

Several hospital-associated infections are measured at the national level and are reported as the number of cases per 1,000 acute occupied bed days:

- *Staphylococcus aureus* bacteraemia (including MRSA);
- *Clostridium difficile*;
- *Escherichia coli*.

Organization/system level

Organizations and systems could use the metrics described for the national-level data; but they may also include measures that are relevant to their clinical practice.

Here are some examples of local organization and system measures:

- the perspective of patients and their families;
- measures of the reliability of critical safety processes;
- information on practices that encourage the monitoring of safety;
- information on the capacity to anticipate safety problems;
- information on the capacity to respond to and learn from safety data;
- data on staff attitudes, staff awareness, and feedback from staff;
- mortality rate indicators;
- data on predefined standards;
- incident reports and reporting levels;
- reports on excellence.

Each clinical area should define its own measurement strategy as well as that of the organization and of the national system, according to the type of clinical care delivered. (For examples of measures, see Box 12.5; see also the case study in Box 12.6.).

Box 12.5 Selected examples of measures for clinical areas

For an intensive care:
- ventilator-associated pneumonia
- central line infections
- tissue viability
- unplanned extubation

For a medical ward
- falls
- pressure ulcers
- staffing levels
- staff well-being
- fragmentation of care
- medication harm
- peripheral line infections

Surgical ward
- surgical site infections
- excessive starvation before surgery
- return to the operating room
- pressure ulcers
- urinary tract infections

Box 12.6 Case study: Scottish Patient Safety Programme (SPSP)

SPSP is a unique national initiative launched in January 2008 that aims to improve the safety and reliability of health and social care and to reduce harm whenever care is delivered. SPSP is led and co-ordinated nationally; its implementation is supported within NHS boards through local teams in hospitals, GP practices, mental health inpatient units, and community pharmacies.

Each level of the system sets locally specific aims against an existing baseline.

Nationally, SPSP set a long-term aim of reducing HSMR by 15% by the year 2013, and then by 20% by December 2015.

- The NHS board or organizational level set local aims and patient safety data that are available across the system.
- This empowers local teams to assess their patient safety data and trial improvements.
- The activity of local teams in wards across Scotland has reduced the harms from deterioration, sepsis and acute kidney injury, falls, and pressure ulcers.
- Through this whole system approach, teams at all levels can benchmark again and learn from one another.

Learning from patient safety data

[illegible]

Summary box

Top tips

- [illegible]
- [illegible]
- [illegible]
- [illegible]
- [illegible]
- [illegible]
- [illegible]
- [illegible]
- [illegible]
- [illegible]
- [illegible]

Further reading

[illegible]

[illegible]

[illegible]

[illegible]

[illegible]

[illegible]

Learning from patient safety data

Ideally, frontline safety data should contribute significantly to systematic, organizational, and national measures of patient safety. Benchmarking for patient safety is extremely challenging, except at the high levels outlined in national metrics.

Summary box

Top tips

- Measures must be easy to collect.
- Measures must be relevant to both patients and staff.
- Harm must be recorded in real time.
- Have several measures that reflect the function of the system.
- Focus on what works well as well as on what does not.
- Measures must tell you how the system is working.
- Display measures openly and in a way that can be understood.
- To enable assessment and learning, data can be displayed in different ways.
- Safety crosses are a visual demonstration of the incidence of a designated harm.
- Run charts as time series analysis.
- Use statistical process control charts for statistical analysis.
- Discuss data daily, at safety huddles or meetings.

Further reading

Berwick, D. M. et al. *A Promise to Learn—A Commitment to Act*. London: Crown copyright, 2013. https://www.gov.uk/government/uploads/system/uploads/attachment_data/file/226703/Berwick_Report.pdf.

Borzecki, A. M. and Rosen, A. K. Is there a 'best measure' of patient safety? *BMJ Quality & Safety* 29.3 (2020): 185–8. doi: 10.1136/bmjqs-2019; https://doi.org/10.1136/bmjqs-2019-009730.

The Health Foundation. *The Measurement and Monitoring of Safety*. Spotlight 2013. https://www.health.org.uk/sites/default/files/TheMeasurementAndMonitoringOfSafety_fullversion.pdf.

Hibbert, P. D. et al. The application of the Global Trigger Tool: A systematic review. *International Journal for Quality in Health Care* 28.6 (2016): 640–9. https://doi.org/10.1093/intqhc/mzw115.

OECD. Measuring patient safety. 2018. https://www.oecd.org/health/health-systems/Measuring-Patient-Safety-April-2018.pdf.

Vincent, C., Burnett, S., and Carthey, J. Safety measurement and monitoring in healthcare: A framework to guide clinical teams and healthcare organisations in maintaining safety. *BMJ Quality & Safety* 23 (2014): 670–7. http://dx.doi.org/10.1136/bmjqs-2013-002757.

Measuring patient safety on the front line

Key points

- Clinical teams can improve outcomes only if they measure their own day-to-day performance.
- The Vincent framework for measuring and monitoring safety gives clinical teams, managers, and executives the opportunity to measure performance in a way that can improve the safety of care.
- The framework is used daily by teams.
- The model assesses the safety of care from the perspective of reliability, human factors, and resilience theories.
- Harm can be measured in several ways and is represented on tools such as the safety cross, on run charts, and on statistical control charts.

Why measure safety on the front line?

In healthcare, measurement systems are typically designed to serve the needs of administrators, regulators, academics, and others, who use data for billing, assurance, or research. Frontline staff gathers and uploads data that it may never see again, although occasionally these data are used to judge or admonish staff members.

An alternative view of measurement, proposed by patient safety science, is founded on the belief that data are critical to understanding problems and to guiding their solutions. This view also suggests that no one is better positioned to benefit from measurement for improvement than the people working on the front line of healthcare.

A good frontline safety measurement system requires just enough data to inform users in a timely way about important processes, cultural indicators, and outcomes. It should also be able to provide rapid feedback on the "tests of change" that are required to design and improve care. (Improvement Chapter 14)

Ideal frontline measurement systems are co-produced with those staff members (and, where applicable, service users) who input and extract data, ensuring that measures are usable and useful. A good design principle for an effective frontline measurement system is that it should be easy to use; the ease with which one can gather, input, display, and interpret the data is important.

Another feature is that the data should reach those who make day-to-day changes as quickly and clearly as possible. Later on these data can be repackaged to meet regulatory purposes, if required. To maximize reach and impact, the outputs of such measurement systems should be shared openly and transparently, including with the patients and their families.

What should be measured?

What should be measured?

There is no single metric that can fully express the complexity of safety, so a portfolio of measures is required if we want to give an accurate picture.

Traditionally safety has been measured by the absence of harm. While harm may indicate a deficit in safety, this is not the only measure of safe care. Considering safety as something that an organization *does* rather than *has* suggests that measuring safe practices and their outcomes is important.

Safe practices—for example care bundles for the prevention of central line infections or for team communication—can be measured and used to predict safe outcomes. It is also possible to examine the shared beliefs and attitudes of practitioners and the culture of safety, all of which influence the way people behave (Safety Culture Chapter 3).

Organizational knowledge of safe practice and culture obtained from measurement and feedback also supports learning and guides improvement efforts. This broader view of safety measurement allows us to ask not only whether we *have been safe* but also whether we *are safe* now and *will we be safe* in the future.

The Health Foundation's framework for measuring and monitoring patient safety, also known as the Vincent framework (see Figure 13.1), suggests a portfolio of five measures:

1. study of past harm;
2. reliability of key clinical processes;
3. sensitivity (awareness) to operations;
4. anticipation of problems that may arise; and
5. integration of learning.

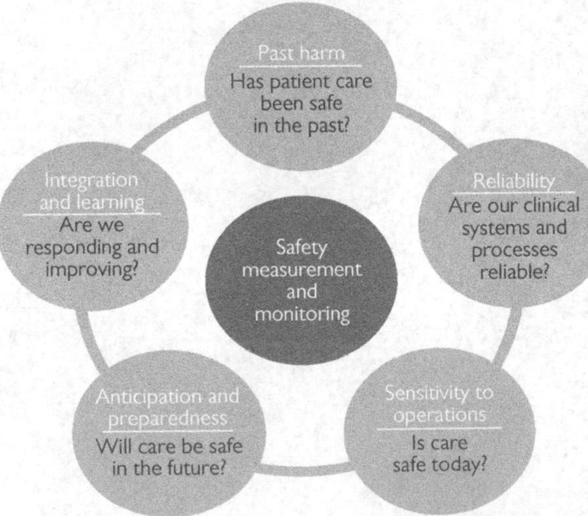
Past harm
Has patient care been safe in the past?
Reliability
Are our clinical systems and processes reliable?
Sensitivity to operations
Is care safe today?
Anticipation and preparedness
Will care be safe in the future?
Integration and learning
Are we responding and improving?
Safety measurement and monitoring

Figure 13.1 Vincent framework for measuring and monitoring safety.

Reproduced with permission from The Health Foundation; Measuring and Monitoring of Patient Safety https://www.health.org.uk/sites/default/files/TheMeasurementAndMonitoringOfSafety_fullversion.pdf

The goal of the framework is not only to provide assurance (a goal related to past harm) but also to address potential harm through a *proactive* management (reliability, sensitivity) of risk rather than a *reactive* management of incidents. The key approach is real-time action (anticipation and preparedness) and learning (integration), prompted and guided by the data collected in each part of the framework.

Past harm: Have we been safe?

Harm is a measure that it is essential to quantify and understand, because this is the feature of safety that matters most to patients. It is important, however, to acknowledge that not all harm is preventable and that it is not always possible, or wise, to determine whether harm was preventable, because there are difficulties with hindsight. Yet reducing harm, regardless of the cause, remains the goal of patient safety and its measurement is critical to this ambition.

It is important that staff and patients on the front line recognize harm in order to measure it. Defining harm from the point of view of the patient, where possible, and creating opportunities to discuss it helps to build shared understanding and contributes to a culture of safety. A good practice is to normalize these discussions by including a review (not necessarily documented) of harm over the previous twenty-four hours at handovers, huddles, or safety pauses on a daily basis.

Another helpful practice is to create openness and to use language that facilitates the discussion of harm to staff—not only physical but psychological and emotional harm, too. All this requires a high level of psychological safety for teams to feel comfortable as they articulate and discuss problems. (Situation Awareness Chapter 8). It is best to link this form of openness with discussions about "what we've done well" and "good catches" in order to remind staff members that most of what they do is successful.

When planning improvement interventions, it is important to have shared operational definitions for specific harms and for grading their severity—for instance those offered by the categories in the MERP tool for medication harm (Medication Safety Chapter 20). Recognizing that not every fall necessarily results in physical injury allows us to consider which falls do so and how these can be measured and ameliorated. Thus we can measure the factor of risk.

There are multiple sources of data, routinely collected from the front line, that contain information about harm. Where it is possible to avoid replication, these data can be used to guide safety interventions. Apart from recording harm from these sources, the staff should become aware of the narrative behind the episodes recorded, as this is likely to contain rich additional information. In Box 13.1 potential sources of data are provided.

Knowledge of past harm is important for the provision of assurance, but it is also a valuable means for frontline teams to understand harm and generate ideas for improvement. Rather than looking at individual harm events for preventability, looking across all events for common risks and themes helps to understand the processes of care involved and what potential solutions there are. Tools such as root cause analysis (RCA) and the 5 WHYs may be helpful in this endeavour, but need to be used cautiously (Clinical Incident Chapter 16).

Box 13.1 Potential sources of data about harm

- *Incident reporting*. Staff should be encouraged to report all incidents and near misses of harm, because low rates of reporting do not accurately reflect safety. On the other hand, targeted incident reporting (e.g. falls or specific medication errors) designed to address a known safety issue over a defined period may be even more useful.
- *Never events*. These are rare incidents with potentially tragic consequences. e.g. wrong site surgery. Often safety practices are in place to prevent them.
- *Mortality statistics*. Examples are the hospital standardized mortality rates (HSMR) and, more recently, the summary hospital mortality indicator (SHMI).
- *Clinical coding databases*. These can be used to identify safety indicators, for example post-operative wound dehiscence. However, the accuracy of clinical coding often varies.
- *Risk registers*. These are records of potential safety issues. They use a standard matrix with action plans in order to mitigate the risks.
- *Trigger tools*. As indicated in Chapter 13, a trigger tool is a case note review that looks for defined events (triggers) and may indicate that an adverse event has occurred. An example of a trigger is the administration of a rescue medication such as flumazenil or naloxone, which suggests that a medication injury may have occurred (e.g. benzodiazepine or opiate overdose). The trigger tool allows for the identification of harm that may not have been reported elsewhere. As suggested earlier, the process of performing the case note review provides insights into safety practices and the safety culture.
- *Safety thermometer*. This is a way to measure and convey the idea of "harm-free" care, that is, the percentage of patients who did not have any of the common harms expected in a clinical area. Data on the high volume of potential patient safety issues can be collected on a single day, each week or month, by reviewing records and speaking to patients and carers. In the UK, the NHS safety thermometer measures pressure ulcers, falls in care, catheter urinary infections, and the treatment for venous thromboembolism (there is also a paediatric version that focuses on deterioration, extravasation, pain, and skin integrity). The goal is to have as many patients as possible complete an episode of care without experiencing any of these four harms, in other words have a reliably safe care.

Reliable processes (Reliability Chapter 10): Can we be sure we are safe?

The effectiveness of clinical care is underpinned by high-quality evidence from medical research. Where such evidence exists, reliable adherence to clinical guidelines and standardized process is the key to obtaining good outcomes. Understanding the smallest deviation from critical processes creates knowledge that can help to achieve high reliability.

There are numerous examples of individual and combined practices that improve safety. One approach is that of care bundles, which are collections of up to five key clinical processes that have—both independently and in combination—an evidence base for improving outcomes. There are many evaluated care bundles, designed for instance to reduce infection from peripheral and central venous cannulation, urinary catheters, ventilator-associated pneumonia, and surgical site infections.

Implementing and improving the reliable use of bundles can be helped with tools such as a reliability matrix (Figure 13.3), which samples and calculates adherence to bundle elements and the reliability of the bundle as a whole. This approach can also be used for learning and feedback when teams are trying to reliably embed new practice habits such as communication (ISBAR) or debriefing (the four steps of an after-action review). These data can be displayed and further analysed using run charts (Figure 13.4) or SPC charts (Figure 13.5).

Sensitivity to operations: Is care safe now?

Real-time measurement and analysis of the current state of safety are essential to ensuring the proactive management of risk. Frontline clinical teams can use the lens of human factors and assess safety from different dimensions, as we have seen in the SEIPS model. (Human Factors Chapter 9) Here are some of the questions one should ask:

- What is the composition of the clinical team?
- Who are the patients and what are their clinical needs and their views on safety?
- Is the team able to complete the required tasks?
- Does the team have the tools and the equipment needed to complete the tasks?
- Is the environment conducive to safety?
- What is the team's culture and what are its members' views on safety? (Culture Chapter 2)

Measuring safety practices such as the reliable use of early warning systems or situation awareness shared through huddles and team communication serves to enhance operational sensitivity.

At a system level, safety walkrounds by senior staff can allow clinical teams to report their views on patient safety, so that there is an alignment of the understanding of real-time safety. It is important to be able to measure and act on this safety intelligence in a timely way, which effectively benefits the local department.

Anticipation and preparedness: Will care be safe in the future?

This is a key element of proactive risk management and is essential to mitigating potential harm on the basis of real-time sensitivity to what's happening. For example, an awareness of staffing levels can lead to the proactive mitigation of future risk; an early warning score that moves in the wrong direction can allow one to predict harm and to escalate care so as to prevent deterioration.

Other measures might involve the degree of preparedness, as in assessing the membership and availability of rapid response teams, or the presence and utility of emergency guidelines. Simulation can be used not only in training but also to assess the readiness of emergency plans.

Integration and learning: Are we responding to, and improving from, safety information?

The measurements discussed so far add value and benefits for clinical teams and, ultimately for patients, if there is reflection on and learning from what the data are saying. In this way reliable safe care can develop and spread throughout a system.

Learning also needs qualitative measures that take into account the views and experiences of staff, patients, and families. Qualitative data can provide information on their own; they may help in triangulation with other, more objective measures or they lend emotional weight to the reasons why addressing safety is important. Such effects can be achieved through storytelling or through structured narratives such as after-action reviews (AARs), where collective experience and sense-making are used to understand events.

Another approach comes from the learning from excellence community (Learning from success Chapter 15), which has pioneered the reporting of excellence from the front line in order to elevate episodes of good practice, kindness, and positive action as events to be celebrated and learned from. Learning from what works well and measuring it is crucial: teams learn how a certain process generates a certain result, and thus they get to replicate it.

Tools for measuring and reporting safety

[illegible]

Tools for measuring and reporting safety

Front line measurement does not need to be complicated. Technology may be useful in the gathering, analysis, storage, and display of information, but it is by no means essential and should be considered only for its additional value.

As important as measuring is, the means by which data are analysed and communicated is more crucial and will determine its impact. Box 13.2 contains some examples of effective measurement and reporting tools, which can be deployed on paper or used in conjunction with some rudimentary information technology, to share information that can influence decisions and shape behaviour.

Box 13.2 Tools that illustrate safety measurement

The **safety cross** presents data in a cross-shaped matrix that represents a calendar month of recording a selected metric, such as medication errors or falls. Additional information, for example severity, is displayed through colour or shading. This tool offers real-time incidence data that raise a team's awareness of the incidents tracked in this way.	Figure 13.2
A **reliability matrix** is a simple tool for recording elements of a care bundle (CB) or any set of processes where the goal is to deliver all the elements every time. The matrix can be used for small samples and simple measures if each element has been delivered. It allows for simple calculations—such as the performance of each CB element, which helps to decide where to focus quality improvement (QI) efforts, and the full bundle delivery (i.e. how many patients received all the CB elements they should have received) as a measurement of the reliability.	Figure 13.3
A **run chart** is a time series analysis that visually demonstrates variation in processes or outcomes. In small samples (e.g. the daily or weekly number of line infections or medication errors), data are plotted over time, to demonstrate the process performance. There are four common rules for highlighting non-random variation: a shift (six or more consecutive data points, all above or all below the mean), a trend (five or more consecutive data points, all going up or all going down), too many or too few runs, and astronomical points (obviously very different from the other values). For rare events (i.e. events in which 50% or more of the data points represent extreme values of the scale), days in between events may be more useful.	Figure 13.4
A **statistical process control chart (SPC)** adds statistical limits to the run chart. This allows one to differentiate between a normal, common cause of variation in the system and a special cause (as shown in Figure 13.5), which is the result of some atypical event or influence and requires a specific response.	Figure 13.5

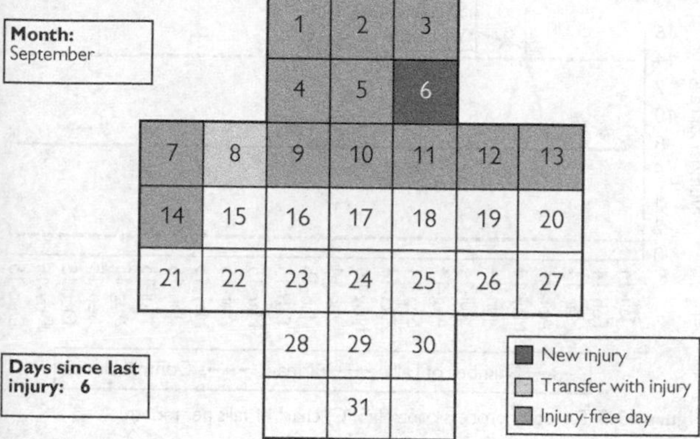

Figure 13.2 Safety cross.

	Patient number					Reliability	
Care Bundle Element	1	2	3	4	5	Fraction	%
A	×	✓	✓	✓	×	3/5	60%
B	✓	✓	✓	✓	✓	5/5	100%
C	✓	×	✓	✓	✓	4/5	80%
D	✓	×	✓	✓	✓	4/5	80%
E	✓	✓	✓	✓	✓	5/5	100%
F	✓	✓	✓	✓	×	4/5	80%
Bundle Elements (✓/6)	5/6	4/6	6/6	6/6	4/6	25/36	69%
Full Care Bundle (6/6)	×	×	✓	✓	×	2/5	40%
Care Bundle Reliability Matrix							

Figure 13.3 Reliability matrix for a care bundle.

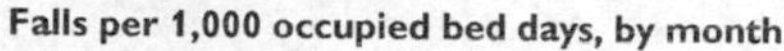

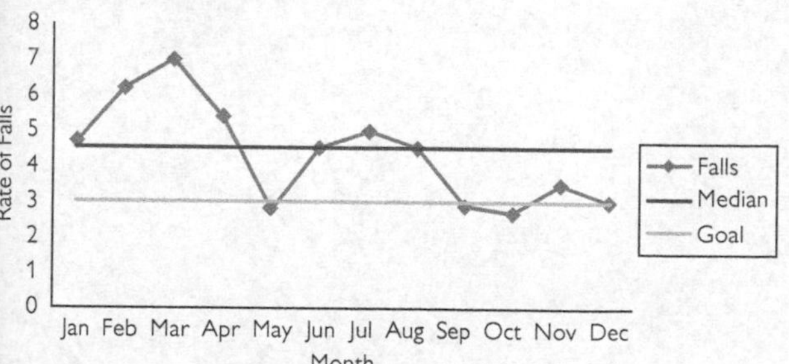

Figure 13.4 Run chart of falls per month.

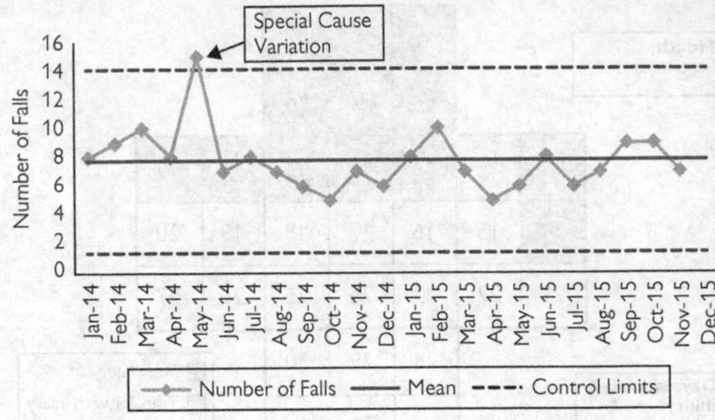

Figure 13.5 Statistical process control (SPC) chart of falls per month.

[illegible]

Summary box

- Measurement of safety in real time by clinical teams can make a difference.
- It is important for safety measurement systems to benefit people who work on the front line, so they can design improvements.
- The importance of measuring harm and error is evident.
- The measurement of what was learned from the successful practice of patient safety guides learning at the front line.

Reference

The Health Foundation. *The Measurement and Monitoring of Safety*. Spotlight 2013. https://www.health.org.uk/sites/default/files/TheMeasurementAndMonitoringOfSafety_fullversion.pdf.

Further reading

Borzecki, A. M. and Rosen, A. K. Is there a 'best measure' of patient safety? *BMJ Quality & Safety* 29 (2020): 185–8. https://qualitysafety.bmj.com/content/qhc/29/3/185.full.pdf.Chapman, S. M. et al. Prevalence and severity of patient harm in a sample of UK-hospitalised children detected by the Paediatric Trigger Tool. *BMJ Open* 4.7 (2014): e005066. https://doi.org/10.1136/bmjopen-2014-005066.

Chatburn, E. et al. Measurement and monitoring of safety: Impact and challenges of putting a conceptual framework into practice. *BMJ Quality & Safety* 27 (2018): 81826. https://doi.org/10.1136/bmjqs-2017-007175.

Hibbert, P. D. et al. The application of the Global Trigger Tool: A systematic review. *International Journal for Quality in Health Care* 28.6 (2016): 640–9. https://doi.org/10.1093/intqhc/mzw115.

Lachman, P. et al. Developing person-centred analysis of harm in a paediatric hospital: A quality improvement report. *BMJ Quality & Safety* 24.5 (2015): 337–44. http://dx.doi.org/10.1136/bmjqs-2014-003795.

Macrae, C. The problem with incident reporting. *BMJ Quality & Safety* 25 (2016): 71–5. https://qualitysafety.bmj.com/content/25/2/71.

Peerally, M. F. et al. The problem with root cause analysis. *BMJ Quality & Safety* 26 (2017): 417–22. https://qualitysafety.bmj.com/content/26/5/417.

Perla, R. J., Provost, L. P., and Murray, S. K. The run chart: a simple analytical tool for learning from variation in healthcare processes. *BMJ Quality & Safety*, *20*(1) (2011): 46–51. https://doi.org/10.1136/bmjqs.2009.037895

Vincent, C., Burnett, S., and Carthey, J. Safety measurement and monitoring in healthcare: A framework to guide clinical teams and healthcare organisations in maintaining safety. *BMJ Quality & Safety* 23 (2014): 670–7. http://dx.doi.org/10.1136/bmjqs-2013-002757.

Chapter 14

Practical approaches to safety improvement

Key points

- To improve the safety of clinical processes optimally, an understanding of improvement methodology is required.
- Combining theories of patient safety (such as human factors, reliability, and resilience) with the methods of improvement science can create conditions for the improvement of safety.
- Engaging the clinical team and patients is the first step.
- Studying the process, as well as measuring process and outcomes, will provide opportunities to improve.
- Through the use of small tests of change, learning and improvement can take place.

Why is understanding improvement theory and methodology important?

It is often assumed that clinicians will improve care as part of their professional duties. This view fails to recognize the complexity of improvement and the need to be skilled in the theories of improvement and implementation science. Frontline clinicians have a critical role in providing reliably safe care (Reliability Chapter 10) through their every action and interaction.

By using a structured and methodological improvement approach, every clinician can overcome these challenges to make improvement part of his or her daily work.

What is the safety improvement issue?

Healthcare systems are complex and adaptive. Failures resulting in unsafe care may be the result of complex interactions between human and environmental factors. Learning from failure and from success is essential to improving safety. We must always keep in mind that a failure to keep a patient safe reflects on the entire system, its people and processes, and can create an opportunity for improvement. Learning from success shows what is possible and how we replicate it.

All healthcare professionals have a role to play in ensuring that health services are safe and of a high quality. This requires an understanding of how outcomes are achieved. A learning organization (or clinical team) will measure its outcomes over time and continually improve in order to provide ever more reliable care. Meaningful and lasting change requires that all those involved in healthcare, at every level—clinicians, patients, managers, researchers, and planners—work together to transform care systems for the benefit of patients and providers. Effectively improving quality requires the understanding and application of improvement methodology.

Eight steps to improve patient safety

Identify the problem

Safety problems can be identified by measuring outcomes, e.g. measuring medication adverse events or harm. In the previous chapter the Vincent framework for measurement and monitoring safety was introduced (see also Vincent, Burnett, and Carthey, 2013). By using this framework, safety areas in need of improvement can be identified.

We can list issues, for example, [illegible] that is specific to a clinical area:

- adverse drug events
- hospital-acquired pressure ulcers
- central line bloodstream infection (CLABSI)
- ventilator-associated pneumonia (VAP)
- [illegible] urinary tract infections
- falls
- missing [illegible]
- [illegible] deterioration.

These measurements can be taken during a defined period, such as the previous twenty-four hours. [illegible] over time [illegible] SPC [illegible] [illegible] the stability of [illegible] variation [illegible] improve.

Using [illegible] approach [illegible] [illegible] [illegible] the first two steps and [illegible] information [illegible] time [illegible] among the team.

[illegible] the improvement process [illegible] team [illegible] sustained and [illegible] This is an essential part of improving care [illegible] to engage the team.

[illegible] improvement process [illegible] the problem [illegible] through the following steps.

Engage the people in the system and build an improvement team

Once the problem has been identified, the next step is to engage members of the team. This is the most important step in the improvement process. It is important to understand the motivation of the people who deliver care, their attitudes and belief systems, and how these affect the underlying safety culture. Such understanding allows you to identify the barriers and the facilitators to change, as well as the champions and the naysayers who can [illegible] [illegible] the improvement [illegible] [illegible] spent on this step assists in building will and the sustainability of the improvement process.

Complex systems involve many people. Carefully consider the stakeholders in the process: patients, clinicians, and support staff. It is useful to have a clear communication plan in order to engage people and ensure that you can have the people [illegible] for the proposed improvement.

In this step the will and the desire for change [illegible] The [illegible] [illegible] design of solutions [illegible] to frontline staff [illegible] [illegible] with patients and families will lead to more [illegible] outcomes.

Eight steps to improve patient safety

Identify the problem

Safety problems can be identified by measuring outcomes e.g. measuring medication adverse events or harm. In the previous chapter the Vincent framework for measurement and managing safety was introduced (see also Vincent, Burnett, and Carthey 2013). By using this framework, safety areas that need to be improved can be identified.

We can measure, for example, past harm that is specific to a clinical area:

- adverse drug events;
- hospital acquired infections,
- central line bloodstream infection (CLABSI),
- ventilator-associated pneumonia (VAP),
- sepsis, urinary tract infections;
- falls;
- pressure ulcers;
- unexpected deterioration.

These measurements can be taken during a defined period, such as the previous twenty-four hours. To measure over time, use a run chart, SPC chart, or a safety cross. Evaluate the reliability of clinical processes, as variation presents an opportunity to improve.

Using a human factors and resilience approach, assess whether you are safe now and whether the service will be safe in the future. This is best achieved by completing the first two steps and gathering information in real time so as to develop situation awareness among the team.

Appraise the learning process and how knowledge is managed and transferred. This is an essential part of improving care, as well as an opportunity to engage the team.

To aid the improvement process, further definition of the problem occurs through the following steps.

Engage the people in the system and build an improvement team

Once the problem has been identified, the next step is to engage members of the team. This is the most important step in the improvement process. It is important to understand the motivation of the people who deliver care, their attitudes and belief systems, and how these values affect the underlying safety culture. Such understanding allows you to identify the barriers and the facilitators to change, as well as the champions and the motivators who can take frontline ownership of the improvement process. Valuable time spent on this step assists in building will and the sustainability of the improvement process.

Complex systems involve many people. Carefully consider the stakeholders in the process; patients, clinicians, and support staff. It is useful to have a clear communication plan in order to engage people and ensure that you can have the required buy-in for a proposed improvement.

In this step, the will and the desire for change are built. The co-production and co-design of solutions gives ownership to frontline staff; and co-producing safety improvement with patients and families will lead to more person-centred outcomes.

It is important to constantly assess how people in the system view the issues and where attention needs to be directed to achieve sustained improvement.

Study the work system

In order to achieve the desired improvement, it is necessary to have a detailed understanding of how the work system functions (see SEIPS Chapter 9). Every work system is different, and appreciating its unique context is vital for a successful safety improvement project. A human factors approach to understanding the work system involves the following features:

- People in the system. How do they behave and interact? For example, do they follow standing operating procedures reliably or not? Do they measure performance? Time spent engaging the team will facilitate this step (see the previous step).
- Patients receiving care and their specific needs. Often improvement projects "do" things to patients rather than working with them to improve the process.
- The environment within which people work and its impact on safety. These components are important. Interventions should be tested and adapted to the specific context in which they will be applied.
- The tasks that are completed and how they are undertaken.
- The tools and technology required to perform a given task and their effect on how work is done.
- The way the work system is organized. Does it measure performance? Is there a common purpose, in other words is it the case that everyone knows what the purpose is and how they must work to achieve desired outcomes? This feature is determined by leadership within the team.

Useful tools to build understanding include the fishbone diagram. Broad and deep understanding can in turn be used to develop the aim statement and the theory of change, as represented in a driver diagram.

See the care process through the eyes of the patient

Patient care is a process. Studying the process of care helps us to identify opportunities to improve. Follow and map a real patient journey. View the tasks that are completed and their sequence carefully. Use this observation to map the process. Look for steps that add value to the outcome and for steps that lead to waste. Some steps are essential and rate-limiting, while others may be unnecessary or of minimal value.

Measure variation

Measurement is a key aspect of understanding processes and their outcomes, that is, what happens to a patient or member of staff. Measurement over time allows dynamic and ongoing understanding throughout the improvement process. It is important to start by measuring the baseline, so that you can assess the extent of improvement when you implement a change. Baseline measurement can begin with a clinical audit, either when you identify the problem (the first of our eight steps) or when you study the work system (the third step).

Careful study and measurement of a process facilitates the identification of unwarranted variation. Variation in the process creates unreliable and often unsafe care; a few examples are:

- variation in the way we prescribe antibiotics;
- variation in the way we assess deterioration or sepsis;
- variation in the way we prevent pressure injuries or falls;
- variation in the way we observe hand hygiene.

A key part of improving outcomes is to improve the reliability of the process. Process variation can be studied and analysed using a run chart or SPC chart.

Sometimes a specific patient condition may require variation. This is then warranted variation.

Design the future state

Most processes need to be redesigned in order to achieve new and more desirable outcomes such as safer care. This requires innovation and learning that is co-designed and co-produced with the clinical staff, as well as with patients and their families.

Many improvements in patient safety have been pioneered elsewhere, hence it can be useful to examine what has worked in other settings and see how it can be adapted to a new context. Design thinking is inherent in the theories and methods of human factors and reliability.

Undertake tasks that are required to implement improvement and test the desired changes

Once the system that produces unsafe care has been studied, undesirable variation has been identified, the beliefs, attitudes, and motivations of the people who operate within the system have been recognized and understood, and baseline measurements have been undertaken, a stable foundation for improvement is established.

Improvement often requires tasks designed to prepare for change (e.g. drawing a up checklist), and then a change method designed to test ideas of change in the real world (e.g. seeing how the checklist performs in a real clinical setting).

The model for improvement provides a framework for practical improvement (Figure 14.1).

- The aim of an improvement initiative is defined by asking: 'What are we trying to accomplish?'. The answer to this question directs the desire and will to change; 'what' is the thing that needs to be improved. Aims need to be SMART, that is *specific* with regard to what is to be improved, *measurable*, *achievable*, *relevant* (i.e. answer 'why' the change is needed) and *timebound* (i.e. specify by when date the improvement will be achieved).
- The question 'How will we know that a change is an improvement?' captures measurement as a foundation of improvement. Its answer incorporates the baseline and progress in processes and outcomes over time (see the step on measure variation).
- The third question, 'What changes can we make that will result in improvement?', captures the point where your understanding of the work system (the third step) allows the identification of potential tasks to perform and changes to test.

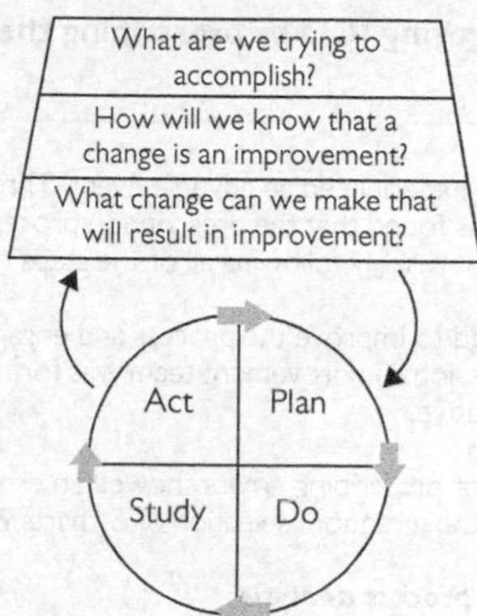

Figure 14.1 Model for Improvement

Reproduced with permission from Associates in Press Improvement; http://www.apiweb.org/

The cycle plan, do, study, act (PDSA) provides the answer to the 'how' question: it tells us how change is made. PDSA cycles use small, rapid cycle changes designed to test and measure impact, then test again, in a much faster and more proactive manner than the traditional audit cycle. While the PDSA cycle may initially appear unfamiliar to the practising clinician, it is essentially similar to the differential diagnosis and management plan within clinical practice. The 'plan' phase is derived from the differential diagnosis and the theory of the possible illness the patient may have. This leads to a planned treatment. The 'do' phase consists of implementing the treatment plan or the solution to be tested. The 'study' phase consists of determining whether the treatment plan or the solution (or test) has worked. And finally the 'act' phase is the point where we determine whether to continue with our treatment plan and solution or we try something new: we choose between adopt, adapt, or abandon.

Hardwire the changes into the system and spread the learning

The improvement that is achieved is unlikely to be sustained until it is hardwired into the system—that is, until it becomes the way work is done by everyone involved. To achieve sustainability, the new process must be relatively advantageous to the patient and to the clinical staff and must not be more difficult to do. Sustainability depends on having local champions, as well as an ongoing measurement of the process and of its outcomes. It is important to pay attention to the fidelity of the change-in other words to register whether the improvement was due to specific changes and how they were implemented.

It is important for successful change projects to be spread, so that others with the same problem can learn from your experience and adapt it to their own context. Successful improvement in one area and the methodology used can help with the design of future change and facilitate improvements in other areas.

Case study: Improving ICU by prescribing the use of a 'sterile cockpit'

Problem

In an ICU, a patient experienced an adverse event. Through root cause analysis (RCA) it was found that the prescription process was unsafe, as prescribers were not reliably following all of the steps required.

Engagement

A consultant decided to improve the process and engaged the clinical team. A multiprofessional improvement team was formed that included a patient representative.

Baseline measures

Baseline measures of prescribing errors showed an error rate of 30% over a 1-week period; a random selection of 5 charts were assessed every day.

Work system and process analysis

The improvement team analysed the work system using the SEIPS model:

People: the prescribers were doctors, ranging from junior to senior trainees. Several nurse practitioners also had prescribing privileges.

Patients: the patients ranged from the elderly to relatively fit young adults, all with different pharmacokinetics.

Environment: the environment was busy and noisy, as prescribing took place anywhere on the unit.

Tasks: the drugs were complex and not all staff members felt comfortable prescribing.

Tools: the tools required were a calculator, a formulary, a list of commonly used drugs, and standard operating procedures.

Organization: patient safety was identified as being important, but prescribing was not seen as a priority.

Design idea

Using a human factors concept, it was decided to adopt a 'sterile cockpit' in which all prescribing would take place. It was envisaged that all the tools for prescribing would be available and that interruptions would not be allowed once a prescriber was in the defined area.

- The aim was to make all prescriptions 100% accurate by December 2021.

Tasks and tests

The new prescribing area was defined and fully equipped. This was the task.

Tests were then undertaken. The aims were to learn through implementation, to decrease the frequency of interruptions, and to improve prescribing accuracy.

These tests revealed that some members of staff required additional reminders about avoiding interruptions and that all new staff needed to undergo 'sterile cockpit' training.

Sustainability

Using a structured improvement approach, the aim was achieved: prescribing errors were eliminated and the number of days between adverse events was increased.

What are the challenges?

[illegible]

What are the challenges?

There are many challenges to safety improvement (Table 14.1):

Table 14.1. Selected challenges and solutions

Challenge	Solution
Absence of an organizational or team safety culture	The foundation of improvement is a learning culture; leadership is essential
Difficulty in convincing people that there is a problem	Develop the 'why' for an improvement; engage others by sharing stories and data in combination
Insufficient recognition and understanding of the complexity of the problem, or difficulty in demonstrating that there is a problem	Study and measure the work system producing variation (in processes and outcomes) and display it using a run chart to demonstrate 'what' needs to improve
Lack of improvement knowledge and skills	Adopt a theory and method of improvement – the 'how' to improve
Setting ambitious goals for improvement projects beyond the capability of the team or organization	A system can produce only the results for which it is designed, so you may need to redesign a process in order to improve it
Tribalism and lack of engagement by team members owing to competing interests	Make engagement of staff the first step and part of understanding the system before changes are implemented; then allow others to 'test' the changes
Securing sustainability of any intervention after the improvement 'project' ends	Build sustainability into improvement from the start, not as an afterthought

Summary box

Practical tips for using improvement methodology to improve safety:

- Use structured tools to increase the depth of your understanding of the problem. Examples include process mapping, 5 WHYs, fishbone diagram or RCA, and patient stories (Tools guide, Chapter 38).
- Improvement methodology works best by appealing to hearts over minds. Tap into intrinsic motivations to do a better job and the reasons why clinicians value their work of caring for people.
- Use data and measurement to influence behaviour. Display data in a dynamic and an easy to understand format that clearly shows variation over time. Examples of useful formats are run charts and SPC charts (Tools guide, Chapter 38, and Measurement, Chapter 13).
- No change is too small to be tested with a PDSA cycle. Testing quickly allows for rapid learning, and by testing cumulative small changes and adopting the ones that work the job of complex change can be done in bite-size, manageable, and acceptable chunks, 'owned' by those who test the changes and generate new knowledge.
- It is best to partner with patients to co-produce improvement (Patient-centred safety, Chapter 4). Patients are the only element of the system with a 360-degree view of their own care journey. This insight, alongside a commitment to be accountable to patients as partners in improvement, can be an immensely valuable lever for change.
- You should seek out other improvers and generate momentum for change together. It only takes two to make a movement. Effective improvers tend to be resilient, creative, systems-thinking, and ever-learning, or; influencers who think broadly and borrow good ideas from wherever they can find them—in healthcare and in other fields.

Reference

Vincent, C., Burnett, S., and Carthey, J. The measurement and monitoring of safety. Health Foundation, April 2013. https://www.health.org.uk/publications/the-measurement-and-monitoring-of-safety.

Further reading

Canadian Patient Safety Institute. *A Guide to Patient Safety Improvement: Integrating Knowledge Translation and Quality Improvement Approaches*. Edmonton, Alberta; CPSI 2020. https://www.patientsafetyinstitute.ca/en/toolsResources/A-Guide-to-Patient-Safety-Improvement/Documents/A%20Guide%20to%20Patient%20Safety%20Improvement.pdf.

Holden, R. J. et al. SEIPS 2.0: A human factors framework for studying and improving the work of healthcare professionals and patients. *Ergonomics* 56.11 (2013): 1669–86. https://doi:10.1080/00140139.2013.838643.

Langley, G. L. et al. *The Improvement Guide*. San Francisco, CA: Jossey-Bass, 2009.

Chapter 15

Learning from success to become safer

Key points

- We have more good care than harmful care.
- Learning can be achieved by looking from the 'bright spots' of success just as much as by looking from clinical incidents.
- Learning from excellence can build psychological safety and resilience.
- Techniques such as appreciative inquiry can assist in developing a learning organization.

What is the safety issue?

Considering safety only in terms of failure

The limitations of a failure-based approach to patient safety

Safety is typically considered to be a condition in which as few things as possible go wrong.

In consequence, efforts to improve safety tend to focus on failure (error and harm) rather than on success.

While the failure-based approach to safety may be helpful in identifying and mitigating error and harm, it also has theoretical limitations:

- Failure is rare by comparison with success (Figure 15.1), and therefore presents fewer learning opportunities.
- Processes for the investigation of failure in healthcare (e.g. root cause analysis) often assume linear causality and are not well suited to application in complex socio-technical systems such as healthcare (see Chapter 12).
- Applying learning and system changes in response to rare failures such as 'never events' is difficult and may result in the introduction of new and unexpected risks.
- When the scrutiny of failure is the sole direction of enquiry, this may adversely impact the staff's well-being and contribute to a blame culture in which staff members are fearful of the patient safety process.

An alternative approach is to consider safety as a condition in which as many things as possible go right (Safety 2).

This view draws attention to success as well as to failure.

Theoretical advantages of looking at success as well as failure

- Success is more prevalent than failure, and therefore offers more learning opportunities.
- Considering success alongside failure compels us to examine the *whole spectrum of work* rather than just the rare occurrences where things go wrong.
- Drawing attention to success can create opportunities for positive feedback and for morale uplift among the staff.

Figure 15.1 graphically illustrates the consequence of defining safety in terms of failure. In this hypothetical illustration, the failure rate is 10% (which is consistent with some healthcare safety research). While significant, failure is a much less frequent outcome than success, so its rate is lower. Despite this, the prevailing endeavours to improve safety focus on the domain of failure.

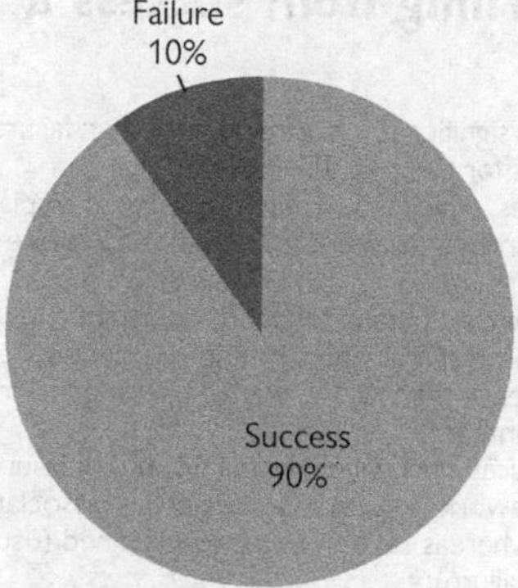

Figure 15.1 The consequence of defining safety in terms of failure.

Why is learning from success a challenge?

Although success is significantly more prevalent than failure, it can be harder to identify. Reasons for this paradox include:

- the negativity bias, which is a human tendency to display higher sensitivity and stronger awareness in relation to failure than in relation to success;
- habituation, which is a human tendency to become less sensitive to events or phenomena that occur frequently: since success is a more frequent occurrence than failure, we have a tendency not to notice it or to take it for granted;
- the fact that failures are defined, classified, and measured as part of a regulatory framework (e.g. fall rate, healthcare associated infection rate, never events), whereas success is not well defined (usually it is seen as the absence of failure);
- the nature of work in healthcare, which is to diagnose and treat illness: this 'find and fix' approach is naturally translated to patient safety and quality improvement.

How can one be safe?

What is known to work?

There is growing interest in a 'strengths-based' enquiry designed to identify success in healthcare. This would be a methodology *complementary* to the prevailing failure-based approach to patient safety.

Several methodologies are available, as indicated in Box 15.1.

Box 15.1 Methods that can be used in order to learn from success

Appreciative inquiry

This is a strengths-based approach to organizational development and is based on a semi-structured interview protocol. An example of interview protocol will follow.

Learning from excellence

This is a strengths-based approach to incident reporting and investigation. Excellence reports are voluntarily filed by staff (and/or by patients and their families); they identify episodes of excellent practice (process or outcome) for the purposes of

- establishing what works well, and therefore can inform system improvements;
- providing positive feedback to staff after excellent practice.

Selected reports are investigated in more depth using the appreciative inquiry approach.

Exnovation

This is a process by which staff members demonstrate and discuss day-to-day practices, uncovering 'hidden competence' within a system for the benefit of shared learning.

Positive deviance

This is the identification of unusually successful behaviours within a community. It generates and tests hypotheses about the cause of success, and this is followed by wider dissemination across the community.

Resilient healthcare and Safety-II methodologies

This is a method of building resilience, as described in Chapter 11.

Practical approach to learning from success

Practical applications of strength-based approaches typically follow the following steps:

1. Identification of an episode of success or excellence. This may be an *outcome* (such as a rapid time-critical patient transfer) or a *process* (such as a positive behaviour or a non-technical action).
2. Enquiry through semi-structured conversations, interviews, or storytelling between frontline staff members.
3. Dissemination of data and learning points to the wider community, where applicable. This may take the form of a bulletin, or some other form of written communication in which the story is re-told along with insights for wider application and adoption.
4. Measurement of impact through changes in a relevant pre-defined metric.

Examples of practical approaches

Learning from success can be employed by following these steps in several settings, as described in Boxes 15.2–15.6.

Box 15.2 By an individual practitioner during daily work

- Identify one episode that went well during routine work (either witnessed or performed by yourself). This can be done in the moment or at the end of a period of work.
- Describe this episode in a reflective document (e.g. in professional development portfolio) or in a conversation with a colleague.
- Include the following points in your reflection:
  a. What happened? Tell the 'story' in detail.
  b. What are the conditions that allowed for success?
  c. How could I (we) replicate or amplify this success?

Box 15.3 Within a team or group

- Regularly identify success and excellence in your own team. This can be done in the moment or at the end of a period of work.
- Provide feedback to colleagues, describing what went well and why it was perceived to be excellent.
- Consider following up with a planned conversation (e.g. an Appreciative Inquiry (AI) interview or discussion) in order to consolidate learning, enhance positive feedback, and generate new improvement ideas.

Box 15.4 Within a quality improvement or safety team project

- Identify a problem in the context of a patient's safety.
- Reframe the problem as an opportunity (see examples of reframing in Table 15.1).
- Develop a project aim that is based on a positively framed opportunity and devise strengths-based QI interventions that are based on the recognition and appreciation of success.
- Implement these strengths-based QI interventions alongside deficit-based interventions, as a complementary approach.

Box 15.5 Debriefing after a real-life or simulated clinical scenario

- Use Appreciative Inquiry (AI), or other positive questioning to understand what went well in the scenario (see AI questions later).
- Build on what worked and what we could do better

Box 15.6 Departmental or organizational level

- Promote a culture of recognition and appreciation of success as a complementary approach to improving patient safety.
- Reframe risks as opportunities.
- Support frontline strengths-based initiatives, such as excellence reporting.

How to use reframing when planning safety and QI projects

Table 15.1. Examples of possible uses of reframing

Failure-based approach Focused on system *weaknesses*		Success-based approach Focused on system strengths	
Problem	Intervention	Opportunity	Intervention
How can we *reduce rates of harm* (HCAI, falls, extravasations, pressure ulcers, etc.)?	Identify and prevent poor adherence to care bundles	How can we *increase rates of harm-free* care episodes?	Identify and reinforce good practice around care bundles
How can we *reduce noise* in our intensive care unit?	Identify and prevent episodes of noisy activity	How can we *increase quiet* in our intensive care unit?	Identify and reinforce episodes of silence and quiet
How can we *decrease rates* of burnout in our staff?	Identify and prevent triggers of psychological morbidity	How can we *increase flourishing and wellbeing* in our staff?	Identify and amplify conditions associated with well-being
How can we *decrease staff attrition* rate?	Identify and mitigate reasons why staff leave	How can we *increase staff retention*?	Identify and amplify, or promote, reasons why staff chose to stay
How can we *reduce medication error rate*?	Identification and prevention of factors associated with medication errors	How can we *increase rates of gold-standard* prescribing and administration of medication?	Identification and promotion of factors that allow prescribing and administration to occur perfectly

Example of Appreciative Inquiry (AI) protocol

The following protocol comprises a series of recommended questions, which can be used to stimulate and provoke strengths-based discussion in a number of settings:

- Tell me what happened, in as much detail as possible.
- What was it about you or the team that allowed this to happen?
- Was there anything that surprised you?
- Does it normally work like this? If not, why not?
- What could have gone worse?
- What didn't go wrong on this occasion?
- What would need to change in order to make this success or excellence occur every time?
- What steps would you (we) need to take to make that happen?
- What resistance or hurdles would we come across if we tried to implement these steps?
- How might we overcome these hurdles?

Summary box

What is the theoretical basis for learning from success?

- The evidence base for various approaches to patient safety (success-based or failure-based) is limited, as most approaches have not been tested in rigorous trials in multiple settings.
- However, supporting evidence for the strengths-based approach can be gathered from other settings.
- Positive feedback, alongside reinforcement, is a more potent learning stimulus than negative feedback.
- Recognition for successful work is associated with increased staff engagement in multiple settings.
- Increased engagement of staff is associated with a number of improved outcomes in healthcare, including overall quality of services and quality of financial performance.

Signpost

Learning from Excellence https://learningfromexcellence.com/

Further reading

Kelly, N., Blake, S., and Plunkett, A. Learning from excellence in healthcare: A new approach to incident reporting. *Archives of Disease in Child* 101 (2016): 788–91.

Smaggus, A. Safety-I, Safety-II and burnout: How complexity science can help clinician wellness. *BMJ Quality & Safety* 28 (2019): 667–71.

Chapter 16

Investigating and learning from adverse events

Key points

- The main purpose of a clinical incident investigation is to learn from the incident and to implement changes so as to make a difference.
- Clinical incidents are in the main a reflection of how a system works.
- A just culture will hold people accountable, though in a fair way and without blame.
- Patients should be involved in the process, with candour and transparency, as the foundation for investigations.
- Learning from the investigation will require constant feedback to clinical teams and across the system.

Introduction

The aim of investigating adverse events is to understand what has happened, why it has happened, and what can be done to reduce the risk of similar events in the future. Investigations also serve to provide an explanation of adverse events for patients and families.

There are various structured methods for investigating adverse events, but root cause analysis (RCA) is the one most widely used in healthcare. This method aims to determine the timeline of events, identify any root causes and contributory factors, and produce recommendations to reduce future risk.

RCA has faced criticism, partly because there is rarely a single root cause for an adverse event and partly because many RCAs focus disproportionately on the actions of individual clinicians and frontline staff. This risks ignoring the many latent and systems factors that are present in almost all adverse events and contribute to them. When done well, RCA does attempt to explore the deep reasons for an adverse event, and some tools (e.g. fishbone diagrams; see Figure 16.1) may help us to understand its contributory factors.

Other safety-critical industries (e.g. aviation, or nuclear power) have moved away from linear analysis models such as RCA to ones that draw on the knowledge of human factors and on safety science. They recognize that, while a small percentage of adverse events may be attributed to egregious or reckless actions of individuals, most are due to failures in the wider system. These industries have become progressively safer partly because their investigations focus on the wider systems in which human error occurs rather than just on the actions of frontline staff.

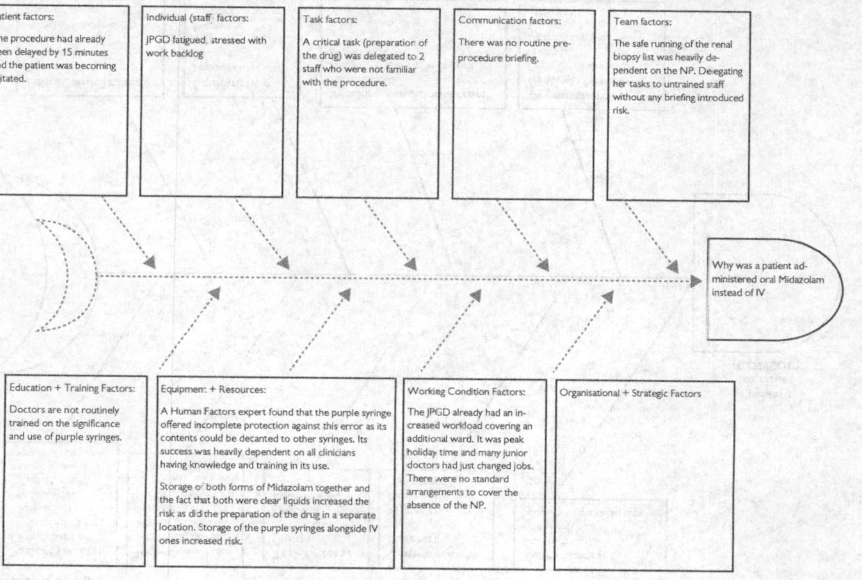
Fishbone Process
Patient factors:
The procedure had already been delayed by 15 minutes and the patient was becoming agitated.
Individual (staff) factors:
JPGD fatigued, stressed with work backlog
Task factors:
A critical task (preparation of the drug) was delegated to 2 staff who were not familiar with the procedure.
Communication factors:
There was no routine pre-procedure briefing.
Team factors:
The safe running of the renal biopsy list was heavily dependent on the NP. Delegating her tasks to untrained staff without any briefing introduced risk.
Why was a patient administered oral Midazolam instead of IV
Education + Training Factors:
Doctors are not routinely trained on the significance and use of purple syringes.
Equipment + Resources:
A Human Factors expert found that the purple syringe offered incomplete protection against this error as its contents could be decanted to other syringes. Its success was heavily dependent on all clinicians having knowledge and training in its use.
Storage of both forms of Midazolam together and the fact that both were clear liquids increased the risk as did the preparation of the drug in a separate location. Storage of the purple syringes alongside IV ones increased risk.
Working Condition Factors:
The JPGD already had an increased workload covering an additional ward. It was peak holiday time and many junior doctors had just changed jobs. There were no standard arrangements to cover the absence of the NP.
Organisational + Strategic Factors

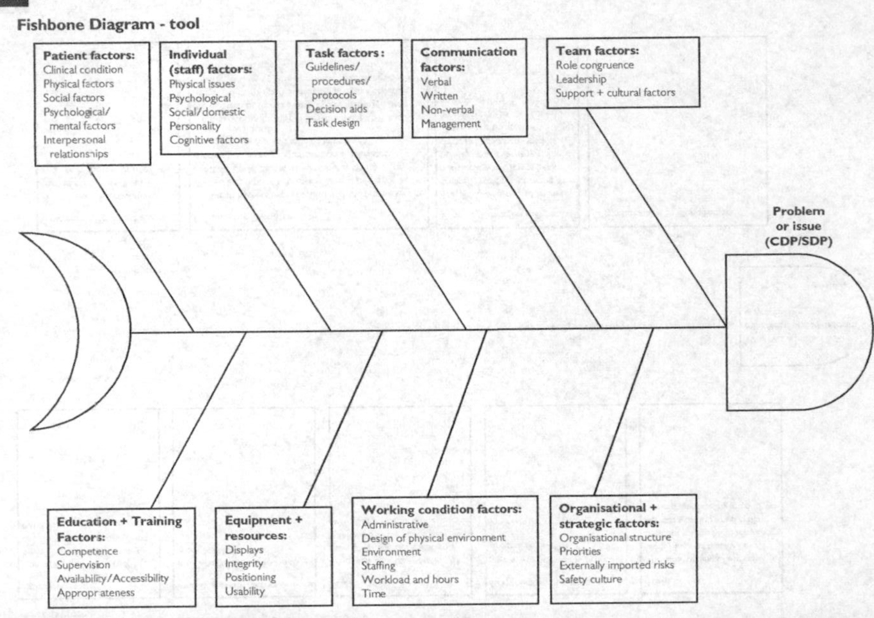

Fishbone Diagram - tool
Patient factors:
Clinical condition
Physical factors
Social factors
Psychological/mental factors
Interpersonal relationships
Individual (staff) factors:
Physical issues
Psychological
Social/domestic
Personality
Cognitive factors
Task factors:
Guidelines/procedures/protocols
Decision aids
Task design
Communication factors:
Verbal
Written
Non-verbal
Management
Team factors:
Role congruence
Leadership
Support + cultural factors
Problem or issue (CDP/SDP)
Education + Training Factors:
Competence
Supervision
Availability/Accessibility
Appropriateness
Equipment + resources:
Displays
Integrity
Positioning
Usability
Working condition factors:
Administrative
Design of physical environment
Environment
Staffing
Workload and hours
Time
Organisational + strategic factors:
Organisational structure
Priorities
Externally imported risks
Safety culture

Figure 16.1 The fishbone diagram

Taxonomy

WHO has commissioned the development of an international taxonomy for patient safety in order to promote greater standardization of terminology and classification. The source for the material presented in this section is WHO 2005.

Adverse event

An adverse event is an injury related to medical management, in contrast to complications of disease (see Reason 1990). Medical management covers all aspects of care, including diagnosis and treatment, failure to diagnose or treat, and the systems and equipment used to deliver care. Adverse events may be preventable or non-preventable.

Incident

An incident is any deviation from usual medical care that causes an injury to the patient or poses a risk of harm. This category includes errors, preventable adverse events, and hazards.

Near-miss

A near miss is a serious error or mishap that has the potential to cause an adverse event but fails to do so through chance, or because it is intercepted.

Error

Error falls into several categories. An error of execution is the failure of a planned action to be completed as intended; an error of planning is the use of a wrong plan to achieve an aim (see Hiatt et al. 1989). Errors may be errors of commission or omission, and usually reflect deficiencies in the systems of care.

Adverse events

International research shows that 10% to 15% of the patients admitted to general hospitals suffer an adverse event, of which around half are thought to be preventable. About 10% of these events cause severe harm or death. Medication errors, problems arising during surgery and procedures, and deficiencies in monitoring and in the processes of care delivery are the most common types.

Primary and community care have been the subject of less research, but existing data suggest that adverse events are common in these settings as well.

Adverse event management

- If an adverse event occurs, a clinician's first actions should be to take whatever immediate steps are necessary to ensure that the patient is safe and that every harm has been dealt with or mitigated.
- The clinician should immediately alert colleagues and superiors and seek help from them if necessary.
- Clear documentation of events and any mitigating action will be helpful for subsequent investigation.
- Any equipment involved in the event (e.g. empty syringes or drug vials) should be collected and retained.
- Debriefing as soon as possible after an adverse event has been shown to be beneficial. It enables risk assessment and management to take place so as to protect other patients from any immediate outstanding risk.
- Clinicians should recognize that they themselves can suffer significant psychological trauma after involvement in an adverse event (the 'second victim' phenomenon). This psychological effect can harm their health and lead to increased risk to patients. If clinicians are concerned about this, they should bring it to the attention of supervisors and colleagues.
- Clinicians have a professional responsibility, and in some jurisdictions a legal one, to offer an apology to patients and their families, with an open and transparent explanation of what happened. This should usually be done by a senior, experienced member of the team.
- An apology does not constitute an admission of legal liability and has been shown to reduce subsequent risk of complaints or litigation.
- Action to reduce the risk of adverse events can be taken only if incidents are reported and investigated. Clinicians involved in adverse events should seek help to report these using whatever local systems exist.

Reporting

- Incident reporting in healthcare has been adapted from an approach used in aviation, where frontline staff are encouraged to report incidents in order to initiate investigations. Sometimes these incidents can be reported anonymously or confidentially.
- Staff members are also encouraged to report near misses and low-harm events, so that serious adverse outcomes may be prevented.
- Reporting of some of the most serious types of events, such as never events, is mandated.
- In aviation, incident reporting is just one component of a much wider safety system, which ensures that there are mechanisms for investigating and improving systems. In many healthcare systems reporting has come to be regarded as an end in itself.
- Healthcare organizations may have local reporting arrangements, and in many countries there are also national bodies for the most serious events (e.g. the England's NHS Learn from patient safety events service. https://www.england.nhs.uk/patient-safety/learn-from-patient-safety-events-service/).
- National systems are useful for understanding events that might be uncommon in individual organizations, or where system-wide action might be needed to remedy the problems.
- Research has shown that incident reporting systems detect only a minority of adverse events. Measuring the number of reported events is therefore largely meaningless, even though this is commonly done in many healthcare systems. Using numbers of reports as a performance measure is counterproductive.
- There are multiple reasons why staff members do not report events. The complexity of the reporting process, the lack of feedback, the absence of obvious changes as a result of reports, and fear of unfair or punitive treatment are the reasons most commonly cited.

Incident reports

Incident reports should include enough information to allow investigators to easily identify both the place of the incident and those involved in it and to retrieve the relevant records. Investigators do not require a comprehensive account or analysis of the event, since this is expected to be done during the investigation.

Useful details to include in incident reports are:

- location, date, and time;
- names of the patient(s) and staff involved;
- a brief account of the event and of the circumstances under which it occurred;
- any equipment involved;
- any information about the local circumstances that may be available to frontline staff but may not be immediately apparent to investigators (e.g. staffing and rosters, patient factors, functioning and availability of IT systems).

The systems approach to safety and the role of contributory factors

While the immediate cause of an adverse event is usually an error or an active failure attributable to a frontline clinician, a systems approach recognizes that the systems in which people work have many inherent weaknesses (latent failures) that create the circumstances in which errors are more likely to occur. Many of these contributory factors arise as a result of decisions made at higher levels of the organization (e.g. staffing, rotas, the procurement of equipment) or externally (e.g. the manufacture of devices). Investigations are unlikely to improve safety unless they capture information on such contributory factors.

There are many approaches to classifying contributory factors the Yorkshire Contributory Factors Framework is one.

Different investigation and analysis models

RCA

The RCA model is adapted from engineering environments and widely used in healthcare. It was originally designed to find causes of equipment and materials failure. It is criticized on the grounds that single 'root causes' are uncommon in patient safety adverse events.

HFACS (Human Factors Analysis and Classification System)

This model, which is based on Jim Reason's Swiss cheese model and adapted from military and aviation investigations, analyses errors on the basis of existing preconditions (either individual or organizational) and supervisory and wider organizational influences.

AcciMap

This is an approach to accident analysis that has been used in a variety of industries. It attempts to illustrate graphically the relationship between the various system factors that contribute to errors in complex sociotechnical systems.

SEIPS (System Engineering Initiative for Patient Safety Human factors, Chapter 9)

This model examines work systems and structures (tasks, technologies, the wider environment, etc.), processes, and outcomes in order to understand the complex factors that contribute to adverse events.

The Yorkshire Contributory Factors Framework

This model has been developed in healthcare from the analysis of reports of adverse events. It classifies contributory factors into situational ones (namely factors related to individual clinicians, the team, the task, and the patient), local working conditions, organizational factors, external influences, and culture or communication.

Just culture

[illegible]

[illegible]

[illegible]

The role of patients and families in investigation

[illegible]

[illegible]

Just culture

Many investigations focus exclusively on the actions of frontline staff and ignore the wider system issues that underlie most adverse events. As a result, a disproportionate number of investigations end up in punitive actions towards individuals (disciplinary process, suspension, re-training, regulatory or even legal action). Not only is this unlikely to reduce similar events in the future, but it fosters a blame culture where the staff are afraid to report incidents, anticipating that its members or others would be unfairly punished.

Calls to replace this kind of environment with a 'no blame' culture are misplaced: professionals have to be accountable for their actions because reckless or egregious behaviour by individuals puts patients at risk, even if this is a factor only in a very small proportion of the totality of adverse events. Sidney Dekker, an international safety expert, has coined the term 'just culture' to describe the ideal approach (see Dekker 2016).

A just culture admits that individuals will make 'honest mistakes' because of multiple systems issues that are beyond their control. If there is deliberately reckless or egregious behaviour on their part, then they should be held accountable for it. Honest mistakes should be investigated in order for us to understand the circumstances in which an individual made a mistake. Human error is a symptom, not a diagnosis.

A just culture approach has been incorporated into investigations in many safety-critical industries, but unfortunately is not yet widely practiced in healthcare.

The role of patients and families in investigation

Patients and families frequently report feeling excluded from the investigation of adverse events. Their reasons include not being fully informed about what has happened, not being asked about their own recollection of events, not being informed about the progress of the investigation, and not being shown the final report. Such lack of transparency compounds the psychological trauma of the event itself, and there is some evidence that it can lead to increased complaints and litigation.

Clinicians have a professional and sometimes a legal obligation to be open with patients and families when things go wrong, but the best approach to involving them in investigations is still unclear. The Healthcare Safety Investigation Branch in the UK is adapting an approach from other sectors whereby the patient and his or her family are routinely interviewed as part of the investigation and their account is used as evidence, alongside the accounts of clinicians and others.

Investigation recommendations

[illegible]

[illegible]

Figure 16.2 Hierarchy of recommendations

[illegible]

What is different about investigations in other industries

[illegible]

[illegible]

Investigation recommendations

Many investigations in healthcare unfortunately continue to produce weak recommendations. A recent Australian study found that only 8% of recommendations from RCAs into serious events had strong recommendations; the recommendations from many RCAs in all healthcare systems focus on (Institute for Safe Medication Practices, 2013) increased vigilance, raised awareness, enforcing policies, or training.

Recommendations are most likely to be effective if they can change the system in which individuals work (see Figure 16.2). The strongest recommendations focus on system change, the weakest on individual behaviour.

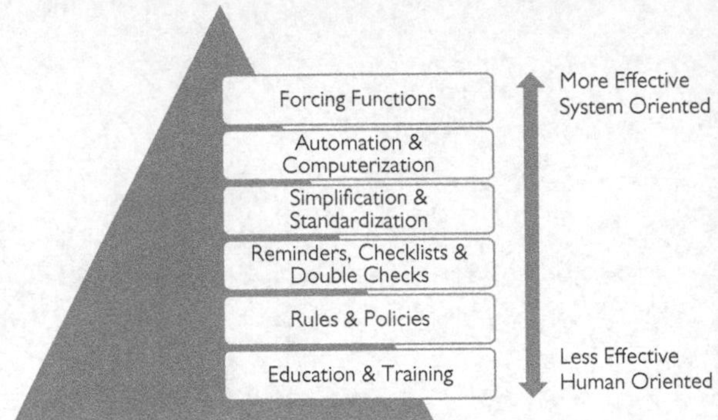

Figure 16.2 Hierarchy of recommendations

A forcing function is one of the strongest. This is a design feature of a piece of equipment or software that makes it impossible, or at least more difficult, to do the wrong thing. For example, some electronic prescribing systems incorporate a forcing function that does not allow drugs that have serious interactions with each other to be prescribed together. Some equipment is designed to prevent dangerous processes (e.g. injection by the wrong route), although this does not always offer complete protection (see the case history in our case study here). Standardization and automation are also strong system-oriented recommendations. The more 'human-oriented' recommendations are, the more likely they are to fail; so, while training has a place among other measures, on its own it is unlikely to improve systems.

What is different about investigations in other industries?

Safety-critical industries, such as aviation and nuclear energy, include rigorous ergonomics, human factors, and systems analysis in their investigations. They do not rely on a single approach such as RCA. Investigations are likely to produce more recommendations that focus on strong, systemic safety improvements and fewer that focus on individuals.

Other industries tend to have dedicated teams of professionally trained investigators who are separate from management process, and these carry out investigations. This distribution is intended to separate the investigation process from the process of determining accountability or blame. Safety investigators are thereby separated from the individuals who determine liability or accountability and may be required to attribute blame. In some circumstances there are legal protections for evidence given to a safety investigation, so that it cannot be used for other purposes.

In some sectors it is common to investigate near misses and low-harm events in order to determine what actions might be taken to prevent the occurrence of a harmful incident. In healthcare, low-harm events are rarely investigated.

Case study

The following case study demonstrates application of the principles of investegation. (Case history adapted and modified from a similar incident investigated by the Healthcare Safety Investigation Branch. www.hsib.org.uk)

The case

A 9-year-old child attended hospital for a renal biopsy. This was to be done on the side room of the day case ward by the consultant, using IV Midazolam as sedation. The consultant was usually assisted in these procedures by a senior postgraduate doctor in training (SPGD) and an experienced nurse practitioner (NP). The NP usually prepared the IV Midazolam in the procedure room. On this occasion the NP was on leave, so a more junior postgraduate doctor in training (JPGD) who was covering the wards was asked to help.

The patient was prepared as normal. The SPGD wrote a prescription for IV Midazolam and sent the JPGD to fetch this from the ward. Being unable to find a nurse to help on that ward, the JPGD went to another ward. The nurse there read the prescription but inadvertently prepared Midazolam liquid for oral use rather than IV. (This was stored alongside the IV preparation.) This was checked by the JPGD against the prescription but neither noticed the discrepancy. The nurse drew the drug up into a purple syringe, marked 'for enteral use' and the JPGD brought it to the side room. The procedure had already been delayed by about 15 minutes and the patient was becoming agitated.

When the SPGD attempted to connect the purple syringe to the IV cannula it wouldn't connect; the syringe has been designed this way to prevent inadvertent IV administration of medication for oral use. However, believing that the preparation was the IV one that had been prescribed and being unfamiliar with the purple syringe, the SPGD decanted the drug from the purple to an IV syringe and administered it. After a few mls had been given he realized that something was wrong and stopped.

The patient suffered no immediate harm but was very distressed and required an overnight stay for observation and a general anaesthetic for the biopsy. The patient's parents were fully informed of events but were so distressed that they refused to have any further treatment at that hospital. While this patient did not suffer lasting harm, the inadvertent administration of an oral medication into a vein can have very serious adverse consequences and can sometimes be fatal. Purple enteral/oral syringes that are incompatible with IV cannulae were designed to eliminate this risk. They are coloured purple to highlight the difference.

The findings

The investigation found that:

1. The inadvertent administration of the oral Midazolam was a 'knowledge-based mistake': the SPGD did what he had intended to do, but he was not aware that the liquid he had been given was the oral preparation because he did not know the significance of the purple syringe.
2. The JPGD was not aware of the significance of the purple syringe either. Neither doctor had received training on its use. All the nurses received such training and they assumed that doctors did as well.
3. The policy for administering medication was not followed. This was a 'necessary violation', since the ward nurse could not leave the ward and the SPGD could not leave the procedure room, so they could not check with each other.
4. The JPGD had no previous experience of the procedure. There was no pre-procedure briefing.
5. Neither the ward nurse nor the JPGD noticed a discrepancy between the prescription and the drug that was prepared. This is a "lapse", usually due to distraction, fatigue, stress etc.
6. The ward nurse had never prepared IV Midazolam before as only the oral preparation was used on her ward. She was not familiar with the process for renal biopsy. She assumed that the JPGD knew the significance of the purple syringe.
7. It was peak holiday time. The JPGD was covering for a colleague who was on leave, as well as for the absent NP. He was fatigued and stressed and had a work backlog.
8. The team was working under time pressures, as the delay led to the patient becoming more agitated.

The analysis

An analysis of this event using the Yorkshire Contributory Factors Framework found the following contributory factors:

1. Team factors. The safe running of the renal biopsy list was heavily dependent on the NP. Delegating her tasks to untrained staff without any briefing introduced risk. There was no routine pre-procedure briefing.
2. Individual staff factors. The JPGD was fatigued and stressed and had a work backlog.
3. Task characteristics. A critical task (preparation of the drug) was delegated to two staff members who were not familiar with the procedure.
4. Workload and staff factors. The JPGD already had an increased workload—had to cover an additional ward. It was peak holiday time and many junior doctors had just changed jobs. There were no standard arrangements to cover the absence of the NP.
5. Training factors. Doctors are not routinely trained on the significance and use of purple syringes.

6. Equipment design, layout, and physical environment. A human factors expert found that the purple syringe offered incomplete protection against this error, as its contents could be decanted to other syringes. Its success was heavily dependent on all clinicians having been trained and knowing how to use it.
7. Storage of both forms of Midazolam together, and the fact that both were clear liquids, increased the risk, as did the preparation of the drug in a separate location. Storage of the purple syringes alongside IV ones increased risk.

Investigation recommendations that would be likely to reduce risk of recurrence

A written standard operating procedure for renal biopsy should include the following points:

1. Arrangements to be made for covering absent colleagues with appropriately trained and available staff.
2. A pre-procedure briefing should be introduced.
3. Storage and preparation of Midazolam to be undertaken in the same location where it is administered.
4. Structured communication techniques that allow junior staff to voice concerns or uncertainty should be implemented.
5. Oral and IV Midazolam and oral and IV syringes should be stored separately and clearly labelled.
6. Standardized training in the purpose and use of purple enteral syringes to be introduced for all health professionals.
7. A review of scheduling of routine procedures should be made, so that, where possible, they are not undertaken when key members of staff are absent or at other high-risk times.
8. A national review of the design of enteral syringes should include redesign intended to make decanting more difficult. Any changes need to be evaluated by human factors experts.

Recommendations that are unlikely to help, or that could be counterproductive

1. Disciplinary processes or other sanctions against the ward nurse or the JPGD and SPGD doctors.
2. Reminders to increase vigilance or pay more attention.
3. Audit of checking or prescribing processes.

References

Dekker S. Just Culture: Restoring Trust and Accountability in Your Organization, Third Edition. London: CRC Press, 2016.

Hiatt, H. et al. A study of medical injury and medical malpractice: An overview. *New England Journal of Medicine* 321.7 (1989): 480–4.

Reason, J. *Human Error*. Cambridge: Cambridge University Press, 1990.

WHO. *World Alliance for Patient Safety: WHO Draft Guidelines for Adverse Event Reporting and Learning Systems*. 2005. WHO, https://apps.who.int/iris/bitstream/handle/10665/69797/WHO-EIP-SPO-QPS-05.3-eng.pdf?sequence=1&isAllowed=y.

Further reading

Conway, J. et al. *Respectful Management of Serious Clinical Adverse Events*, 2nd edn. Cambridge, MA: Institute for Healthcare Improvement, 2011.

HSIB. Lessons from never events in England. 2021. https://www.hsib.org.uk/documents/272/HSIB_Never_Events_-_analysis_of_HSIBs_national_investigations_Report_V09.pdf.

Institute for Safe Medication Practices. Designing effective recommendations. ISMP, 2013. www.ismp-canada.org/download/ocil/ISMPCONCIL2013-4_EffectiveRecommendations.pdf

Janet, E. et al. Using Safety-II and resilient healthcare principles to learn from never events. *International Journal for Quality in Health Care*, 32.3 (2020): 196–203, https://doi.org/10.1093/intqhc/mzaa009.

Kok, J., Leistikow, I., and Bal, R. Patient and family engagement in incident investigations: Exploring hospital manager and incident investigators' experiences and challenges. *Journal of Health Services Research & Policy* 23.4 (2018): 252–61. https://doi.org/10.1177/1355819618788586.

Leistikow, I. et al. Learning from incidents in healthcare: The journey, not the arrival, matters. *BMJ Quality & Safety* 26 (2017): 252–6. https://qualitysafety.bmj.com/content/26/3/252.

McDonald, T. B. et al. Responding to patient safety incidents: The 'seven pillars'. *Quality & Safety in Health Care* 19.6 (2010): e11. https://doi.org/10.1136/qshc.2008.031633.

Parker, J. and Davies, B. No blame no gain? From a no blame culture to a responsibility culture in medicine. *Journal of Applied Philosophy* 37 (2020): 646–60. https://doi.org/10.1111/japp.12433.

Vincent, C. et al. Safety analysis over time: Seven major changes to adverse event investigation. Implementation Science 12.1 (2017 Dec 28). https://doi.org/10.1186/s13012-017-0695-4.

Weaver, S., Stewart, K., Kay ,L. Systems-based investigation of patient safety incidents. *Future Healthc J*. 2021;8(3):e593–e597. doi:10.7861/fhj.2021-0147

Wiig, S., Hibbert, P. D., and Braithwaite, J. The patient died: What about involvement in the investigation process? *International Journal for Quality in Health Care*, 32.5 (2020): 342–6. https://doi.org/10.1093/intqhc/mzaa034

Wiig, S. et al. Next of kin involvement in regulatory investigations of adverse events that caused patient death: A process evaluation. *Journal of Patient Safety* (2019). https://doi.org/10.1097/pts.0000000000000630.

Chapter 17

Open disclosure

Key points

- Open Disclosure is the process of the patient and the family coming to understand what happens.
- The aim is to exercise a duty of candour and to include the patient and the family in the understanding of what has happened.
- The process is to acknowledge the incident, not to speculate about the cause, and to show inclusion and information sharing as the investigation proceeds.
- The key is to listen to the patient and his or her family.
- Support for the clinical staff is essential.

What is open disclosure?

Open disclosure is defined as *the open discussion, with the patient, the family, and the carers, of any adverse events that result in harm to a patient while receiving healthcare.*

The elements of open disclosure are:

- an apology or expression of regret, which should include the words 'I am sorry' or 'we are sorry';
- a factual explanation of what happened;
- an opportunity for the patient, the family, and the carers to relate their discussion of the potential consequences of the adverse event;
- an explanation of the steps taken to manage the adverse event and to prevent its recurrence;
- open disclosure is not a one-way provision of information but a discussion between two parties and an exchange of information that may take place in several meetings over a period of time.

Why is open disclosure important?

- Approximately 1 in 10 patients admitted to hospital will suffer unintended harm, most of which will not be caused by individual error (the clinician's). Therefore the compassionate management of patient disappointment that arises from such harm is a significant component in maintaining an effective clinician–patient relationship.
- Honest and transparent communication from clinicians can facilitate patient and family acceptance and recovery from the emotional and physical consequences of unintended harm.
- Clinicians have ethical and legal responsibilities to respect their patients' autonomy, and this requires patients and their families to be informed about important elements of their treatment, including the impact and consequences of unintended harm arising from their care. In some jurisdictions this is referred to as a 'duty of candour'.
- To act autonomously, a patient requires sufficient information to make decisions about future care that aligns with his or her beliefs and values. Failure to provide information about unintended harm can deny the patient that autonomy.
- The requirement 'first do no harm' extends to the care administered after unintended harm. Honesty and transparency can decrease the risk of additional emotional distress and grief caused by ignorance of the facts or by the loss of trust in those who provide care.
- The patient's insights and feedback as a result of open disclosure conversations can assist in informing the system's response so as to prevent recurrences.
- Planning and preparing for open disclosure acts as a conduit to ensure that the clinician's experience of anxiety or concerns after unintended patient harm can be supported.
- The absence of open and honest conversations after unintended harm can lead to:
    - loss of trust by patients and their families in clinicians, organizations, and the system;
    - additional distress and suffering for the patient;
    - increased risk of the patient's misplaced or ill-directed efforts to seek redress or to hold to account individual clinicians and organizations on the basis of erroneous assumptions that an error has been made;
    - a culture of secrecy and cover-up, which in turn may lead to unwillingness to report critical near misses and system faults. Such underreporting can threaten system learning and increase the risk of recurrence.

How to undertake open disclosure

Important legal considerations

- Expressing regret for a patient's experience is an appropriately empathic response to suffering and is not the same as admitting an error.
- Apologizing for one's own actions (or for those of another) as the cause of the harm can be an admission of liability.
- Many jurisdictions have legal protections for expressions of regret or apologies given *before* a patient commences a legal action against a clinician or a hospital.
- Before apologizing for an action or decision that may have led to unintended harm, it is wise to seek advice from your employer or indemnifier in order (or both), to ensure that your admission is based on fact and not on conjecture or speculation.
- The wording of any expression of regret or apology should be written into the patient record or some other appropriate repository.
- Clinicians are required to disclose unintended harm to a patient when knowledge of the harm is required for subsequent decisions that the patient needs to make about his or her care; when there is a statutory duty in the jurisdiction in which you practice; or when the patient and the family have an expectation that disclosure would occur.

Preparation

- Prepare (and even rehearse) the wording of information and support that will be provided.
- Involve the most senior clinician in the team where possible.
- Ensure privacy and patient comfort.
- Consider accessing formal advice on any legal and regulatory implications.
- Reflect on whether the conversation should be witnessed and by whom (noting the identity of these witnesses in the medical record).

Conducting the conversation

- Welcome the patient's request for a supporting person to be present.
- Express regret or sorrow about the patient's experience.
- Provide as much time as needed to listen attentively and empathetically to the patient's concerns and questions.
- Confine yourself to facts in the information and answers you give to the patient; avoid speculation at all times.
- Where factual answers cannot be provided at the time of the conversation, offer to supply them once the problems have been elucidated.
- Never comment on the quality of the care provided by other clinicians without their permission.
- Avoid arguing with the patient and balance the need to correct any misperceptions with expressions of understanding and concern for the distress he or she is experiencing.
- Use a model such as the open disclosure response (see Box 17.1) in conducting the conversation. This will assist in managing patient expectations.
- Agree on a plan for future care and further information giving—including the results of any investigations into the causation of the unintended harm.

Follow-up after an open disclosure discussion

- Document the discussion and lodge any mandatory reports.
- Follow through on the plan of care agreed with the patient.
- Complete all investigations or inquiries into causation and bring the results to the patient and his or her family.

Box 17.1 The open disclosure response

- Acknowledge the personal impact of the incident.
- Provide an appropriate apology.
- Provide factual information regarding the event.
- Listen to the patient's experience and perspective.
- Answer the patient's questions honestly.
- Inform the patient how 'lessons will be learnt'
- Agree on an appropriate plan for future care.
- Consider the financial impact and respond where possible.
- Ensure continued patient engagement.

Common pitfalls in conducting open disclosure

Box 17.2 Common pitfalls

- doing too much talking and not enough listening;
- arguing with the patient and the family;
- speculating on causation without sufficient evidence;
- failing to agree on a plan for future care that addresses the patient's concerns;
- commenting on the care provided by other clinicians without their knowledge or the full facts;
- allowing different clinicians to give conflicting information that leads to perceptions of a cover-up;
- failing to follow through on an agreed plan, including the provision of further information on causation as it is uncovered;
- failing to check in with the patient on his or her welfare and satisfaction with how things progress.

Caring for the clinicians who undertake open disclosure

- Clinicians who look after a patient can experience significant emotional and psychological distress when unintended harm occurs to that patient.
- Particularly in cases where clinicians believe they may have made an error, common feelings can include:
  - guilt/shame;
  - anxiety/worry;
  - self-doubt;
  - isolation;
  - depression.
- Clinicians may also fear facing litigation, possible sanction, loss of reputation and harsh judgment from their colleagues.
- Recognizing these strong emotions and fears in oneself should prompt one to seek collegial and professional support.

Box 17.3 Common sources of support

- the family doctor;
- a senior, trusted colleague;
- an occupational physician;
- the in-house employee support programme;
- an indemnifier or a trade union;
- a professional college or association;
- a doctor's health advisory service.

Summary box

- Open disclosure assists in the resolution of clinical incidents.
- Open disclosure fulfils the requirement for a duty of candour.
- Open disclosure requires a careful process and clinicians need training in how to implement it.
- Support is required for clinicians involved in an incident, and this will facilitate open disclosure.
- Open disclosure reflects the culture of safety of an organization.

Further reading

Australian Commission on Safety and Quality in Health Care, *Australian Open Disclosure Framework*. ACSQHC, Sydney. 2013. https://www.safetyandquality.gov.au/our-work/open-disclosure/the-open-disclosure-framework.

Bismark, M. et al. Accountability sought by patients following adverse events from medical care: The New Zealand experience. *Canadian Medical Association Journal* 175.8 (2006): 889–94. https://doi.org/10.1503/cmaj.060429.

de Vries, E. N. et al. The incidence and nature of in-hospital adverse events: A systematic review. *Quality and Safety in Health Care* 17.3 (2008): 216–23. https://doi.org/10.1136/qshc.2007.023622.

Friele, R. D and Sluijs, E. M. Patient expectations of fair complaint handling in hospitals: Empirical data. *BMC Health Services Research* 6.106 (2006). https://doi.org/10.1186/1472-6963-6-106.

Gallagher, T. H. et al. W. Patients' and physicians' attitudes regarding the disclosure of medical errors. *JAMA* 289.8 (2003): 1001–7. https://doi.org/10.1001/jama.289.8.1001.

Gallagher, T. H. et al. US and Canadian physicians' attitudes and experiences regarding disclosing errors to patients. *Archives of Internal Medicine* 166.15 (2006)

Helmchen, L. A., Richards, M. R., and McDonald, T. B. How does routine disclosure of medical error affect patients' propensity to sue and their assessment of provider quality? Evidence from survey data. *Medical Care* 48.11 (2010): 955–61. https://doi.org/10.1097/mlr.0b013e3181eaf84d.

Institute for Healthcare Improvement. *Shining a Light: Safer Health Care through Transparency*. Boston, MA: National Patient Safety Foundation, 2005. http://www.ihi.org/resources/Pages/Publications/Shining-a-Light-Safer-Health-Care-Through-Transparency.aspx.

Openness and honesty when things go wrong: The professional duty of candour, 2015. Joint NMC and GMC guidance. https://www.nmc.org.uk/globalassets/sitedocuments/nmc-publications/openness-and-honesty-professional-duty-of-candour.pdf.

Sirriyeh, R. et al. Coping with medical error: a systematic review of papers to assess the effects of involvement in medical errors on healthcare professionals' psychological well-being. *Quality and Safety in Health Care* 19.6 (2010): e43. https://doi.org/10.1136/qshc.2009.035253.

Smith, K. M. et al. Lessons learned from implementing a principled approach to resolution following patient harm. *Journal of Patient Safety and Risk Management* 24.2 (2019):83–9. https://doi.org/10.1177%2F2516043518813814.

Chapter 18

Caring for the caregivers: The second victim

Key points

- A clinical incident has an impact on the patient and family who are the first victims.
- The clinician or clinical team involved the incident can suffer psychological harm because of the incident and are termed the second victim
- Early intervention to support the clinicians involved in a clinical incident decreases the impact on their wellbeing and their clinical performance.
- A safety system will address the needs of the first victim through open disclosure, a transparent investigation process and support for the clinicians involved.

Background

Medical error is a major public health challenge. One in ten of hospitalized patients are involved in a patient safety incident (PSI) of which nearly 50% are preventable. A PSI is defined by the WHO as 'any deviation from usual medical care that either causes an injury to the patient or poses a risk of harm, including errors, preventable adverse events and hazards" (WHO, 2020, p14).

Unfortunately, there may be more than one victim after a PSI (Chapter 4). The first victim is the patient. Alongside the patient, it is his or her family and social network that are the most important victims. However, the healthcare professionals involved (second victims) and the healthcare organization and their management (third victims) can also suffer in the aftermath of a PSI (Figure 18.1). In this chapter, the focus will be on the second victims.

What is a second victim?

The fact that healthcare professionals can also suffer in the aftermath of a PSI has been described over the last two decades. Scott et al. (2009, p326) defines a second victims as 'healthcare providers who are involved in an unanticipated adverse patient event, in a medical error and/or a patient related injury and become victimized in the sense that the provider is traumatized by the event. Frequently, these individuals feel personally responsible for the patient outcome. Many feel as though they have failed the patient, second guessing their clinical skills and knowledge base.'

Recently there has been some criticism of the term 'second victim' and patient communities have questioned why the concept of second victim has become embedded in patient safety. Some patient communities have suggested abandoning this term. As an alternative name has yet to be determined, we will still use 'second victim' in this chapter.

Almost 85% of healthcare professionals report being emotionally affected in the aftermath of a PSI, at least once in their career.

How does a second victim feel?

How does a second victim feel?

After a PSI, second victims develop symptoms that affect both their personal well-being and their professional functioning.

Box 18.1 Possible symptoms of a second victim (see also Figure 18.2)

- hypervigilance
- stress
- anxiety
- shame
- flashbacks
- fear
- guilt
- frustration
- anger
- feeling inadequate
- risk avoidance
- insomnia
- unhappy and dejected
- self- doubt about knowledge and skills,
- difficulty concentrating

The symptoms may have a serious impact on individual and team performance, with consequences for the safe provision of quality of care. Second victims may feel uncomfortable within the team and may report significantly higher work-home interference. Second victims are at a greater risk of burnout with higher levels of intention to leave their job.

The prevalence ratio of these symptoms increases the higher the degree of patient harm reported, namely running from no harm to temporary harm, permanent harm and death. The reaction of the healthcare professional also depends on the degree of personal responsibility assumed for the PSI. In Figure 18.2, the duration of the top six symptoms and the level of harm is visualized.

Finally, it is important to know the duration of these symptoms after a PSI, as second victims are at risk for post-traumatic stress disorder (PTSD). If these symptoms persist for more than one month, the phenomenon may be indicative of a stressor-related disorder (e.g. PTSD, according to the criteria in DSM 5).

Understanding the symptoms and their duration can help organizations decide how to support second victims in a caring, compassionate, and effective way.

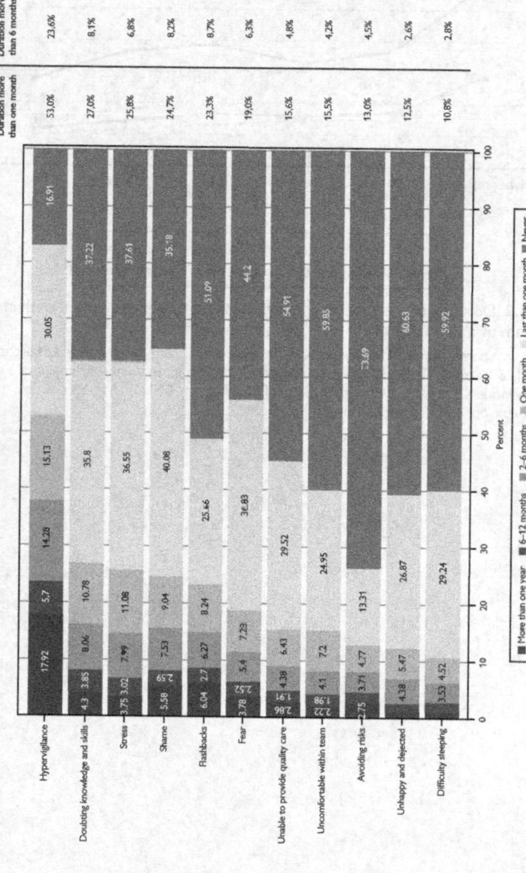

Figure 18.1 Overview of the reported symptoms.
Reproduced with permission from Vanhaecht et al. 2019

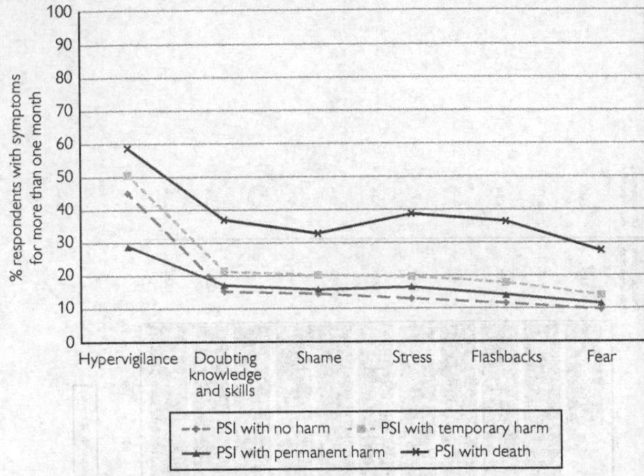

Figure 18.2 Duration of the top six symptoms that last longer than one month in the aftermath of a PSI.

Reproduced with permission from Vanhaecht, K. S., D., Schouten, L., Bruyneel, L., Coeckelberghs, E., Panella, M., & Zeeman, G. (2019). Duration of second victim symptoms in the aftermath of a patient safety incident and association with the level of patient harm. BMJ Open http://dx.doi.org/10.1136/bmjopen-2019-029923

Long-term impact

It has been shown that not responding to a PSI in a timely and effective manner can have a significant impact on the second victims and healthcare organizations. This impact can take the form of absence of healing, loss of trust, lack of learning, or lack of improvement. It may also increase the likelihood of legal action and patient complaints.

The impact on doctors or nurses in training can be immense, as it can increase the risk of a future PSI. Young clinicians who perceive that they have made patient errors in the past demonstrate less empathy. They are then at risk for subsequent errors. Those with associated depression are twice as likely to make an additional error in the future.

What can be done by the clinical team and the organization to support a second victim?

[illegible]

[illegible]

Preventive action

[illegible]

[illegible]

[illegible]

Support for the second victim

[illegible]

[illegible]

[illegible]

What can be done by the clinical team and the organization to support a second victim?

The support given in the aftermath of a PSI is crucial, not only for the second victim but also for the individual who provided the support. This is required not only in the aftermath of a PSI but also for healthcare professionals who are involved in a complaint or in a lawsuit, as the emotional impact is more severe in such cases.

Hospitals have started to accept that they have a role in providing an institutional support system to meet the needs of second victims. However, there is a gap between the needs of second victims and the level of support offered by their organization. In addition, individuals within the organization can play a role in supporting second victims.

Preventive action

In general, organizations should aim for a positive patient safety culture and psychological safety, as this is associated with lower psychological impact and faster recovery for the healthcare professionals involved in an adverse event.

The patient safety culture should reflect a non-punitive attitude to errors. This may encourage supportive actions and openness to discuss error and to mitigate the negative effects of a PSI. The perception of managerial support and the provision of information about the rights of a second victim are positively associated with well-being and can reduce defensive practices in healthcare professionals who are involved in complaint investigations.

A key preventive intervention is to educate and train healthcare professionals about the second victim phenomenon as part of their professional and post graduate training. Work based learning includes both immediate support in the aftermath of a PSI and monthly team meetings dedicated to sharing best practices.

Support for the second victim

The well-being of the healthcare professional is directly correlated to patient outcomes. A support program is most effective if it is part of the response process to PSIs. To ensure the success of the support system, support should always be available 24/7.

Team meetings can provide emotional support to second victims. This can be done either in support groups, where the PSI is discussed by those involved in the incident, or at morbidity and mortality meetings.

A more comprehensive supportive approach is shown in Box 18.2.

An adapted version of Scott's three-tiered emotional support system was developed by the University of Leuven (Figure 18.3), with the addition of emotional and cognitive support to each tier.

Box 18.2 Scott's three-tiered emotional support system

1. Make sure that the second victim is okay and is provided immediate emotional first aid. This support is sufficient for 60% of the participants.
2. Make sure that support is given to the second victim by peers trained in the second-victim phenomenon. This will meet the needs of a further 30% of participants.
3. Secure referral to professional counselling. This is required for 10% of participants.

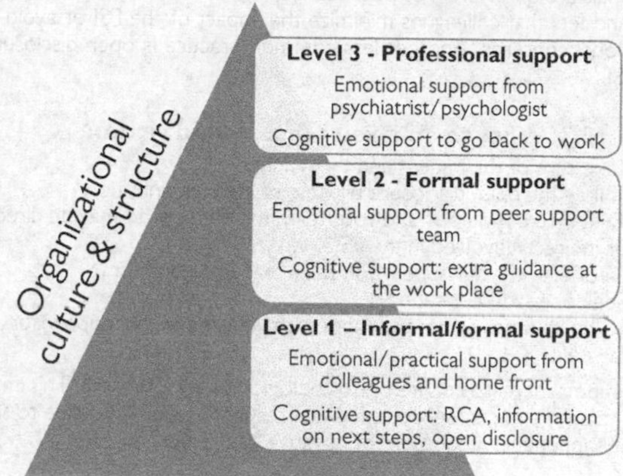

Figure 18.3 Adapted version of Scott's three-tiered emotional support system

Adapted with permission from Van Gerven E, Bruyneel L, Panella M, Euwema M, Sermeus W, Vanhaecht K. Psychological impact and recovery after involvement in a patient safety incident: a repeated measures analysis. BMJ Open. 2016;6(8):e011403. https://doi.org/10.1136/bmjopen-2016-011403

How can you support each other?

Individual support can be perceived positively or negatively by the healthcare professional involved in the aftermath of a PSI and can also reduce the likelihood of being involved in a future PSI. Colleagues can be supportive by discussing what went wrong. For this reason, a trusting relationship is important. When healthcare professionals accept criticism, they also perceive more support.

Family members and friends are less able to provide the needed support. Supervisors can support second victims by emphasizing their continued trust in them. However, this is not common practice, as healthcare professionals are often afraid of potential damage to their professional reputation and feel that colleagues minimize the impact of the PSI or avoid their emotional concerns. Another less common practice is open disclosure of the PSI.

Box 18.3 What to do if you are a second victim?

1. Take care of the patient and the family.
2. Follow the open disclosure process of your organization.
3. Take care of yourself and your team members, who may be directly or indirecty involved in the PSI.
4. Debrief with your supervisor, team leader, or mentor.
5. Seek peer-to-peer support.
6. If you have any symptoms, approach your mentor or supervisor for help.

It is important that a culture of psychological safety is present. This implies that team members feel accepted and respected. They feel safe to share what happened, without fear of negative consequences.

Summary box

Key points

- Organizations should be prepared and know how to support a second victim.
- Each second victim requires an individual approach, which should be based on their needs and on symptoms and their duration.
- Teams should be able to support their members.
- Support on how to cope with the symptoms in the aftermath of a PSI, complaint, or lawsuit is essential, as these can profoundly affect an individual's personal well-being, professional performance, and teamwork.
- Early intervention is required to minimize long-term sequelae, as the duration of the symptoms after a PSI is underappreciated.

References

WHO. Patient safety incident reporting and learning systems: technical report and guidance. Geneva: World Health Organization; 2020. Licence: CC BY-NC-SA 3.0 IGO. https://www.who.int/publications/i/item/9789240010338

Scott, S. D. et al. The natural history of recovery for the healthcare provider 'second victim' after adverse patient events. *Quality & Safety in Health Care* 18.5 (2009): 325–30. https://doi.org/10.1136/qshc.2009.032870.

Van Gerven, E. et al. Psychological impact and recovery after involvement in a patient safety incident: A repeated measures analysis. *BMJ Open* 6.8 (2016): e011403. https://doi.org/10.1136/bmjopen-2016-011403.

Vanhaecht, K. S. et al. Duration of second victim symptoms in the aftermath of a patient safety incident and association with the level of patient harm. *BMJ Open* 9.7 (2019). http://dx.doi.org/10.1136/bmjopen-2019-029923.

Further reading

Conway, J., Federico, F., Stewart, K., & Campbell, M. (2011). Respectful management of serious clinical adverse events. IHI Innovation Series white paper. *Cambridge, Massachusetts: Institute for Healthcare Improvement*, (Available on www.IHI.org).

Mira JJ, Lorenzo S, Carrillo I, et al. Lessons learned for reducing the negative impact of adverse events on patients, health professionals and healthcare organizations. Int J Qual Health Care. 2017 Aug 1;29(4):450–460. https://doi.org/10.1093/intqhc/mzx056

Panella, M. et al. The determinants of defensive medicine in Italian hospitals: The impact of being a second victim. *Revista de Calidad Asistencial* 31 Suppl 2 (2016). https://doi.org/10.1016/j.cali.2016.04.010.

Seys, D. et al. Supporting involved health care professionals (second victims) following an adverse health event: A literature review. *International Journal of Nursing Studies* 50.5 (2013): 678–87. https://doi.org/10.1016/j.ijnurstu.2012.07.006.

Seys, D. et al. Health care professionals as second victims after adverse events: A systematic review. *Evaluation & the Health Professions* 36.2 (2013): 135–62. https://doi.org/10.1177/0163278712458918

Van Gerven, E., et al. Increased risk of burnout for physicians and nurses involved in a patient safety incident. *Medical Care* 54.10 (2016): 937–43. https://doi.org/10.1097/mlr.0000000000000582.

Wu, A. W. Medical error: The second victim. *Western Journal of Medicine* 172.6 (2000): 358–9. https://doi.org/10.1136/ewjm.172.6.358.

Zeeman, G. et al. Prolonged mental health sequelae among doctors and nurses involved in patient safety incidents with formal complaints and lawsuits. *European Journal of Public Health* 30.4 (2020): 777–9. https://doi.org/10.1093/eurpub/ckz138.

Part 3

Translating theory into clinical practice

Chapter 19

Patient safety and information technology

Key points

- Safety is dependent on the provision of reliable services.
- Digital solutions can assist in the achievement of safer processes.
- Electronic health records and computerized provider order entry systems both allow for the standardization of processes by using human factors and reliability theories to achieve safety.
- The digitalization of processes needs to be implemented within a learning environment and a culture of safety.
- New opportunities in diagnostics, monitoring, and telehealth can facilitate safer care.

Providing the context

When caring for patients in the healthcare setting, new clinicians will use their best judgement and reasoning on the basis of their education, experience, pathways, and collaborations with other team members. Recent advances in technology and information services have added tools and stressors to clinicians that will both challenge and support them in the work they do to ensure the best quality, safety, and outcomes for their patients.

Furthermore, the evolution of innovative approaches and technologies designed to address day-to-day healthcare challenges creates opportunities to achieve better patient safety and quality outcomes. This chapter will provide an overview of the current state of affairs in this field and some considerations related to it.

Electronic documentation and ordering

Documentation of clinical activities has been a long-standing and important part of healthcare activities, whether for payment purposes or for the linear tracking of a patient's health. In recent years, technology has created additional mechanisms designed to increase efficiency, to improve the sharing of data across multiple providers and sites of care, and ideally to enhance quality and safety within the clinical settings. Similarly, technology can be more efficiently used to order more tests, medication, follow-up care, and other important patient-related activities that will enhance overall clinical outcomes.

Electronic health records (EHR)

The Healthcare Information and Management Systems Society (HIMSS) has defined the electronic health record (EHR) as 'a longitudinal electronic record of patient health information generated by one or more encounters in any care delivery setting. Included in this information are patient demographics, progress notes, problems, medications, vital signs, past medical history, immunizations, laboratory data and radiology reports. The EHR automates and streamlines the clinician's workflow. The EHR has the ability to generate a complete record of a clinical patient encounter—as well as supporting other care-related activities directly or indirectly via interface—including evidence-based decision support, quality management and outcomes reporting' (Atherton, 2011, 186).

Not all countries or clinical settings are fully integrated into an EHR, and there is often a mix of paper-based and electronic medical records used in clinics, hospitals, or health systems. This is not ideal, as mixed environments create opportunities for error owing to cross-referencing multiple platforms, illegibility challenges, misinterpretation, lack of visibility into a common view of historical and current activities, and supplementary time needed to ensure that providers are able to have a complete picture of the care they are offering. Moving to a common platform is an important priority for those responsible for creating the best clinical environment for clinical practitioners and their patients.

Effectiveness of electronic records

The adoption of EHRs in the clinical setting has been steady over the past few decades; however, perceptions about its effectiveness for productivity and quality outcomes have been mixed. A 2018 survey of primary-care physicians (PCPs) in the United States by Stanford Medicine and the Harris Poll found increased satisfaction among physicians about their use of EHR (66%), with recognition that the EHR has led to improved patient care in general (63%). A frequent complaint among practitioners who use EHRs or similar technology is that it takes away from the personal attention they are able to offer the patient, as they are now looking at a screen instead of engaging directly with their patient.

Patients, similarly, have described this process as frustrating, necessitating a focus by practitioners to mitigate this perception as much as possible when they provide and document the care. The Stanford/Harris study (Stanford Medicine 2018) found that increasing amounts of time are spent with the EHR at the expense of the patient, 69% of participants agreeing that the use of the EHR takes 'valuable time away from the patient'. Additionally, while physicians are generally pleased with the ability to keep patient information all in one place in order to help improve care (for ease of access, increased ability to provide medical records to patients, increased ability to share information with other providers across the care continuum), the study found that half of respondents agree that 'using an EHR detracts from their clinical effectiveness'. Further, the EHR has not yet met their satisfaction of 'facilitating better patient–provider interaction' (50% satisfied), 'co-ordinating care for patients with complex conditions' (56%), or 'identifying high-risk patients' (52%).

Computerized provider order entry (CPOE)

Computerized provider order entry (CPOE) has been a companion technology to the EHR, with increasing implementation and presence across care environments. Intending to make care safer and more efficient, this technology allows for practitioners to enter and send orders for medications, studies, tests, and so on via computer. Often the CPOE will be used in combination with e-prescribing systems that can detail the patient's current and past medications, allergies, and so on. A prime reason behind the adoption of CPOE is to ensure better patient safety outcomes by addressing the problem of illegible ordering or by correcting the errors that may occur in the transcription of orders written by providers. Its usage has also been linked to increased efficiency and processes that result in reduced length of stay.

Other important aspects of CPOE include:

- the provision of feedback to the provider about possible conflicts with orders,
- facilitating behind-the-scenes compliance checks with regulatory guidelines,
- reporting on effectiveness of the system to the management, to enable improvements to increase efficiencies and flows,
- connecting with mobile devices to ensure seamless and integrated use by providers.

Often the CPOE is integrated in the EHR, which makes the combination a powerful tool for providers.

Initially the adoption of CPOE was challenging: many physicians embraced this new tool, but most resisted it in the early phase. A broader adoption occurred once EHRs established a stronger presence and support in clinical settings. A common goal of health systems or hospitals is to ensure that up to 90% of orders are entered via CPOE. This is an implicit admission that a 100% adoption rate is difficult in view of the nature of some of the orders: some of them (e.g. cancer-related medication) are too complex to be entered via this method.

Challenges to the introduction of digital solutions

The transition to a digital interface is challenged by a host of unintended problems that are difficult to solve. Here are some examples:

- complex flow of navigating the electronic screens and systems within platforms;
- requirement to enter passwords multiple times for privacy protection;
- the frequent inability to customize the process of entering information;
- alert fatigue;
- disconnect between the clinical workflow and the electronic system workflow: this state may cause further errors, wasted time, or distractions.

Interoperability

A major factor that will impact the success of these systems is interoperability, which continues to be a challenge across platforms, vendors, health systems and other settings. As defined by HIMSS interoperability is ' the ability of different information systems, devices and applications (systems) to access, exchange, integrate and cooperatively use data in a coordinated manner, within and across organizational, regional and national boundaries, to provide timely and seamless portability of information and optimize the health of individuals and populations globally.' (HIMSS, 2021, https://www.himss.org/resources/interoperability-healthcare). As more systems, devices, and access points for information are developed, the ability to address interoperability will become increasingly important for ensuring the best patient safety possible. The advent of digital healthcare in the COVID pandemic has already started this process.

New technologies and innovation to improve outcomes and patient safety

Technology in healthcare settings is evolving at a fast pace, beyond just 'at the elbow' tools like the EHR and CPOE. Newly developed technologies have created unimagined opportunities to impact patient outcomes, including increased patient safety, improved clinical outcomes, better adherence, equity of care, and broader access to care. As health systems were unable to successfully address all the existing challenges in the delivery of care, they have often looked outside traditional environments for innovative solutions, which have accelerated the application of these new technologies and the impact they will have on patient care.

However, it is important to recognize that the sources of this innovativeness can be clinicians at the bedside, venture-funded startups external to the health system, and many other individuals, companies, and partnerships. The importance of health systems embracing these new innovations is equalled by the importance that physicians and other clinical providers place on working with these solutions in order to inform their development, test their impact on patient safety, and ensure they are truly able to make a difference to the delivery of care.

There is a spectrum of new innovations and technologies that will be helpful to patient care in the future. For example a focus on 'citizen health', artificial intelligence, virtual reality, blockchain, patient-controlled testing, cognitive computing, wearables, ingestibles, absorbables, sensor activations, and patient-created devices.

There are thousands of examples globally that illustrate both the importance of trying new solutions and the significant effect they can have on patient safety and quality in healthcare settings.

These brief examples, picked out of thousands, demonstrate the power of the possibilities that innovation and new technologies can create when addressing conditions within healthcare.

A final note: these technologies, once created and used, will add to the demands of the healthcare provider and other clinicians, as will the need to address genetic, microbiomic, and other -omic data in the care of patients in the future. More data will create a more informed view of patients, but will also lead to other challenges, such as those related to interpreting and interfacing with all these data in meaningful ways for clinicians to be successful in application, diagnosis, and treatment.

Box 19.1 Examples of the possible impact of new technology

Machine learning has created the ability for computers to read faster and more accurately through hundreds or thousands of studies or tests (e.g. imaging studies) and to diagnose issues appropriately. The nature of this technology allows for the computer to learn continuously and to get more accurate each time.

Virtual reality has been used to help surgeons to find new approaches to hard-to-visualize areas in complex organs and systems (e.g. the intricacies of the heart) provided by traditional imaging. Additionally, it has been used in creative ways to assist patients in coping with various conditions. For example it can create a 'snow world' that helps burn patients cope with their injuries.

Biomonitoring tracking 'tattoos' have been created to allow for the monitoring of vital signs and other data. These are bioelectronic stickers that interface with the human epidermis and collect electrophysiological data.

A sensor activation reminder system for caregivers to wash their hands is a proven way to prevent hospital-acquired infections (HAI). This technology uses a sensor on clinicians who care for patients and a wall-mounted base that emits an audible reminder message for caregivers when they pass by it. This technology has demonstrated improved outcomes in the initial hospitals where it has been deployed, including reducing HAIs by 66% and saving nearly $10M per year in direct costs.

Solutions designed to address the diabetic condition

- A contact lens was being developed to monitor blood sugar levels via patient's tears. It aimed to the patient through a red light when levels are too high or too low.
- The tracking of glucose levels via mobile apps and smart watches has enabled patients with diabetes to detect and address more effectively changes in these levels, also allowing parents of young children with diabetes to monitor them from a distance.
- A patient has spearheaded a movement to create a do-it-yourself technology that will allow for a better monitoring and treatment of diabetes through an artificial pancreas.

COVID-19 and the rise of telehealth

External factors can sometimes force healthcare providers to adopt new technologies in an effort to become more agile. During 2020, the global pandemic ushered in an increased use of telehealth to connect patients and physicians for care.

While around for decades, telehealth had not been widely adopted or used consistently as a tool until COVID-19 forced new ways of interacting with patients on the basis of 'stay-at-home' orders, lockdowns, and social distancing. By mid-2020, US providers had rapidly scaled their telehealth offerings and via this technology increased the number of patients seen per unit time than seen previously with in person consultation. Similar adoption rates have been experienced globally.

In the future, telehealth will probably be used much more than it was in the past; however, there will be greater variability in the frequency of its use. Society has realized the benefits of this technology and consumers may now prefer this option for care.

Additionally, telehealth has proven to be of great benefit in addressing challenges systems have faced for years (healthcare equity, access, etc.). As healthcare providers identify the best ways to engage with patients in delivering care, telehealth will probably be an ongoing option; with appropriate patients and settings and for specific conditions, it can add immense value. Telehealth will have to be thoughtfully balanced with both traditional and future means of providing care to patients. Additionally, more focus on new technology and digitization has led some organizations to create Chief Digital Officer positions which have been instrumental in shaping this space.

Technology partners for change in health systems

Within the clinical setting and within healthcare environments, there are several key individuals who will partner with providers in order to enhance their ability to be effective with the technologies described in this chapter. The chief information officer (CIO) will work closely with caregivers, providers, and employees across the healthcare setting to ensure that both the hardware (computers) and the systems (e.g. the EHR and CPOE) function optimally and support clinical activities.

Many organizations are now hiring chief medical informatics officers (CMIOs), whose primary responsibility is to bridge the information services and provider worlds. The critical nature of these physician roles cannot be understated: CMIOs have often been both key champions for physicians, as they adopted new technology in effective ways, and representatives of the administration and of the CIO in implementing new systems (such as the EHR and CPOE). The CMIO will often have a direct link to and partnership with the chief quality officer, as they both ensure that quality outcomes are achieved.

Finally, chief innovation officers (CIxO) have become more prevalent in health systems, as they begin to recognize the critical need to drive change through approaches that have not been tried in the past. Their partnership with the providers, who often serve as champions for innovative technology trials and for proof of concept, implementation, and scaling, is another means by which patient safety can be secured, namely through the introduction of new technologies such as the ones exemplified in this chapter. It is important to establish strong, collaborative relationships that will help to leverage technology in the right way and to deliver exceptional patient care.

Summary box

The use of the new ways of documenting and communicating medical information, both in real time and retrospectively, has increased healthcare practitioners' ability to improve the quality of outcomes and to ensure the best patient safety in our health systems globally.

Supporting hospitals, health systems, and practitioners in their work of implementing and using new technology, many countries and organizations have established guidelines and support mechanisms.

The SAFER Guides, established by the US government (www.HealthIT.gov), constitute such an example. This is a corpus of nine guides that aim to guarantee base practices for the safe use of health information technology, specifically the electronic health record. They offer self-assessment tools designed to identify possible risks and the ways to mitigate them. Another example is the work carried out by the World Health Organization (WHO) in providing structure, recommendations, and guidelines for digital interventions, eHealth, and innovations—all towards rendering these new technologies and their governance helpful in the delivery of safe healthcare for all.

There is no doubt that the use of technology in healthcare will help to create a safer experience for patients and communities, while improving quality and reducing the rate of medical error.

Even with all these additional efforts to support providers and practitioners in their day-to-day work, one will always have to be vigilant and make efforts both to minimize the unintended consequences of this technology and to realize its true benefit for all patients.

The movement from paper to electronic documentation and ordering has led to the following positive outcomes (among others):

- decreased medication errors;
- improved adherence to applicable care pathways and guidelines;
- aligned and coordinated care across care providers;
- renewed focus on improving patient safety;
- improved satisfaction for physicians, nurses, and other clinical professionals.

Signpost

The following websites have good information on information technology.
Digital Health Australia https://www.digitalhealth.gov.au/
Digital Health Canada https://digitalhealthcanada.com/
E-Health Ireland https://www.ehealthireland.ie/
NHS Digital https://digital.nhs.uk/
US Government https://www.healthit.gov
World Health Organisation https://www.who.int/ehealth/en

References

Artherton J. Development of the Electronic Health Record *Virtual Mentor*. 13(3) (2011): 186–189. doi:10.1001/virtualmentor.2011.13.3.mhst1-1103.

Healthcare Information and Management Systems Society (HIMSS). What is Interoperability? https://www.himss.org/resources/interoperability-healthcare

Stanford Medicine. White paper: The future of electronic health records. 2018. www.med.stanford.edu/content/dam/sm/ehr/documents/SM-EHR-White-Papers_v12.pdf.

Further reading

Bestsennyy, O. et al. Telehealth: A quarter-trillion dollar post-COVID-19 reality? McKinsey. 29 May 2020. https://www.mckinsey.com/industries/healthcare-systems-and-services/our-insights/telehealth-a-quarter-trillion-dollar-post-covid-19-reality

Cresswell, Kathrin, Bates, David, and Sheikh, Aziz. Ten key considerations for the successful optimization of large-scale health information technology. *Journal of the American Medical Informatics Association* 24.1 (2017): 181–7. https://doi.org/10.1093/jamia/ocw037.

Neves, A. L. et al. Impact of providing patients access to electronic health records on quality and safety of care: A systematic review and meta-analysis. *BMJ Quality & Safety* 29 (2020): 1019–32. http://dx.doi.org/10.1136/bmjqs-2019-010581.

Niazkhani, Z. et al. Barriers to patient, provider, and caregiver adoption and use of electronic personal health records in chronic care: A systematic review. *BMC Med Informatics & Decision Making* 20.1 (2020), article 153. https://doi.org/10.1186/s12911-020-01159-1.

Page, N., Baysari, M. T., and Westbrook, J. I. A systematic review of the effectiveness of interruptive medication prescribing alerts in hospital CPOE systems to change prescriber behaviour and improve patient safety. *International Journal of Medical Informatics* 105 (2017): 22–30. https://doi.org/10.1016/j.ijmedinf.2017.05.011.

Rumball-Smith, J., Ross, K., and Bates, D. W. Late adopters of the electronic health record should move now. *BMJ Quality & Safety* 29 (2020): 238–40. http://dx.doi.org/10.1136/bmjqs-2019-010002.

Sarkar, U. and Lyles, C. Devil in the details: Understanding the effects of providing electronic health record access to patients and families. *BMJ Quality & Safety* 29 (2020): 965–7. http://dx.doi.org/10.1136/bmjqs-2020-011185.

References

[illegible]

[illegible]

[illegible]

Further reading

[illegible]

[illegible]

[illegible]

[illegible]

[illegible]

[illegible]

[illegible]

Chapter 20

Enabling medication safety

Key points

- A safe medication management system comprises of four key processes: prescribing, dispensing, administration, and reconciliation.
- Each process requires reliablity and standardization to ensure safety and to mitigate the risk of harm
- Polypharmacy is a challenge with the increasing complexity of the healthcare
- Methods to improve health literacy can decrease medication harm.

What is the safety issue?

Medications are the most common intervention in healthcare. No matter the setting of care, it is likely that a patient will be prescribed, or will receive, a medication. As a result, medications are associated with a high rate of medication errors and medication-related harm. It is estimated that annually as many as 1.5 million Americans experience harm as a result of medication errors. The WHO reports that globally the costs associated with medication errors have been estimated at $42 billion USD per annum.

Why is it a challenge?

Medication management is complex because it involves prescribers, pharmacists, nurses, patients, and other care providers. All these manage multiple medications with various routes of administration and with potential for causing harm when used incorrectly.

Some patients experience harm even when a medication is used correctly. Many interventions to improve medication safety are poorly implemented or may not include systems thinking or a human factors analysis in their development.

Common terms

A few common terms are defined in Box 20.1.

Box 20.1 Common terminology

Medication safety	The appropriate use of medication that does not cause harm to the patient.
Medication errors	Any preventable event that may cause or lead to inappropriate medication use or patient harm while the medication is in the control of the healthcare professional, patient, or consumer. (NCC MERPP). Not all medication errors lead to harm.
Medication-related adverse event or harm	An experience of the patient that may or may not be the result of an error.
Adverse drug reactions (ADR)	Unexpected or documented side effects of a medication.
Potential adverse drug events	Those events that under other circumstances might cause harm to the patient but on a given occasion did not.

Classification of medication errors

Medication errors are classified using the NCC MERP Index, as indicated in Figure 20.1. This enables clinical teams to assess all degrees of error and therefore allows for learning and remedial action.

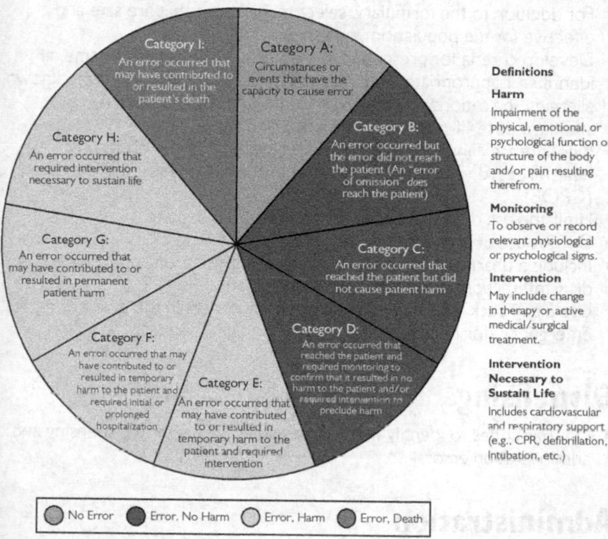

Figure 20.1 NCC MERP Index for categorizing medication errors.

Reproduced with permission by National Coordinating Council for Medication Error Reporting and Prevention,

How can one be safe?

Medication safety requires a system approach for each step of the medication process: prescribing, preparation and dispensing, administration and monitoring.

Leadership for safety

- Identify a multidisciplinary team to work on improving the processes.
- Develop a culture of psychological safety and teamwork.
- Ensure that there is leadership support.
- Understand the root causes of the defects before beginning to design new processes.

Introducing a reliable prescribing process

- Use standardization and simplification, for example protocols, algorithms, and order sets.
- For addition to the formulary, select medications that are safe and effective for the population you serve.
- Develop criteria for prescriptions that include the patient's name, an identifier if appropriate, and information concerning age, weight, known allergies, indications, the generic name of the drug, dosage (using standard doses if possible), frequency, and route.
- Incorporate clinical decision support systems in the electronic health record (EHR) and in the computerized physician order entry (CPOE)
- Limit the use of verbal orders to emergency situations.
- Do not use orders that are sent via SMS (text orders).
- Include a pharmacist's review of the prescriptions for appropriateness, drug interactions and therapeutic duplication.
- Use 'read back' as a way to confirm verbal orders in the event of an emergency (for pharmacists and nurses).

Dispensing

- Use bar codes to identify medications so as to minimize dispensing and administration errors.

Administration

- Provide protected space and time for nurses who administer medications to minimize distractions and interruptions: a 'sterile cockpit' in which interruption is not allowed.
- Ensure proper monitoring of patients after medication administration in order to determine if a patient is experiencing adverse effects.
- Develop nurse-managed protocols for medications such as narcotics and benzodiazepines, so as to be ready to administer reversal agents or rescue medications as quickly as possible in the event of an adverse event.
- Understand the needs and risks associated with the care of different populations such as children, elderly people, obese people, and people with organ dysfunctions.

Measuring medication safety

- Identify and measure the harms experienced by patients in order to determine the safety of a medication system. Methods include the use of full chart reviews, trigger tools, and patient-reported harm.
- Measure medication errors using observation methods, voluntary reports, and pharmacist interventions.

Medications at the interfaces of care (medication reconciliation)

- Collect the best possible list of the medications that a patient is taking on admission to a hospital or during a visit to a clinic or in a doctor's office.
- Use the list to determine whether therapy is to be continued, modified, or discontinued on the basis of the treatment plan for the patient.
- Ensure that changes to patients' medications are communicated with other providers in care and with patients and their families.
- Use digital solutions where available, so as to reconcile medications.

Understanding the level of the patient's health literacy

- Look for signs of low health literacy levels through interactions with the patient.
- Provide instructions at the level of literacy that is appropriate for the patient.
- Use 'teach back' to confirm that the patient has understood the instructions.
- Use 'show back' to confirm that the patient has the ability to execute the use of inhalers and to self-administer medications.

Prevention and reduction of polypharmacy

- Review a patient's medication list for the appropriateness of medications.
- Limit medications to the essential few.
- Involve the patient in developing a treatment plan.
- Use deprescribing guidelines to reduce the number of medications.

The future of medication safety

- Be prepared to manage a larger number of older patients who have more comorbidities and greater need for medications.
- Understand the use of pharmacogenomics and its implications for medication treatment plans and the provision of equitable care.
- Monitor the literature for newly identified drug interactions and adverse events related to medication use.
- IT solutions such as CPOE can be introduced. More recently, blockchain-based systems have been used for the management of electronic health records, including medications; in these systems a decentralized, continuously growing online ledger of the medication record is validated peer to peer by the clinicians, nurses, and pharmacists who work in the system.

Summary box

- Medication errors resulting in adverse events constitute the largest part of patient safety harm.
- Attention to the entire medication process, from prescribing to dispensing and administration, is essential for lowering the possibility of errors that result in an adverse event.
- The study of near misses is important for improving the process.
- Regular medication safety huddles can make a difference to decreasing harm.

Further reading

AHRQ. *AHRQ Health Literacy Universal Precautions Toolkit.* February 2015, last updated September 2020. https://www.ahrq.gov/professionals/quality-patient-safety/quality-resources/tools/literacy-toolkit/index.html.

American Society of Health-System Pharmacists. ASHP guidelines on the pharmacy and therapeutics committee and the formulary system. *American Journal of Health-System Pharmacy* 65 (2008): 1272–83.

Assiri, G. A. et al. What is the epidemiology of medication errors, error-related adverse events and risk factors for errors in adults managed in community care contexts? A systematic review of the international literature. *BMJ Open* 8 (2018): e019101. https://doi:10.1136/bmjopen-2017-019101pmid and http://www.ncbi.nlm.nih.gov/pubmed/29730617.

Farre, A. et al. How do stakeholders experience the adoption of electronic prescribing systems in hospitals? A systematic review and thematic synthesis of qualitative studies. *BMJ Quality & Safety* 28 (2019): 1021–31. http://dx.doi.org/10.1136/bmjqs-2018-009082.

Farrell, B. et al. Reducing polypharmacy in the elderly. *Canadian Pharmacists' Journal* 146.5 (2013): 243–4.

Frankel, A. et al. *Framework for Safe, Reliable, and Effective Care* (White Paper). Cambridge, MA: Institute for Healthcare Improvement and Safe & Reliable Healthcare, 2017.

How-to Guide: Prevent Adverse Drug Events by Implementing Medication Reconciliation. Cambridge, MA: Institute for Healthcare Improvement, 2011.

How-to Guide: Prevent Harm from High-Alert Medications. Cambridge, MA: Institute for Healthcare Improvement; 2012.

Isaacs, A. N. et al. Hospital medication errors: A cross-sectional study. International Journal for Quality in Health Care 33.1 (2020). https://doi.org/10.1093/intqhc/mzaa136.

Koyama, A. K. et al. Effectiveness of double checking to reduce medication administration errors: A systematic review. *BMJ Quality & Safety* 29 (2020): 595–603. http://dx.doi.org/10.1136/bmjqs-2019-009552.

Lambert, B. L. et al. Automated detection of wrong-drug prescribing errors. *BMJ Quality & Safety* 28 (2019): 908–15. http://dx.doi.org/10.1136/bmjqs-2019-009420.

Langer, T. et al. Patient and families as teachers: A mixed methods assessment of a collaborative learning model for medical error disclosure and prevention. *BMJ Quality & Safety* 25.8 (2016): 615–25. http://dx.doi.org/10.1136/bmjqs-2015-004292.

Luetsch, K., Rowett, D., and Twigg, M. J. A realist synthesis of pharmacist-conducted medication reviews in primary care after leaving hospital: What works for whom and why? *BMJ Quality & Safety* 30.5 (2021): 418–30. http://dx.doi.org/10.1136/bmjqs-2020-011418.

Machen, S. et al. The role of organizational and professional cultures in medication safety: A scoping review of the literature. *International Journal of Quality in Health Care* 31.10 (2019): G146–G157. doi: 10.1093/intqhc/mzz111. (Erratum: 804.)

Padula, W. V. and Steinberg, I. What current and missing data can teach us about medication errors. *BMJ Quality & Safety* 30.2 (2020): 89–91. doi: 10.1136/bmjqs-2019-010555.

Rozich, J. D., Haraden, C. R., and Resar, R. K. Adverse drug event trigger tool: A practical methodology for measuring medication related harm. *Quality and Safety in Health Care* 12 (2003): 194–200.

Schnipper, J. L. et al. Effects of a multifaceted medication reconciliation quality improvement intervention on patient safety: Final results of the MARQUIS study. *BMJ Quality & Safety* 27 (2018): 954–64. https://doi:10.1136/bmjqs-2018-008.

Westbrook, J. I. et al. Associations between double-checking and medication administration errors: A direct observational study of paediatric inpatients. *BMJ Quality & Safety* 30.4 (2020). doi: http://dx.doi.org/10.1136/bmjqs-2020-011473.

WHO. *Medication without Harm*. WHO, 15 May 2017. https://www.who.int/initiatives/medication-without-harm.

Wolf, Michael S. The role of health literacy in patient safety. PSNet. 2009. https://psnet.ahrq.gov/perspective/role-health-literacy-patient-safety.

Chapter 21

Safe prescribing in paediatrics

Key points

Medication safety in children has specific challenges.

- Dose is related to age and is calculated by weight.
- Doses therefore change and need to be calculated as appropriate.
- Therapeutic index is narrow and margin of error is small.
- Doses are extrapolated as there are few clinical trials in children.
- Every stage of the medication process carries a risk to medication safety.

What is the medication safety issue in paediatrics?

Paediatric patients are more susceptible to medication errors and are at higher risk of experiencing adverse events related to those errors. The increased risk of medication errors is due to pharmacokinetic differences at different stages of development, dependency on parents and other caregivers to provide medications, and unique epidemiology of medical conditions.

- The rate of potential adverse events has been estimated by Kaushal et al. (2001, 2007) to be potentially three times higher in pediatric patients than it is in adult patients
  - Most errors originates in the prescribing phase.
  - The rate of errors and potential adverse drug events is significantly higher in the neonatal intensive care unit.
- The severity of adverse events in paediatric patients has been shown to be serious or life threatening in up to 35% of events identified (Tham et al. 2011).
- Harm events reported by age show that
  - children aged 0–4 years had the highest proportion of serious event types;
  - children aged 5–14 years had the highest rate of total events and medication errors, specifically (Field et al. 2019).

Therefore medication errors and resultant adverse events are an important safety issue in the paediatric population.

Why is paediatric medication safety a challenge?

[illegible]

Figure 24.1 The medication process

Procurement

[illegible]

Prescribing

[illegible]

Why is paediatric medication safety a challenge?

Achieving medication safety in the paediatric population has significant challenges. These challenges permeate the medication process, from procurement to administration. The medication process is depicted in Figure 21.1.

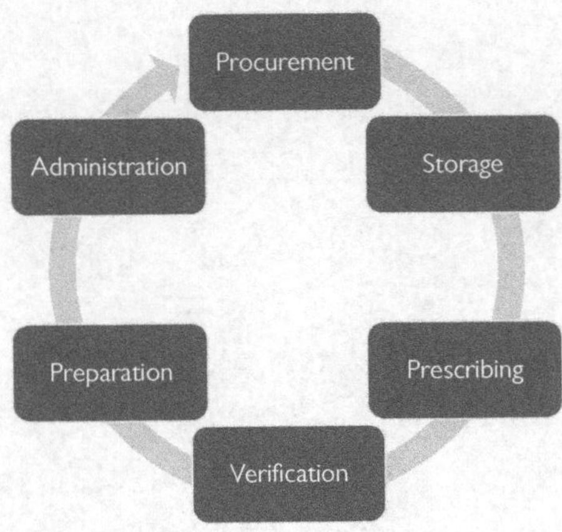

Figure 21.1 The medication process.

Procurement

Acquiring specific paediatric formulations is especially difficult, since most manufactured products do not come in a paediatric dosage format. In addition, in the era of drug shortages, the drug of choice in paediatric patients may no longer be available, and this can lead to errors. Surveys on harm events associated with drug shortages have found that up to 20% of the events reported involve paediatric patients. The lack of published evidence on the use of medications in paediatrics exacerbates the risks associated with drug use in children when the few options that have evidence to support their use are in short supply. Counterfeit drugs pose an even greater risk to paediatric medication safety, as an estimated 10% of medical products in low- and middle-income countries are substandard or falsified, thereby exposing children to even greater risks.

Prescribing

Many medication errors originate in the prescribing phase of the medication use process (see Box 21.1). The dosing of most medications in paediatrics is initially based on adult data. An important factor that contributes to errors is the need for individualized dosing in paediatric patients, as opposed to the 'one dose fits all' approach that may be seen in adults. Children require multistep calculations to individualize doses according to their age and weight, and this can lead to calculation errors. In addition, children have

Box 21.1 Factors to consider in prescribing for children

- lack of paediatric data on prescribing;
- individualization requirements for the child;
- the growth and development of child;
- dose individualization by age and weight;
- consideration regarding ideal vs actual weight;
- rounding the dose up or down;
- prescribing in transitions of care.

pharmacokinetic variation that is based on age and organ system development and that changes rapidly as they grow and develop. Obese children are at higher risk of adverse events if their actual weight rather than their 'ideal weight' is used in medication dosage calculations.

Another factor that may potentiate the risk of error during the ordering phase is risk associated with transitions of care. Increased risk of errors has been shown in paediatric patients during admission, during discharge, and in the outpatient setting. This result is consistent with the fact that adult studies show transitions of care to be a high-risk area. Another factor complicating transitions of care occurs if volumetric rather than weight-based dosing of a drug is used.

The non-standardized approaches to compounding paediatric formulations may further confuse things if a patient is being transitioned to an inpatient setting or moving from one facility to another.

Digital solutions can improve prescribing, if the process is fully understood and a safe prescribing culture is in place (see Box 21.2). However, most of the technology for medication use has been developed for the adult population and requires customization for children.

Box 21.2 Technological ways to improve prescribing

Computerized provider order entry (CPOE) systems have been shown to be safe and efficacious for use in paediatric patients and significantly decrease the rates of medication errors, if a robust review of safety and of the process of prescribing is undertaken before implementation. A human factors and ergonomics approach is essential.

Clinical decision support is essential for safe prescribing. This entails much customization and local support for the maintenance of order sets, order sentences, drug–drug interactions, and more.

Preparation and dispensing

There are several challenges to safe dispensing and these safety issues need to be addressed (Box 21.3).

Many medications must be compounded into a liquid dosage form from the manufacturer's tablets. The way compounded liquids are provided for patients can vary from one institution to another, causing confusion for the clinicians and the patients. The dose that the clinician or the parent is used to drawing up may have changed significantly, depending on how the formulation is compounded.

Box 21.3 Safety issues in dispensing for children

- the preparation of medications from tablets to liquid;
- changes dependent on the preparation of a dose;
- specificity complications related to intravenous preparations;
- adjustment of doses to a measurable form for administration.

The specificity of paediatric doses also complicates intravenous medication preparation. In adult institutions, it is common to batch many doses of the same drug and doses, because many different patients will be receiving it. Paediatric patients have specific dosing requirements, which necessitate much more individualized intravenous (IV) compounds. There is often a need to make different concentrations for very small patients or for patients who cannot handle a very diluted drug. Care must also be taken with rounding doses up or down so that the dose being delivered is in measurable form.

Administration

Dose measurement can become a challenge in adult facilities, for example emergency rooms that may not be equipped with oral syringes of the proper size, which are necessary for measuring smaller doses (1 or 5 mL syringes). In addition, the measurement of doses from outpatient to inpatient or between facilities may be inconsistent, changing from teaspoons to droppers to oral syringes. Interruptions to nurses' work during the medication process increase the risk of error, either in the preparation or in the administration of a dose. These challenges are summarized in Box 21.4.

Box 21.4 Challenges in administration

- dose measurement;
- inappropriate equipment, designed for adults, not for children;
- interruptions;
- the need for monitoring;
- risks in community settings.

As in issues with CPOE, many drug delivery systems were not designed with children in mind. The small doses that are given to children may not fit into a bag for accurate administration and may require a longer infusion than what is possible when pushing by hand.

Owing to narrow therapeutic index medications and to pharmacokinetic variation in children, closer monitoring is required after administration. Administration to a child (or young person) as an outpatient is a safety concern because, as a healthcare provider, you are relying on that child (or young person) or on their caregiver to give medications appropriately at home or at school; and some studies have indicated that the risk may be higher in those settings.

How can paediatric medication safety be improved?

Procurement

A formulary should be in place for all facilities that care for paediatric patients, and oversight of this formulary should be given to a [illegible] committee (e.g. a [illegible]) and [illegible] (see Box 21.1). This group should:

- ensure that drugs are appropriate for use in paediatric [illegible]
- improve clinical [illegible] data [illegible] formulations
- review formulary additions for the possibility of [illegible]
- [illegible] of high-alert drugs.

A drug shortage management plan should be in place to mitigate the risks associated with drug shortages. This management plan should include:

- a practical and timely assessment of [illegible]
- communication plan to healthcare providers of any changes to formulary items or [illegible].

Box 21.1 [illegible] for formularies and [illegible] of medications

- [illegible] associated with [illegible]
- [illegible] management plan [illegible]

Prescribing

The following should be included in the ordering of drugs (see Box 21.1):

- doses calculated in weight [illegible]
- [illegible] the patient's weight [illegible] required [illegible] order entry in CPOE
- standard [illegible] for continuous infusions [illegible]
- [illegible] dose [illegible] always [illegible]
- [illegible] maximum [illegible]
- no abbreviations.

Electronic health records should include CPOE [illegible] with clinical decision support [illegible] the paediatric population:

- dose range checking
- [illegible]
- order sets [illegible] specifically designed for the paediatric patients.

Medication reconciliation is a key process designed to decrease medication errors during transitions [illegible]. [illegible] medication reconciliation has been shown to [illegible]. The medications must be reconciled at every visit, admission, and discharge.

How can paediatric medication safety be improved?

Procurement

A formulary should be in place for all facilities that care for paediatric patients, and oversight of this formulary should be given to an interdisciplinary team such as a pharmacy and therapeutics committee (see Box 21.5). This group should:

- ensure that drugs are appropriate for use in paediatrics;
- approve clinical pathways, protocols, order sets, and dose calculation forms;
- review formulary additions for the possibility of errors;
- ensure procurement of non-counterfeit drugs.

A drug shortage management plan should be in place to mitigate the risks associated with drug shortages. This management plan should include:

- operational and clinical assessment of shortage item; and
- communication plan to healthcare providers of any changes to formulary items or normal processes.

Box 21.5 Key recommendations for the safe procurement of medications

- Develop a pharmacy and therapeutics committee that ensures appropriate use of medications in paediatrics.
- Develop a robust drug shortage management plan to mitigate the risk associated with shortages.

Prescribing

These elements should be included in the ordering phase (see Box 21.6):

- dose, indicated in weight, not in volume (e.g. mg NOT mL);
- entry and verification of the patient's weight (in kilograms, not pounds), required before order entry in CPOE;
- standard dosing style for titratable infusions (e.g. mcg/kg/minute vs mg/kg/hr);
- the calculated dose, always to be entered in orders for paediatrics;
- dose, rounded to measurable units;
- no abbreviations.

Electronic health records should include CPOE and be customized with the clinical decision support specific to the paediatric population:

- dose range checking;
- drug–drug interactions;
- order sets and order sentences specifically designed for the paediatric patients.

Medication reconciliation is a key process designed to decrease medication errors during transitions. Improvement projects have helped to optimize the medication reconciliation process and increase the completion rate; outcomes are not often reported. Medication reconciliation has been shown to increase the identification of medication errors. The medications must be reconciled at every visit, admission and discharge.

Standardized protocols for specific conditions, for example checklists or clinical practice guidelines, can also be used to lower the rate of medication errors during the ordering phase and to improve adherence to proven best practices. These guidelines and protocols should then be monitored for adherence and updated on a regular basis.

Box 21.6 Key recommendations for safe prescribing of medications

- Always indicate the dose in weight and not in volume only.
- Always include the calculated dose with the dose per weight.
- Round the dose to measurable units.
- Apply medication reconciliation.
- Standardize prescribing with order sets, guidelines, and protocols.

Preparation and dispensing

Standardization of preparation and dispensing practices can help to limit medication errors in paediatric patients. Some of the following recommendations can be used (see Box 21.7):

- Standardize and limit the concentrations and dosage strengths of high-alert medications.
- Use only one consistent formula or standard concentration when preparing IV solutions (e.g. epinephrine drip) and avoid practices such as 'the rule of six' to prepare infusions.
- Use commercially available preparations when possible.
- Have the pharmacy prepare all non-commercially available admixtures when available.
- Pharmacists should mathematically double-check all calculated doses.
- Dispense only oral syringes to inpatients with patient-specific doses.
- Use standard concentrations within the health system and nationally, if there is a recommended standard concentration.
- Require pharmacist verification of the components of sterile compounds prior to mixing.
- Employ barcode verification in preparation of IV and oral liquids.

Box 21.7 Key recommendations for the safe preparation and dispensing of medications

- Standardize concentrations and limit dosage strengths.
- Use commercially available products.
- Use national-standard compounded solutions.
- Require pharmacist verification of sterile components prior to mixing.
- Employ barcode verification in preparation of IV and oral liquids.
- Consider the increasing use of dispensing robots that may decrease the frequency of medication errors (e.g. IV sterile preparation robots).

Administration

Some medication errors occurring in the administration phase can be mitigated with the following measures (see Box 21.8):

- Use syringe pumps when applicable.
- Use smart infusion pumps with an activated library for the administration of high-alert medications.
- High-alert medications should require independent double-checking before administration.
- Nurses should mathematically double-check calculated doses.
- Require a bedside barcode scanning system for medications.

The administration of medications at home or in the school setting is less under the control of healthcare providers. However, with proper patient and guardian education, errors at home can be decreased. Improved communication between healthcare providers and parents and improved communication between pharmacists and parents is the best prevention strategy. Clinicians should use methods such as 'teach back' and require parents, before they leave the hospital, clinic, or pharmacy, to show how they will dose a medication. This will demonstrate that the clinician or patient knows exactly how the medication should be given. Caregivers should also be counselled to give doses only with the measuring device that comes with the medicine and not to use household spoons for measuring doses.

Box 21.8 Key recommendations for the safe administration of medications

- Use syringe pumps or smart pumps with activated library.
- Double-check independently for high-alert medications.
- Use bedside barcode scanning.
- Use patient and parent counseling.

Summary box

- Children are at a higher risk of medication errors and adverse events than adults.
- Hospitals and health systems treating paediatric patients should work to increase the detection of medication errors among this population and to identify system improvements that can limit these errors.
- Many of the safety issues concerning paediatric patients stem from the fact that medications and products are [illegible] with the adult patient in mind.
- Major improvements can be made throughout the medication process by focusing on developing a culture of medication safety, [illegible] human factors theory, standardizing medication processes and procedures, and then applying technological solutions.

References

[illegible]

[illegible]

[illegible]

Further reading

[illegible]

[illegible]

[illegible]

[illegible]

[illegible]

[illegible]

[illegible]

[illegible]

[illegible]

Summary box

- Children are at higher risk of medication errors and adverse events than adults.
- Hospitals and health systems treating paediatric patients should work to increase the detection of medication errors in this population and to identify system improvements that can limit these errors.
- Many of the safety issues concerning paediatric patients stem from the fact that medications and medication devices were created with the adult patient in mind.
- Major improvements can be made throughout the medication process by focusing on developing a culture of medication safety, understanding each part of the process, applying reliability and human factors theory, standardizing medication processes and procedures, and then applying technological solutions.

References

Field C, et al. Exploring Vulnerability to Patient Safety Events along the Age Continuum. *Pa Patient Saf Advis* 2019 Mar;16(1).

Kaushal, R. et al. Adverse drug events in pediatric outpatients. *Ambulatory Pediatrics* 7.5 (2007): 383–9.

Kaushal, R. et al. Medication errors and adverse drug events in pediatric patients. *JAMA* 285 (2001): 2114–20.

Tham, E. et al. Sustaining and spreading the reduction of adverse drug events in a multicenter collaborative. *Pediatrics* 128 (2011): e438–e445.

Further reading

ASHP/FDA. Standardize 4 Safety. 2016. https://www.ashp.org/pharmacy-practice/standardize-4-safety-initiative

Donaldson, L. J. et al. Medication without harm: WHO's third Global Patient Safety Challenge. *Lancet* 389.10080 (2017): 1680–1.

Kanjia, M. K. et al. Increasing compliance of safe medication administration in pediatric anaesthesia by use of a standardized checklist. *Paediatric Anaesthesia* 29.3 (2019): 258–64.

Morris, F. H. et al. Effectiveness of a barcode medication administration system in reducing preventable adverse drug events in a neonatal intensive care unit: A prospective cohort study. *Journal od Pediatrics* 154 (2009): 363–8.

Rappaport, D. I. et al. Implementing medication reconciliation in outpatient pediatrics. *Pediatrics* 128 (2011): e1600–e1607.

Ruano, M. et al. New technologies as a strategy to decrease medication errors: How do they affect adults and children differently? *World Journal of Pediatrics* 12.1 (2016): 28–34.

Santell, J. P. and Hicks, R. Medication errors involving pediatric patients. *Joint Commission Journal on Quality and Patient Safety* 31. 6 (2005): 348–53.

Takata, G. S. et al. Characteristics of medication errors and adverse drug events in hospitals participating in the California Pediatric Patient Safety Initiative. *American Journal of Health-System Pharmacy* 65 (2008): 2036–44.

Tyler, L. S. et al. ASHP guidelines on the pharmacy and therapeutics committee and the formulary system. *American Journal of Health-System Pharmacy* 65.13 (2008):1272–83.

White, C. M. et al. Utilising improvement science methods to optimise medication reconciliation. *BMJ Quality & Safety* 20.4 (2011): 372–80.

Prevention of healthcare-associated infections

Key points

- Healthcare-acquired infections (HCAIs) are a major safety risk to people who are receiving care.
- The impact of HCAIs on individuals is significant: increased length of stay in hospitals, increased morbidity, and increased mortality.
- The financial cost is significant—for individuals, for the healthcare system, and for society.
- Many HCAIs can be prevented and many are due to lapses in care.
- The application of reliability methodology such as care bundles, human factors methods in design, and cognitive approaches can decrease or eliminate specific HCAIs.
- A culture of safety is essential to implementing the changes required.

What is the safety issue?

- In high-income countries, 5% to 15% of the hospitalized patients develop healthcare-associated infections (HCAIs) and 9% to 37% end up in ICU.
- Here are some figures for the estimated annual HCAI burden in acute hospitals in Europe (HELICS data):
  - 5 million HCAIs
  - 25 million extra days of hospital stay
  - €13–24 billion extra financial cost
  - 1% attributable mortality (50,000 deaths per year)
- According to the Agency for Healthcare Research and Quality (AHRQ) in USA, HCAI is
  - the most common complication of hospital care; and
  - one of the top ten leading causes of death.
- Of the top ten patient safety interventions with the strongest evidence base (ARHQ 2014), six relate to the prevention of HCAI:
  - bundles for the prevention of central venous catheter-associated infection;
  - real-time ultrasonography for the insertion of central venous catheters;
  - avoidance of urinary catheter-associated infection;
  - bundles for the prevention of ventilator-associated pneumonia;
  - hand hygiene;
  - barrier precautions to prevent HCAI.

Why is it a challenge?

- Prevention and control of HCAI are multifactorial—a 'wicked problem'.
- HCAI, sepsis, and antimicrobial resistance (AMR) are intrinsically linked:
  - Sepsis is frequently due to an underlying HCAI.
  - Antibiotic exposure is a risk factor for HCAI:
    - The selection of microorganisms that are resistant to antibiotics (such as methicillin resistant *Staphylococcus aureus* (MRSA) and resistant Gram-negative bacteria) can cause HCAIs;
    - Vascular access devices used to deliver antibiotics can be a source of infection (e.g. central venous catheters (CVCs)).
    - Secondary infections, such as candidiasis and *Clostridioides difficile* infection, can be a consequence of antibiotic exposure.
- Risk factors for HCAI are increasing in frequency; some of the reasons are as follows:
  - There are more individuals at the extreme ends of the age spectrum.
  - Immunosuppressive therapies are increasingly used.
  - There is increasing use of invasive and implantable devices.
  - The levels of AMR are rising.

How can one be safe?

- Not all HCAIs are preventable; preventable cases [illegible] between 30% and 70% depending on the type of infection.
- Reducing the incidence of HCAIs requires a multifaceted approach (see Figure 12.1).

How can one be safe?

- Not all HCAIs are preventable; preventable cases generally range between 30% and 70%, depending on the type of infection.
- Reducing the incidence of HCAIs requires a multimodal approach (see Figure 22.1).

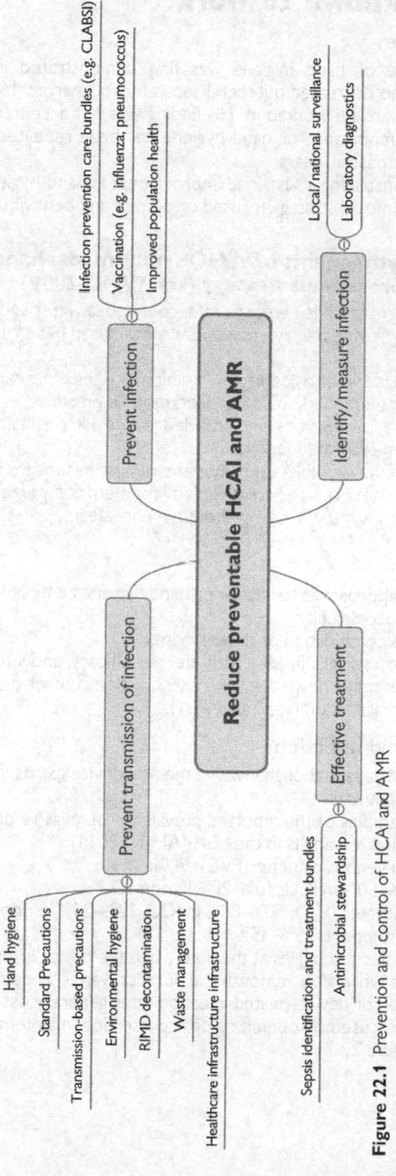

Figure 22.1 Prevention and control of HCAI and AMR

CLABSI = central line associated bloodstream infection; RIMD = reusable invasive medical device

What is known to work?

Hand hygiene

The importance of hand hygiene was first demonstrated in 1847 by Semmelweis who decreased puerperal sepsis mortality from 16% to 3% in the maternity ward he worked in. His finding was not accepted for many years, but the importance of hand hygiene has been repeatedly demonstrated over the past 50 years.

Studies demonstrating a sustained improvement in hand hygiene compliance use a multimodal strategy focused on system and behaviour changes.

Box 22.1 Components of WHO's multimodal hand hygiene improvement strategy (see WHO 2009)

- system change: provide access to safe, continuous water supply, soap, and towels; provide readily accessible alcohol-based hand rub at point of care;
- training/education: provide regular training to all healthcare workers;
- evaluation and feedback: monitor hand hygiene practices, infrastructure, perceptions, and knowledge; provide results of feedback to healthcare workers;
- reminders in the workplace: prompt and remind healthcare workers;
- institutional safety climate: create an environment and perceptions that facilitate awareness-raising about patient safety.

- Behavioural approaches to improving hand hygiene compliance are likely to be successful by:
  - targeting a combination of determinants;
  - focussing on social influence, attitude, self-efficacy, and intention rather than only knowledge, awareness, action control, and behaviour facilitation (see Table 22.1).

Device-related infections

- These can be caused though invasive medical device exposure in hospitalized patients.
- Here are examples of the reported prevalence of invasive device use among hospitalized adults in the USA (AHRQ 2014):
  - peripheral venous catheter (PVC): 90%;
  - CVC: 35%–50% in ICU, 10%–20% in non-ICU;
  - urinary catheter (UC): 50%–80% in ICU, 12%–24% in non-ICU;
  - ventilator support: 25%–45% in ICU.
- The risk of infection begins at the time when the device is inserted and persists for a while after removal (the duration varies by device).
- The reduction of device-related infection rates generally uses bundled approaches focused on optimizing device insertion, maintenance, and removal (Figure 22.2).

Table 22.1. Behaviour change determinants and techniques most likely to improve hand hygiene compliance

Behavioural determinant	Behaviour change technique	Example
Social influence	Provide information about peer behaviour	Information about peers' opinions on correct hand hygiene
Social influence	Provide opportunities for social comparison	Group sessions with peers: discussion and social comparison of hand hygiene practices
Social influence	Mobilize social norm	Exposing the professional to the social norm of important others such as opinion leaders
Attitude	Persuasive communication	Positive consequences of proper hand hygiene
Attitude	Reinforcement of behavioural progress	Praise, encouragement, or material rewards
Self-efficacy	Modelling	Role model demonstrates proper hand hygiene behaviour in group, class, or team
Self-efficacy	Verbal persuasion	Messages aimed to strengthen control beliefs about correct hand hygiene technique
Self-efficacy	Guided practice	Teaching skills and providing feedback. Specific instruction for correct hand hygiene behaviour
Self-efficacy	Plan for coping responses	Identification of and coping with potential barriers
Self-efficacy	Graded tasks, goal setting	Desired hand hygiene behaviour achieved with a stepwise model
Intention	General intention information	Explanation of hand hygiene goals/targets
Intention	Agreement with behavioural contract	Contract/commitment with defined goals

Central line-associated bloodstream infection (CLABSI)

- CLABSI is the commonest cause of preventable healthcare-associated bloodstream infections. It accounts for 10% of HCAI (30% in ICU); it is attributed a 10% mortality rate; and it extends a patient's hospital stay by a median of 13 days.
- There has been considerable reduction in CLABSI thanks to the implementation of central venous catheter (CVC) insertion and maintenance bundles.
  - Many hospital units have achieved more than 90% reduction in CLABSI rates by rigorous adherence to bundles.

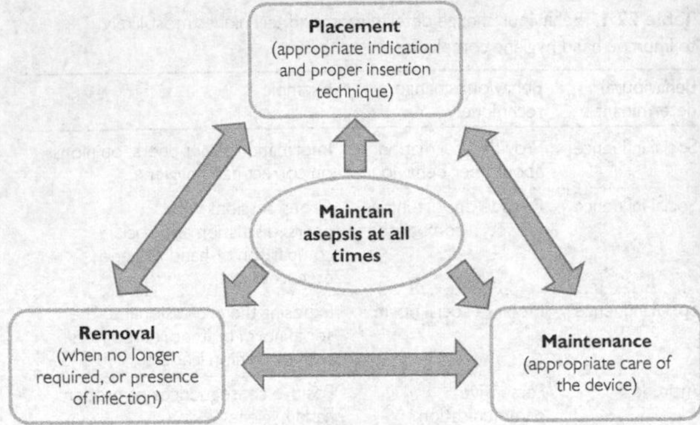

Figure 22.2 Core principles for the prevention of device-related infections

Box 22.2 Typical components of Central Venous Catheter (CVC) care bundles

Insertion bundle

- hand hygiene (with alcohol-based hand gel) before insertion;
- aseptic technique throughout insertion, with maximal sterile barrier precautions;
  - mask, cap, gown, sterile gloves, sterile full-body drape;
- insertion site chosen so as to minimize infectious and non-infectious complications on the basis of the individual patient's characteristics;
  - femoral site to be avoided in obese adult patients;
- choice of CVC with minimum number of ports/lumens required for the individual patient;
- insertion site prepared with 2% chlorhexidine in 70% alcohol;
- sterile gauze, transparent, or semipermeable dressing applied to the insertion site.

Maintenance bundle

- daily review and recording of ongoing requirement for CVC;
- daily checking that the CVC dressing is intact and was changed within the previous 7 days;
- alcohol CVC hub decontamination ('scrub the hub') to be performed before each hub access;
- hand hygiene before and after all CVC maintenance/access procedures;
- use of chlorhexidine 2% in 70% alcohol for cleaning the insertion site during dressing changes;
- daily bathing with chlorhexidine of ICU patients over the age of 2 months.

Box 22.3 Suggested methods for making the delivery of all CVC bundle elements more reliable

- Keep standardized/preferred equipment for CVC insertion stocked in a cart or kit.
- Use an insertion checklist that includes all bundle elements for CVC insertions.
- Empower all the staff involved in CVC insertion to stop the process if element(s) of the bundle are not being executed.
  - Use team-based behavioural change methods to support this (e.g. crew resource management (CRM), TeamSTEPPS, safety pauses).
- Include an assessment for the removal of CVC in daily goal sheets.
- State the line day (e.g. 'line day 6') during rounds, as a reminder of how long the CVC has been in place.
- Ensure hand hygiene materials (e.g. alcohol hand gel dispensers) are readily available at the bedside and ergonomically sited.
- Measure bundle compliance using an 'all or nothing' measurement and share compliance data with the staff.
  - Make feedback as close to real time as possible.

Catheter-associated urinary tract infection (CAUTI)

- UTI is the commonest HCAI (40% of HCAI).
- 60% of CAUTI cases are considered preventable.
  - CAUTI is a preventable cause of healthcare-associated bloodstream infection.
  - There is a 5% increase in the risk for CAUTI with each day of keeping the urinary catheter (UC) in place.
- United States (annually, 2002 data):
  - 13,000 attributable deaths;
  - 2–4 days increased hospital stay;
  - $1200–2400 additional cost per case.

Box 22.4 Typical components of Urinary Catheter (UC) care bundles

Insertion bundle

- Avoid unnecessary catheterization.
- Choose a UC of appropriate size.
- Use sterile items and equipment.
- Insert the UC using a strict, aseptic, non-touch technique.
- Use a closed drainage system.

Maintenance bundle

- Review and record the need for a UC daily.
  - Remove the UC promptly when no longer necessary.
- Use an aseptic technique for daily catheter care.
  - Use hand hygiene and sterile items and equipment.
- Don't break the closed drainage system.
  - If a urine specimen is required, take it aseptically via a sampling port

- Risk factors for CAUTI:
  - prolonged duration of UC use;
  - female sex;
  - older age;
  - diabetes mellitus;
  - UC insertion outside the operating room;
  - breaches in the closed system of UC drainage.

Ventilator-associated pneumonia (VAP)

- This is the most frequent HCAI in ICU.
  - 10% to 20% of patients who are mechanically ventilated for more than 48 hours develop VAP if no prevention bundle is in place.
- VAP doubles the numbers of deaths in ICUs; the mortality attributable to it is around 10%.
- Risk factors for VAP are:
  - increasing age (from 55 years on);
  - chronic lung disease;
  - (micro-)aspiration as a result of being in a supine position;
  - chest or upper abdominal surgery;
  - previous antibiotic therapy, especially broad-spectrum antibiotics;
  - prolonged intubation or reintubation;
  - acute respiratory distress syndrome;
  - frequent ventilator circuit changes;
  - polytrauma, head injury, or both;
  - prolonged paralysis;
  - premorbid conditions (e.g. malnutrition, renal failure, anaemia).

Box 22.5 Typical components of VAP prevention care bundles

- Elevate the head of the bed (30°–45°).
- Schedule a daily sedation interruption and a daily assessment of readiness to extubate.
- Use subglottic secretion drainage.
- Avoid scheduled ventilator circuit changes.
- Change circuit only when clinically indicated (e.g. soiled, faulty).

Clostridioides difficile infection (CDI)

- *Clostridioides difficile* was formerly known as *Clostridium difficile*.
- In 2011, CDI accounted for 12% of HCAIs in the United States.
- Risk factors comprise:
  - antibiotic exposure;
  - gastrointestinal surgery/manipulation;
  - prolonged hospital/residential healthcare stay;
  - any serious underlying illness;
  - immunocompromising conditions;
  - advanced age;
  - proton pump inhibitors;
  - H2-blockers.
- *Clostridioides difficile* is a spore-forming bacterium. It facilitates environmental contamination and person-to-person transmission.
- Prevention bundles: strongest evidence base is for antimicrobial stewardship.

Box 22.6 Typical components of *Clostridioides difficile* infection (CDI) prevention care bundles

- antimicrobial stewardship:
  - facility-wide reduction in antimicrobial consumption;
  - interventions targeting the use of 'the five Cs': cephalosporins, co-amoxiclav, clindamycin, carbapenems, fluoroquinolones ('ciprofloxacin');
  - antibiotics to be stopped where possible, if CDI is suspected;
- hand hygiene and contact precautions:
  - alcohol gel before, soap and water after contact with the patient, as alcohol gel is ineffective on spores;
  - gloves and apron/gown for direct patient contact;
- dedicated patient equipment;
- staff education;
- patient education;
- environmental cleaning;
  - use of chlorine-based disinfectant prior to re-use of room;
- patient isolation;
- proton pump inhibitor stewardship;
  - use to be limited to ICU or specific indications;
- systems and workflow changes.

Surgical site infection (SSI)

- A SSI is an infection that occurs up to 30 days after surgery (or up to one year after implant surgery) and affects the incision or the deep tissue at the operation site.
- SSIs occur overall after 2%–5% of surgical procedures (US data)
  - Some procedures have higher rates (e.g. about 20% after colorectal surgery);
  - SSIs account for about 20% of HCAIs.
- Mortality in patients with SSI is twice as high as mortality in patients without SSI and four times higher in older adults.
- On average, SSI adds 7 to 11 hospital days per patient.
- 60% of cases are considered preventable through the application of evidence-based interventions.
- The onset often occurs after discharge from hospital, for example incidence after discharge is 6% for colon resection and 88% for knee arthroplasty. Therefore accurate SSI measurement requires post-discharge surveillance.
- Prevention bundles incorporate pre-, intra-, and post-operative interventions (see Figure 22.3)
  - SSI bundle components with the strongest evidence base are:
    - appropriate skin preparation (clipping rather than shaving);
    - guideline-based antimicrobial prophylaxis with appropriate timing, dosing and re-dosing;
    - blood glucose control (especially for cardiac surgery);
    - maintenance of normothermia;
    - optimizing tissue oxygenation;
    - chlorhexidine and alcohol-based skin preparation;
    - plastic wound protector (gastrointestinal and biliary surgery);
    - surgical safety checklist.

Preventing Surgical Site Infections
Key Recommendations for Practice

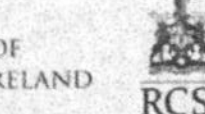

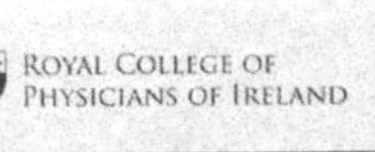

Pre-Op...

1. Avoid hair removal at the surgical site. If hair must be removed use single-patient use clippers and not razors.

2. Wash the patient or make sure that the patient has showered (or bathed/washed if unable to shower) on day of or day before surgery.

3. Use the right drug at the right time for the right duration for antibioloti prophylaxis:
   a. **Right drug:** Prescribe antibiotic prophylaxis according to local antimicrobial prescribing guidelines
   b. **Right time:** Ensure that the antibiotic is given at induction - Within 60 minutes before skin incision. In surgery where a tourniquet is to be applied, a 15 minute period is required between the end of antibiotic administration and tourniquet application.
   c. **Right duration:** Single dose only, unless otherwise indicated[1]

Intra-Op...

1. Use 2% chlorhexidine gluconate in 70% isopropyl alcohol solution for skin preparation. If the patient is sensitive or allergic use povidone-iodine.[2]

2. Make sure that:
   a. The patient's body temperature is maintained above 36°C during the perioperative period (Excludes cardiac patients)
   b. The patient's haemoglobin saturation is maintained above 95%, or as high as possible if there is underlying respiratory insufficiency
   c. If the patient is diabetic, that the glucose level is kept at <11mmol/l throughout the operation

3. Give an additional dose of antibiotic if the surgical procedure is prolonged[3] or there is major intra-operative blood loss (>1.5 litres in adults or 25ml/kg in children) - otherwise the duration of surgical prophylaxis should be a single dose.

4. Cover the surgical site (wound) with a sterile dressing prior to removal of drapes at the end of surgery.

Post-Op...

1. Do not tamper with or remove the wound dressing for 48 hours post-op unless clinically indicated.

2. Use aseptic (no touch) technique[4] for wound inspection and/or wound dressing changes.

3. Hand hygiene is mandatory before and after every time the wound is inspected or the dressing is changed.

1. With the exception of a very small number of surgical indications (see supporting documentation), the duration of surgical prophylaxis should be a SINGLE dose.
2. Allow skin to dry thoroughly, avoid pooling of disinfectant and drape patient after skin is dry (see supporting documentation).
3. A supplementary intraoperative antibiotic dose may be warranted in two circumstances:
a. Blood loss – fluid replacement: Serum antibiotic concentrations are reduced by blood loss and fluid replacement, especially during the first hour of surgery when antibiotic levels are high. In the event of major intra-operative blood loss (>1.5 litres) additional doses of prophylactic antibiotic should be considered after fluid replacement
b. Prolonged surgical procedures: Many antibiotics, such as cephalosporins like cefuroxime, are short acting and therefore an additional dose should be administered during the surgery if the procedure lasts longer than 4 hours. The re-dosing time will vary depending upon the half-life of the drug in question, and the patient's underlying renal and hepatic function.
4. Aseptic (no touch) technique aims to prevent microorganisms on hands, surfaces or equipment being introduced to a surgical site (wound). Use no touch technique with clean or sterile gloves, where appropriate, for any change or removal of surgical site (wound) dressings.

Developed by the Joint RCSI/RCPI Working Group on Prevention of Surgical Site Infection (2012)

Figure 22.3 Example of an SSI prevention bundle

Source: Joint RCSI/RCPI Working Group on Prevention of Surgical Site Infection. https://rcpi-live-cdn.s3.amazonaws.com/wp-content/uploads/2016/01/Preventing-Surgical-Site-Infections-Care-Bundle.pdf

How do you measure your safety?

Outcome measures	
Device-related infection rates (number of episodes per 1,000 device days)	Need clear and easily applied laboratory and clinical criteria for defining episodes. Robust surveillance case definitions produced by CDC (US), ECDC (Europe), WHO.
Daily device ward census (number of patients with device at given time each day) provides acceptable denominator	Also raises awareness of who has a device in place each day.
Process measures	
Hand hygiene compliance	Observational audits (WHO methodology): people prone to the Hawthorne effect
Alcohol gel consumption (e.g. litres per 100 bed days)	Surrogate marker of hand hygiene
Monitors of adherence to the process	1. % compliance with insertion bundle 2. compliance with maintenance bundle 3. audit of indication for device insertion 4. percentage of devices with at least one documented and agreed indication 5. median duration of device placement (days) 6. device prevalence (percentage of patients with device in place each day, averaged over week or month)

Summary box

The best interventions to try

- Local audit and feedback:
  - Provide teams and units with tools for rapidly collecting and analysing their own data on hand hygiene compliance, device-related infections, etc.
- Simple ethnography:
  - Observe practices at the point of care, in collaboration with the frontline team or unit staff.
- Co-design of local interventions:
  - Use the findings of local audit and ethnographic observations.
  - Use collaboration techniques such as Liberating Structures (http://www.liberatingstructures.com) with teams or unit staff to develop local solutions.
  - Focus on behaviour change and human factors-based solutions.
- Develop locally agreed indications for the insertion and use of invasive devices.
- Develop and provide a pre-assembled standardized kit containing all materials required for the insertion of the targeted invasive devices.

References

AHRQ (Agency for Healthcare Research and Quality). Healthcare-associated infections program. 2014. https://www.ahrq.gov/professionals/quality-patient-safety/hais/index.html.

WHO. The WHO multimodal hand hygiene improvement strategy. 2009. https://www.who.int/gpsc/5may/Guide_to_Implementation.pdf

Further reading

Huis et al. A systematic review of hand hygiene improvement strategies: a behavioural approach. *Implementation Science* 7 (2012), article 92. http://www.implementationscience.com/content/7/1/92

Institute for Healthcare Improvement. Measures to prevent healthcare-associated infections. IHI, n.d. http://www.ihi.org/resources/Pages/Measures/MeasurestoPreventHAIs.aspx.

Society for Healthcare Epidemiology of America et al. *Compendium of Strategies to Prevent Healthcare-Associated Infections in Acute Care Hospitals: 2014 Update*. SHEA, 1 May 2014. https://www.shea-online.org/index.php/practice-resources/41-current guidelines/417-compendium-of-strategies-to prevent-healthcare-associated-infections-in-acute-care-hospitals-2014-update.

Chapter 23

Sepsis and antimicrobial stewardship

Key points

- Sepsis is associated with high levels of morbidity and mortality
- Sepsis-related mortality can be reduced through early recognition and prompt protocolized therapy
- Antimicrobials are life-saving drugs, but are associated with adverse drug events, secondary infections, and selection of antimicrobial resistance
- Antimicrobial stewardship is a balance between early effective therapy and avoiding unnecessary antimicrobial use
- Care bundles methodology can improve the reliability of processes relating to sepsis management and antimicrobial stewardship

What is the safety issue?

Sepsis

- Sepsis is defined as a life-threatening organ disfunction caused by a dysregulated immune response to infection.
- It has a rate of 15% to 24% attributable mortality among hospitalized adults.
- It has a long-term impact on survivors, causing cognitive and functional impairment, sustained inflammation and immune dysfunction, reduced health-related quality of life, and increased mortality.
- Early recognition and treatment of sepsis can decrease mortality.

Antimicrobial stewardship

- 20%–40% of antimicrobial therapy is considered inappropriate.
- 20% of patients receiving antimicrobials have an adverse drug event.
- Infections caused by antimicrobial resistant organisms could become the commonest cause of death.
    - About 10 million deaths per year are projected worldwide by 2050.
- Both mortality and financial costs are doubled for infections caused by resistant versus sensitive bacteria.
- Antimicrobial stewardship programs reduce mortality, morbidity, and financial costs, while reducing the selective pressure for antimicrobial resistance.

Why is it a challenge?

Sepsis

- Sepsis has been described as 'the perfect storm of immense public health burden combined with unexplained practice and outcomes variation' (Walkey and Lindenauer 2017: 1019)
- Sepsis is a heterogeneous syndrome, comprising multiple subtypes.
  - Variation in prognosis and response to therapy between sepsis subtypes may explain the failure to demonstrate improved survival in randomized control trials (RCTs).
- Clinicians may fail to recognize sepsis in the absence of supportive tools, and its diagnosis is variable and can be subjective.
- Overtreatment of sepsis leads to unnecessary antimicrobial exposure, investigations, and healthcare resource use.
- Both the rational management of sepsis and the rational use of antimicrobials are influenced by behavioural biases.
- Projects focusing on improved sepsis recognition tend to look at patients with lower illness severity.
  - Lower mortality may be due to sepsis intervention, changes in the casemix, or a combination of both.
  - Reporting outcomes only for patients with a final diagnosis of sepsis may miss unintended consequences for patients with alternative final diagnoses.

Antimicrobial stewardship

- Antimicrobial prescribing is a complex task, comprising multiple subtasks.
- Prescribers often lack knowledge of key aspects of antimicrobial use, such as:
  - spectrum of activity of the antimicrobial;
  - pharmacokinetics/pharmacodynamics of the antimicrobial;
  - antimicrobial susceptibility data at individual patient and unit/institution level;
  - propensity for selection for antimicrobial resistance;
  - frequency and type of associated adverse drug events.
- Antimicrobial prescribing is often reflexive and based on local habits and culture.
- Lack of access to or availability of rapid diagnostics to identify pathogens to guide initial antimicrobial prescribing decisions can result in incorrect choice of antibiotic
- Management of infection, including sepsis, is often seen as an immediate or individual patient care issue.
  - Antimicrobial resistance and other adverse effects of antimicrobials are often seen as longer-term societal issues.
- The duration of antibiotic courses is rarely evidence-based.
  - This duration is often based on 'magic numbers' (multiples of 5 or 7).
  - Antibiotics are continued after the infection is cured or ruled out.
    - This practice reflects inertia, habit, or the lack of a planned stop date.

How can one be safe?

- An effective recognition and management of sepsis and rational antimicrobial use share some common features:
  - understanding behavioural biases, the local culture, and the context;
  - understanding the role of human factors and ergonomics;
  - getting access to laboratory diagnostics;
  - getting access to the relevant experts in the field;
  - using measurement and feedback of data for improvement;
  - using care bundles, checklists, and other cognitive support tools.

What is known to work?

Sepsis

- Sepsis care bundles are mostly aimed at the early recognition and immediate management of the condition.
- They are closely linked to early warning systems for the recognition of illness severity or deterioration.

Box 23.1 Components of the 2018 Surviving Sepsis campaign 'Hour-1 Bundle' for the immediate resuscitation and management of sepsis *(see http://www.survivingsepsis.org/Pages/default.aspx)*

- Measure the lactate level; re-measure if >2 mmol/L.
- Obtain blood cultures before giving antibiotics.
- Administer antibiotics.
- Give 30 mg/kg crystalloid for hypotension or lactate ≥4 mmol/L.
- Give vasopressors if patient remains hypotensive despite fluid resuscitation.

- Each care bundle element involves multiple subtasks.
  - Delivery within the time limit requires considerable coordination and streamlining of processes.
- Methods that have proven successful in delivering sepsis care bundles include:
  - using ethnographic observation to understand the process flow at the ward or unit level;
  - simulating sepsis scenarios (with direct or video observation);
  - redesigning work areas and equipment storage spaces so as to facilitate the delivery of care bundle elements in time;
  - developing and providing a 'sepsis pack' that contains all necessary equipment for the delivery of care bundle elements;
  - gamification.

Antimicrobial stewardship

Antimicrobial stewardship in acute hospitals

- Persuasive approaches are most likely to deliver sustained improvement and culture changes in relation to antimicrobial use.
- Examples of persuasive approaches:
  - audit and feedback of prescribing data to prescribers;
  - academic detailing:
    - peer-to-peer educational outreach;
    - meetings with prescribers targeting specific aspects of antimicrobial use;
  - 'handshake' stewardship:
    - rounding-based review of prescribed antimicrobials;
    - face-to-face feedback to prescribers by a pharmacist–physician team.
- Restrictive approaches are most likely to deliver quick wins, but may not be sustainable.

  - They work only for antimicrobials that are targeted for restriction.
  - They may lead to 'squeezing the balloon': prescribers may overprescribe non-restricted agents.
- Examples of restrictive approaches:
  - formulary restrictions:
    - only selected antimicrobials are available on the hospital formulary;
  - requirement for authorization by infection specialists before prescribing specified agents:
    - resource intensive;
    - can be an opportunity for the infection specialist to deliver academic detailing or handshake stewardship.
- Antimicrobial care bundle 'Start Smart, then Focus' (see Figure 23.1):
  - 'Start Smart' reflects the initial diagnostic uncertainty and the need for empiric prescribing.
  - 'Then Focus' reflects the ability to make an informed antimicrobial decision in light of the diagnostic information and clinical course.
- Behavioural 'nudges' can drive desired changes in prescribing practice.
- Examples of successful antimicrobial stewardship nudges:
  - suppressing susceptibility results for selected antimicrobials on microbiology reports;
  - provision of relevant clinical/prescribing advice on microbiology reports;
  - replacing suggested therapy duration in prescribing guidelines with specific guidance as to when to stop antimicrobial;
  - provision of laminated cards with common antibiotic indications to attach to ID badges;
  - reminder stickers in charts/prescription records (Figure 23.2), or pop-up dialogue boxes on electronic healthcare records.

Antimicrobial stewardship in ambulatory care

- Greater role for public, patient, and family education than in hospital settings;
- Public, patient, and family educational targets:
  - duration of common, self-limiting illnesses;
  - not wasting antibiotics (ecological messaging);
  - promotion of self-care for self-limiting illnesses:
    - key role for community pharmacists;
    - web-based (e.g. www.undertheweather.ie);
- Prescriber education:
  - focus on the psychology of patient–prescriber interaction;
  - focus on clinical risk rather than on bacteria versus viruses;
- Feedback of prescribing data:
  - comparison with national and regional averages;
  - initial focus on 'preferred antibiotics':
    - narrow spectrum; compliance with prescribing guidelines;
- Alternatives to immediate antimicrobial prescription:
  - provisional ('only if') prescription:
    - only to be filled if there are specified new symptoms or there is lack of improvement within a specified time;
    - supports patient or parent involvement in care decisions;

Start Smart, Then Focus

An Antibiotic Care Bundle for Hospitals

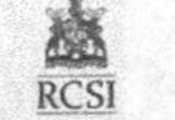

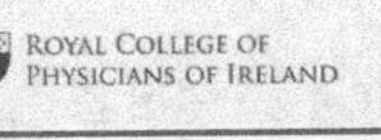

Day 1: Start Smart...

1. Start antibiotics only if there is clinical evidence of bacterial infection
   -If there is evidence of bacterial infection, prescribe in accordance with your local antibiotic guidelines and appropriately for the individual patient (see notes below)
2. Obtain appropriate cultures before starting antibiotics
3. Document in both the drug chart and medical notes:
   - Treatment indication
   - Drug name, dose, frequency and route
   - Treatment duration (or review date)
4. Ensure antibiotics are given within four hours of prescription
   - Within 1 hour for severe sepsis or neutropenic sepsis

When deciding on the most appropriate antibiotic(s) to prescribe, consider the following factors:
- History of drug allergy (document allergy type: minor (rash only) or major (anaphylaxis, angioedema))
- Recent culture results (e.g. is patient colonised with a multiple-resistant bacteria?)
- Recent antibiotic treatment
- Potential drug interactions
- Potential adverse effects (e.g. *C. difficile* infection is more likely with broad spectrum antibiotics)
- Some antibiotics are considered unsafe in pregnancy or young children
- Dose adjustment may be required for renal or hepatic failure

Consider removal of any foreign body/indwelling device, drainage of pus, or other surgical intervention

For advice on appropriate investigation and management of infections, consult your local infection specialist(s) (microbiologist, infectious disease physician and/or antimicrobial pharmacist)

... then Focus (Day 2 onwards)

At 24–48 hours after starting antibiotics, make an **Antimicrobial Prescribing Decision**
- Review the clinical diagnosis
- Review laboratory/radiology results
- Choose one of the five options below
- Document this decision

Options

1. Stop antibiotic(s)
   - no evidence of bacterial infection, or infection resolved
2. Switch from intravenous to oral antibiotic(s)
   - if patient meets criteria for oral switch
3. Change antibiotic(s)
   - narrower spectrum, if possible; broader spectrum, if indicated
4. Continue current antibiotic(s)
   - review again after further 24 hours
5. Outpatient parenteral antibiotic therapy
   - consult with local OPAT team

Developed by the RCPI Hospital antimicrobial Stewardship Working Group (2012)
Adapted, with permission, from the UK Department of Health "Start smart, Then Focus" hospital antimicrobial stewardship programme

Figure 23.1 'Start Smart, Then Focus': The antibiotic prescribing bundle.

Source: RCPI Hospital Antimicrobial Stewardship Working Group. Adapted, with permission, from the UK Department of Health's 'Start Smart, Then Focus' hospital antimicrobial stewardship programme

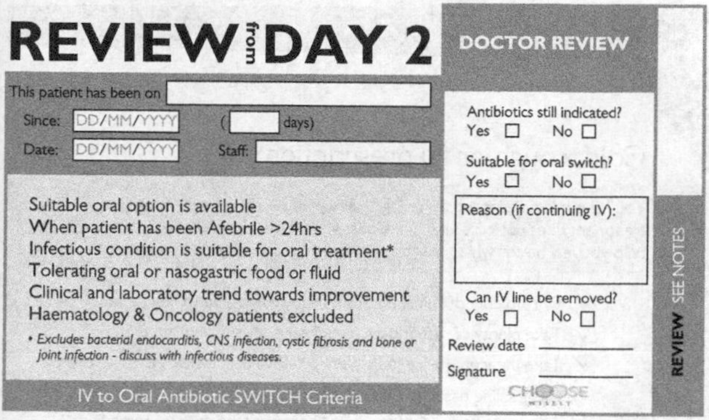

REVIEW from DAY 2

This patient has been on

Since: DD/MM/YYYY (days)

Date: DD/MM/YYYY Staff:

Suitable oral option is available
When patient has been Afebrile >24hrs
Infectious condition is suitable for oral treatment*
Tolerating oral or nasogastric food or fluid
Clinical and laboratory trend towards improvement
Haematology & Oncology patients excluded

• Excludes bacterial endocarditis, CNS infection, cystic fibrosis and bone or joint infection - discuss with infectious diseases.

IV to Oral Antibiotic SWITCH Criteria

DOCTOR REVIEW

Antibiotics still indicated?
Yes ☐ No ☐

Suitable for oral switch?
Yes ☐ No ☐

Reason (if continuing IV):

Can IV line be removed?
Yes ☐ No ☐

Review date ________

Signature ________

CHOOSE WISELY

REVIEW SEE NOTES

Figure 23.2 Example of sticker inserted into clinical notes to support the 'Then Focus' antibiotic decision

Reproduced with permission of Chris Little Capital and Coast District Health Board New Zealand

- 'wellness' pack:
  - provision of a pack containing self-care advice and materials (symptomatic remedies, tissues, etc.);
- non-antibiotic 'prescription' (Figure 23.3);
- Reminders/pop up messaging within primary care practice management software;
- Academic detailing:
  - face-to-face antimicrobial stewardship workshops with GPs;
  - reflection on antibiotic prescribing, guidance, clinical scenarios, strategies to improve prescribing, demonstration of patient-facing resources, audits, educational resources.

Antimicrobial stewardship in long-term care facilities

- This is often a mixture of what works in acute hospital and ambulatory care settings.
  - The degree of overlap varies according to the level of care provided by the facility.
- Audit and feedback may be effective, but may be more difficult to implement than in hospital and ambulatory settings.
- Frequently reported interventions include:
  - academic detailing on indications for antimicrobial use;
  - agreement on local prescribing guidelines;
  - interventions to reduce misdiagnosis of infection (e.g. reducing the use of urine dipsticks);
  - interventions to prevent infections (e.g. urinary catheter and respiratory care bundles);
  - resident or family education and involvement in stewardship-related decisions;
  - provision of access to expertise.

Cold, cough or flu prescription

You have been diagnosed as having an illness caused by a virus. Antibiotic treatment does not cure viral infections. The treatments prescribed below will help you feel better while your body's own defenses are defeating the virus.

- ✓ Drink plenty of fluids, hot drinks should help you to feel better
- ✓ Take plenty of rest and avoid excessive physical exertion
- ✓ Take paracetamol or ibuprofen to relieve headaches, pain and fever.
- ✓ Use a saline nasal spray to relieve congestion.
- ✓ Ask your pharmacist for advice about over the counter remedies.

Specific medicines to take ______________________________

Use medicines as directed by your doctor, pharmacist or package instructions.
Stop the medication when the symptoms get better.

Follow up:
If not improved in ____ days, if new symptoms occur, or if you have other concerns, please call or return to the office for a recheck. If you have a cough it is normal for it to continue for up to three weeks.

Signed: Dr. ______________________________

Antibiotics are wasted on colds and flu

For more information visit:
www.hse.ie/go/antibiotics

Figure 23.3 Example of a non-antibiotic 'prescription' to promote self-care of viral respiratory tract infections

Reproduced with permission of Fidelma Browne, Health Services Executive, Dublin, Ireland.

How do you measure your safety?

Sepsis

- Process measures:
    - % compliance with sepsis care bundle elements
    - It may start with one or two key elements (e.g. time to ordering/completion of blood cultures/antimicrobials)
    - Time to completion of the bundle elements
        - Important to define 'time 0' clearly
- Outcome measures:
    - Number or rate of sepsis cases detected
    - Hospital mortality, ICU admission, length of stay of patients with discharge ICD code; [illegible] Note the potential bias of detection of less severe cases

Antimicrobial stewardship

- Process measures:
    - % compliance with elements of the antimicrobial [illegible]
    - Compliance with local prescribing guideline plus documentation of indication in the [illegible] notes; [illegible] review
- Measurement of antimicrobial consumption:
    - Days of therapy (DOT) per 1000 bed days:
        - Accurate measure [illegible]
        - Difficult to obtain without electronic health record (EHR) or e-prescribing system
    - Defined daily dose (DDD) per 1000 bed days:
        - Underestimation of [illegible] use of low doses (e.g. paediatric or renal failure)
        - [illegible] doses used; [illegible] recommend [illegible] (DDD) [illegible]
    - Point prevalence surveys (PPS) are an alternative [illegible]:
        - [illegible] of baseline data for [illegible] and subsequent surveys may be the most feasible measurement [illegible]
- Outcome measures:
    - Clostridioides difficile infection (CDI) rates are useful for antimicrobial stewardship, as they target broad spectrum antibiotics, particularly fluoroquinolones and other agents associated with high CDI rates
    - Antimicrobial resistance:
        - It is difficult to define a standard to measure overall antimicrobial resistance
        - Usually you should target a specific local antimicrobial resistance issue (e.g. rate of infections caused by extended-spectrum beta-lactamase (ESBL)-producing Gram-negative bacilli)
    - Antimicrobial-related adverse drug events:
        - Accurate measures may require post-discharge follow-up
        - Usually you should target a specific local issue of drug events (e.g. AKI [illegible] nephrotoxic [illegible])

How do you measure your safety?

Sepsis

- Process measures:
  - % compliance with sepsis care bundle elements:
    - start with one or two key elements (e.g. time to guideline-compliant antibiotic administration);
  - time to completion of care bundle elements:
    - important to define 'time 0' clearly.
- Outcome measures:
  - number or rate of sepsis cases detected;
  - hospital mortality, 30-day readmission, length of stay among patients with discharge ICD code for sepsis. Note potential bias due to detection of less severe cases.

Antimicrobial stewardship

- Process measures:
  - % compliance with elements of the Start Smart, then Focus (SSTF) bundle.
  - Combined compliance with local prescribing guideline plus documentation of indication for therapy is a useful initial measurement for improvement.
- Measurement of antimicrobial consumption:
  - days of therapy (DoT) per 100 bed days:
    - accurate measure of antimicrobial use;
    - difficult to obtain without electronic health records (EHRs) or an e-prescribing system;
  - defined daily dose (DDD) per 100 bed days:
    - underestimation of antimicrobial use if low doses used (e.g. paediatrics, kidney failure)
    - overestimation if high doses used (e.g. guidelines recommend increased individual dose for a given condition: number of doses stays the same, but DDD increases);
  - point prevalence surveys (PPSs) of antimicrobial use:
    - provision of baseline data for improvement. Frequent rapid surveys may be the most feasible measurement in long-term care settings.
- Outcome measures:
  - *Clostridioides difficile* infection (CDI) rates are useful for antimicrobial stewardship, as they target a broad spectrum of antibiotic use (particularly fluoroquinolones and other agents associated with high CDI rates).
  - Antimicrobial resistance:
    - It is difficult to define a standardized measure of antimicrobial resistance.
    - Usually you should target a specific local antimicrobial resistance issue (e.g. rate of infections caused by extended spectrum beta lactamase (ESBL)-producing Gram-negative bacilli).
  - Antimicrobial-related adverse drug events:
    - Accurate measurement may require post-discharge follow-up.
    - Usually you should target a specific local adverse drug event (ADE) issue (e.g. acute kidney injury related to nephrotoxic antimicrobials).

Summary box

Best interventions to try

Sepsis

- Develop a sepsis pack that contains all necessary equipment for delivering care bundle elements.
- Make ergonomic adjustments to work flows and equipment, on the basis of the observation of simulated sepsis clinical scenarios.

Antimicrobial stewardship (hospital)

- Establish weekly audits of compliance with prescribing guidelines and documentation of indication for antimicrobial therapy, with feedback to prescribers.
- Co-design guidelines and reminder cards with prescribers.
- Use reminder stickers to encourage 'Then Focus' bundle components.

Antimicrobial stewardship (ambulatory care)

- Offer regular feedback of antimicrobial prescribing rates, with comparison to national and regional averages.
- Provide tools for self-assessment of prescribing practice (audit against prescribing guidelines).
- Co-design the use of alternatives to immediate prescription (e.g. wellness packs)

Antimicrobial stewardship (long-term care)

- Adopt care bundles for the prevention and management of specific infections (e.g. urinary tract infection).
- Use automatic stop dates for antimicrobials (to reduce excessive duration or unnecessary long-term prophylaxis).
- Use behavioural nudges to reduce unnecessary testing of urine samples (e.g. moving urine dipsticks to a locked cupboard).

References

Walkey, A. J. and Lindenauer, P. K. Keeping it simple in sepsis measures. *Journal of Hospital Medicine* 12.12 (2017): 1019–20. doi:10.12788/jhm.2873.

Further reading

Davey P, et al. Interventions to improve antibiotic prescribing practices for hospital inpatients. Cochrane Database of Systematic Reviews 2017, Issue 2. Art. No.: CD003543. doi:10.1002/14651858.CD003543.pub4.

Fitzpatrick et al. Sepsis and antimicrobial stewardship: Two sides of the same coin. *BMJ Quality & Safety* 28 (2019): 758–61. https://qualitysafety.bmj.com/content/early/2019/04/24/bmjqs-2019-009445.info.

Ivers, N. et al. Audit and feedback: Effects on professional practice and healthcare outcomes. Cochrane Library, 13 June 2012. https://www.cochranelibrary.com/cdsr/doi/10.1002/14651858.CD000259.pub3/full.

O'Neill J. et al. Tackling drug-resistant infections globally: final report and recommendations: he Review on Antimicrobial Resistance. 2016, London. Wellcome Trust. https://wellcomecollection.org/works/thvwsuba/items

Rhee, C. et al. Diagnosing sepsis is subjective and highly variable: A survey of intensivists using case vignettes. *Critical Care* 20.89 (2016). https://doi.org/10.1186/s13054-016-1266-9.

Chapter 24

Preventing and limiting deterioration on the medical wards

Key points

- Patients can deteriorate unexpectedly and needlessly die.
- Situation awareness of all the factors and anticipation of deterioration can improve outcomes.
- Risk of deterioration must be managed proactively.
- This includes the use of early warning systems, the assessment of family concerns, and having a high level of awareness.
- Other risks to patients, such the risk of falls, pressure injuries, and hospital acquired or healthcare associated infections (HAIs), must be anticipated.

Deterioration

The definition of clinical deterioration has evolved over time, as methods of describing adverse events have moved from end events (mortality) to describing discrete complications (ICU admission, cardiac arrest) in the currently prevailing framework, which uses parameters of physiological instability to predict risk of deterioration. The United Kingdom's National Early Warning Score 2 (NEWS2) calculates an aggregated score and, when a predetermined threshold is reached, a predefined response is triggered (i.e. a review by a clinician). Delayed recognition of deterioration is a commonly identified safety event.

Why is it a challenge to prevent deterioration?

The recognition of and response to the deteriorating patient presents multiple barriers and can be challenging. Patient safety initiatives to [illegible] the response to the deteriorating patient [illegible] recognized that delay in critical care and treatment can lead to suboptimal results. The challenges in preventing deterioration can be categorized into three key areas:

Assessment

- Not knowing the patient well; the need for a thorough handover; the use of structured handover tools such as ISBAR (Identify, Situation, Background, Assessment, Recommendation) has been shown to improve communication and confidence about recognizing deteriorating patients, which is essential for improvement in patient safety.
- The importance of using family members, carers, and relatives of the patient [illegible] to recognize subtle signs of deterioration and subtle changes in behaviour.
- Some evidence suggests that critical care outreach teams (CCOTs) or rapid response teams assist with the early management and improve the care of deteriorating patients. They may also improve the confidence of ward staff. Other reviews reported that there is no strong evidence of improved outcomes; the unintended consequence of [illegible] implementation of such teams may deskill the ward staff.
- [illegible] have been found to have a significant role in [illegible] the ability to recognize subtle signs and deterioration (Parfitt and King 2012).

Why is it a challenge to prevent deterioration?

The recognition of and response to the acutely unwell patient provides multiple barriers and can be challenging. Patient safety is integral to escalation and to the response to the deteriorating patient. It is recognized that a delay in time-critical care and treatment can lead to suboptimal results. The challenges in preventing deterioration can be categorized into three key areas:

Assessment

- Not knowing the patient well: the need for appropriate handover: the use of structured handover tools such as ISBAR (introduction, situation, background, assessment, recommendations) has been shown to improve communication and confidence about recognizing deteriorating patients, with subsequent improvements in patient safety.
- The importance of using family members, friends, and relatives of the patients: this practice supports clinicians to recognize soft signs of deterioration and subtle changes in behaviour.
- Failure to recognize and escalate: the NEWS or the paediatric early warning score (PEWS) is normal but the patient looks unwell.
- Delays in escalation: these are delays in the escalation of care secondary to a hierarchical process of escalating through 'the knowledge of skills ladder', often from healthcare assistant (HCA) to junior nurse, ward sister, junior doctor, specialist registrar and appropriate consultants as needed.

Staffing/environment

- Is appropriate equipment available in monitored and non-monitored areas.
- Some studies suggest that medical emergency teams (MET) or rapid response teams assist with the early management and improved care of deteriorating patients. They may also improve the bedside education of ward staff. Others have reported that there is no strong evidence of improved outcomes. The unintended consequence of widespread implementation of such teams may de-skill the ward staff.
- Is there an appropriate nurse staffing ratio and skill mix? Currently there are no mandatory standards, but recommendations are set locally by individual health providers. They vary depending on the setting, for example intensive care (1:2) may be different from A&E (suggested 1:4)—which in turn may be very different in a care home, in a paediatric ward, and so on. The department of health and the Royal College of Nursing have published guidance that can be found at www.rcn.org.uk.
- Overwhelming workload and experience have been found to have a significant role in determining the ability to recognize subtle signs in patient deterioration (Purling and King 2012).

Human factors

- Non-technical skills relate to communication, raising concerns, and having 'gut feelings'. Common themes from incidents regarding missed deterioration or failure to rescue a patient are communication barriers and situational awareness.
- Poor leadership should be eliminated. It has been reported that detecting and limiting deterioration and improving patient safety depends on good role models within the organization.
- Senior clinicians, including ward managers and supervisors, need to ensure an environment where staff members feel able to raise a concern and create a 'no blame' culture. While a 'no blame' culture is important, individuals involved in caring for deteriorating patients need to be supported and educated appropriately.

This third key area of challenge is discussed in Chapter 9. Application of the SEIPS model is helpful to understand the challenges to detect deterioration.

How can one be safe and what is the theoretical basis?

To optimize the ward nurse's response to a deteriorating patient, it is essential to flatten the hierarchical structure of clinical practice. A multidisciplinary response to the deteriorating patient has been shown to improve patient outcomes dramatically, in conjunction with developing the non-technical skills associated with escalation and leadership.

The measurement and documentation of vital signs is often delegated to junior staff members, who often see it as an observation round and as a task-oriented process rather than as a clinical assessment of the trend in the patient's physiology. The observation rounds are an opportunity to include a full physical assessment, encompassing visual prompts and enlisting the aid of touch. The staff may become reliant on technology and scoring systems to trigger concerns about a patient; however, a holistic assessment is equally important.

The National Patient Safety Agency (2004) published *Seven Steps to Patient Safety*, which sets out seven steps that healthcare organizations should take to improve patient safety and to help them to meet their clinical governance and risk management targets.

Seven steps to patient safety

- Build a safety culture.
- Lead and support your staff.
- Integrate your risk management activity.
- Promote reporting.
- Involve and communicate with patients and the public.
- Learn and share safety lessons.
- Implement solutions to prevent harm.

Table 24.1 highlights practical approaches in which individuals and their microsystems, mesosystems, and macrosystems can follow these steps in order to improve patients' safety on the medical ward.

Table 24.1. Practical approaches to improving safety on the medical ward

Individual	Ward/Environment	Hospital
It is estimated that 23,000 in-hospital cardiac arrests in the UK and at least 20,000 unanticipated intensive care admissions may be avoidable with better patient care (National Institute of Clinical Excellence 2011). Individuals must work within their own skill set and know when to ask for help.	Abnormalities of pulse rate, blood pressure, temperature, etc. occur before 79% of in-hospital cardiac arrests, and in 54% of in-hospital deaths and emergency ICU admissions (National Institute of Clinical Excellence 2011). In some cases the deterioration is well documented, but there is little evidence of intervention. In other cases the monitoring of vital signs has been found to be incomplete or inaccurate (ibid.). Access to senior clinicians/consultant presence on the ward may facilitate appropriate and timely escalation. Audits of ward practice where patients have deteriorated may highlight areas of training for the staff.	The National Institute of Clinical Excellence (NICE) requires that all adult patients in hospitals have a clear monitoring plan, whereby vital signs should be recorded, the severity of illness measured using early warning scores (EWSs), and a graded response strategy in place (National Institute of Clinical Excellence 2011). EWSs have been widely demonstrated to improve the recognition of deteriorating patients and the predictions mortality. Use of 'e-obs'—a wireless handheld computer-based system—allows the staff to record these vital signs electronically; it calculates the EWS and provides instructions to bedside staff. These data are integrated so that the staff elsewhere in the hospital is able to access these data instantaneously (ibid.). Trusts that have adopted these 'pocket performance systems' have reported a significant (up to 40%) reduction in hospital standardized mortality ratio (HSMR).
It is essential for individuals to expand on their current knowledge base and recognize where further development and training are required. This may be within their own scope of practice, but in a multidisciplinary team there is also a sharing of knowledge and experience whenever possible.	Visibility of patients to staff, ward layout and location of monitored beds. Visibility of physiology, e.g. NEWS documentation at the end of the bay rather than in a bedside folder (where it may be a case of 'out of site out of mind').	Investing in staff education and training, including non-technical skills and simulation. Statutory mandatory training and induction. Deliberate organizational learning requires organizations to actively integrate new knowledge and insights in order to improve patient outcomes. An approach that the Institute of Medicine states is a necessity for an effective healthcare system.

(Continued)

Table 24.1. *(Contd.)*

Individual	Ward/Environment	Hospital
Participation in good quality handover and 'role-modelling' one's behaviour.	Ensuring safe staffing levels and an appropriate skill mix on each shift, with appropriate rota coordination for junior doctors.	Share learning and information across different specialities—promotion of incident reporting. Structured morbidity and mortality meetings with feedback and learning.
Ensuring that oneself and others have taken appropriate breaks, meals. and rest.	Appropriate side rooms, ensuring availability of protective masks, gowns, hand gel for infection control purposes.	A 'guardian of safe working' should protect patients and doctors, in order to ensure that doctors are not working unsafe hours.
Upholding individual responsibility in maintaining governance, e.g. though self-audit and incident reporting with yearly appraisals.	Safety huddles involve a short briefing between ward staff to identify and discuss any deteriorating patients or to discuss potentially avoidable patient harms per shift, e.g. falls and pressure ulcers. These huddles have been shown to improve patient outcomes and to avoid harm; a good example is the Leeds Teaching Hospitals, as described in the Health Foundation's programme Huddling Up for Safer Healthcare.	Ensuring up-to-date guidelines, policies, and procedures such as antimicrobial stewardship. Use of care bundles in some areas has been demonstrated to improve management, e.g. sepsis, ventilator-associated pneumonia (VAP), acute kidney injury (AKI), and chronic obstructive lung disease (COPD). Executive safety walkabouts have been shown to improve the safety culture within organizations.

Early warning systems

[illegible]

[illegible]

[illegible]

How do you measure safety on a medical ward?

[illegible]

Falls

[illegible]

Pressure ulcers

[illegible]

Hospital-acquired infections

[illegible]

Early warning systems

In 2017 the Royal College of Physicians (RCP) published NEWS2, where it aimed to improve safety for patients with hypercapnic respiratory failure by suggesting a separate oxygen saturation (SpO2) parameter scoring system for such patients. The plan was to have this system adopted by all acute hospitals by March 2019. Similar early warning systems are available in other countries.

The system allows for a common language between the community setting, the ambulance service, and intra-hospital people in order to avoid any potential delays in responding to an unwell patient.

A clinical response is required for NEWS of 5 and above, as this is an indication of a potentially acutely unwell patient. Evidence is growing to support the view that NEWS2 is more sensitive to the identification of sepsis and allows improved management and recognition of patients with hypercapnic respiratory failure.

How do you measure safety on a medical ward?

The top three safety issues reported on medical wards are:

Falls

Falls in the in-patient setting are the most commonly reported patient safety incident type across England and Wales, accounting for 240,000 incidents, as per the consensus statement from Public Heath England, 2017. All in-patients over the age of 65, and those between 50 and 64 years who are considered high falls risk, should be considered for a multifactorial assessment during their in-patient stay. (See Frailty Chapter 34)

Pressure ulcers

The prevalence of pressure ulcers on a general medical ward is estimated to be 4.7% (Thompson, Healey, and Scobie 2007). Estimates for the daily cost of a pressure ulcer are between £43 and £374. Hospital-acquired pressure ulcers extend the length of an in-patient stay by an average of 5–8 days per pressure ulcer (Bennett, Dealey, and Posnett 2004). All adult in-patients should have on admission, a risk assessment designed to determine the likelihood of their developing a pressure ulcer, and those identified as high risk should be treated with preventable measures. (See Frailty Chapter 34)

Hospital-acquired infections

Hospital-acquired infections, also termed healthcare-associated infections, develop either as a result of a medical or surgical intervention or through contact with a healthcare environment. Every year, approximately 300,000 individuals develop a hospital-acquired infection—a prevalence of 6.4% of in-patients across all specialities, as per the Health Protection Agency's annual survey in 2012/13. The most common types of hospital-acquired infection on a general medical ward are respiratory infection, urinary tract infection, including catheter-associated infection, gastrointestinal infection, and blood stream infection. (See HAI Chapters 22 and 23)

Specific tools for measuring safety on a medical ward

Mortality and morbidity meetings are an essential method for measuring and analysing safety. The RCP has developed a National Mortality Case Record Review (NMCRR) toolkit to support trusts to implement a standardized way of reviewing case records in adults who have died in acute hospitals across England and Scotland. The national programme aims to improve understanding and to promote best practice across the NHS. Here are some of the tools:

- audit of medical emergency calls and cardiac arrests;
- survival to discharge following cardiac arrest;
- monitoring escalation to higher levels of care;
- staff turnover and staffing levels;
- patient experience;
- friends and family complaints and feedback to assess satisfaction (in the UK this is part of required reporting);
- serious incidents and monitoring incidents of hospital-acquired infections such as MRSA and *Clostridium difficile*;
- compliance with hand hygiene and monthly audits of practice;
- compliance with sepsis screening and NEWS compliance;
- the NHS safety thermometer is a point-of-care survey instrument designed to provide a 'temperature check' of harm locally. Safety thermometer tools are available for different clinical areas such as mental health, paediatrics, and medication safety. The original tool, which is used on medical wards, involves measuring harm from pressure ulcers, falls, catheter-associated urinary tract infections, venous thromboembolism, and harm-free care;
- mandatory and statuary training: intermediate, advanced, and basic life support (ILS, ALS, BLS);
- completion of the mandatory General Medical Council Survey and learning from its results.

Summary box

Key points for limiting deterioration

- correct and continuous training for staff and appropriate skill mix on all shifts;
- appropriate use of Early Warning Systems, monitors and side rooms;
- good handovers and safety huddles to proactively manage risk;
- dissemination of learning in real time;
- up-to-date guidelines and policies that are reliably applied.

References

Bennett, G., Dealey, C. and, Posnett, J. The cost of pressure ulcers in the UK. *Age Ageing.* 33.3 (2004): 230–5.

National Institute of Clinical Excellence. Improving the detection and response to patient deterioration: Shared learning database. NICE, February 2011. https://www.nice.org.uk/sharedlearning/improving-the-detection-and-response-to-patient-deterioration.

National Patient Safety Agency. *Seven Steps to Patient Safety: An Overview Guide for NHS Staff.* NPSA 2004. https://www.publichealth.hscni.net/sites/default/files/directorates/files/Seven%20steps%20to%20safety.pdf.

Purling, A. and King, L. A literature review: Graduate nurses' preparedness for recognisisng and responding to the deteriorating patient. *Journal of Clinical Nursing* 21.23–24 (2012): 3451–65.

Thompson, R., Healey, F., and Scobie, S. *Safer Care for the Acutely Ill Patient: Learning from Serious Incidents.* Patient Safety Observatory Report. National Patient Safety Agency, 2007. https://www.baccn.org/static/uploads/resources/NPSA_Report.pdf.

Further reading

Ball, C., Kirkby, M., and Williams, M. Effect of the critical outreach team on patient survival to discharge from hospital and readmission to critical care: Non-randomised population based study. *BMJ* 327.7422 (2003), article 1014. doi: 10.1136/bmj.327.7422.1014.

Joint Position Statement on Rapid Response Systems in Australia and New Zealand and the Roles of Intensive Care. ANZICS 2016. https://www.cicm.org.au/CICM_Media/CICMSite/CICM-Website/Resources/Professional%20Documents/IC-25-Joint-ANZICS-and-CICM-Rapid-Response-Systems-Position-Statement.pdf.

Leonard, M., Graham, S., and Bonacum, D. The human factor: The critical importance of effective teamwork and communication in providing safe care. *BMJ Quality and Safety* 13.1 (2004): i85–i90.

Massey, D., Chaboyer, W., and Anderson, V. What factors influence ward nurses' recognition of and response to patient deterioration? An integrative review of the literature. *Nursing Open* 4.1 (2017): 6–23.

Royal College of Physicians. *National Early Warning Score (NEWS)* 2. 19 December 2017. https://www.rcplondon.ac.uk/projects/outputs/national-early-warning-score-news-2.

Thompson, J. et al. Using the ISBAR handover tool in junior medical officer handover: A study in an Australian tertiary hospital. *Postgraduate Medical Journal* 87.1027 (2011): 340–4.

Winters, B. D. et al. Rapid response systems: A systematic review. *Critical Care Medicine* 35.5 (2007):1238–43.

Chapter 25

Preventing and limiting diagnostic error

Key points

- The process of diagnosis commences at the point of deciding whether to investigate or not.
- The process needs to be co-produced with the patient and family.
- Safety challenges occur at every step: ordering, then performing the investigation, interpreting the results, and giving feedback to the patient
- Human factors, reliability, and resilience theories assist in designing a safe process.

What are the key safety issues?

The use of investigation is a key part of the diagnostic process. There are many possible steps in the process that can lead to error or delay in diagnosis, from taking the specimen or ordering the intervention to performing the test, interpreting the results, and acting on the results. In addition, delays to the process may result in harm.

In this chapter we focus on the system that delivers diagnosis rather than on the individual who makes a wrong judgement or overlooks a finding. By identifying the key components of the patient's journey and designing that journey with the patient's safety in mind, the team will mitigate the risks of error.

The adoption of a proactive approach will ensure that every member of staff has a commitment to high-quality safe care at every stage of the process, not only during that part for which he or she has direct responsibility (see Table 25.1).

We have focused on imaging, but apart from the specific safety issues around ionizing radiation, the sequence of the patient's journey and the approaches to reducing the risk of diagnostic error are very similar in any diagnostic service.

Table 25.1. The diagnostic pathway

Decision to undertake the test	Delivery of the test	Post-test and reporting and next steps
Technology/ culture/ system resilience	Technology/ culture/ human factors/ safe design/ reliability/ system resilience	Technology/ culture/ reliability/ system resilience
Referrer's knowledge, including evidence base/ decision support systems	Protocols and their adjustment to maximize diagnostic accuracy	Interpretation errors/ accuracy (HF/ error reporting and review, double reporting, imaging software systems to increase perception)
Referring patient information	Scheduling and prioritization	Reporting/ transcribing errors
Referrer/ diagnostician processes and documentation	Key process reliability and protocol compliance (including radiation dose and accumulative maintenance of equipment and anaesthesia)	Communication between diagnostician and referrer (urgent flagging/ prioritization systems)
Referrer/ diagnostician communication	Team safety culture	Affirmation that necessary next steps are clear to the referrer and that action is taken in the required time scale
Referrer/ diagnostician relationships/ culture of shared responsibility for outcome	Diagnostic department safety culture and systems (e.g. check lists/ ID check/ room safety/ wrong site discipline)	Amount of feedback and learning from errors and near misses, as part of a continuous learning system
Amount of feedback and learning	Amount of feedback and learning	The patient's experience and feedback

Why is it a challenge?

All diagnostic services (including imaging, endoscopy, laboratory, interventional radiology) are complex systems. The risk of error is considerable in these departments and in their interactions with referring clinicians, patients and their families, and the organization at large.

How do you measure safety?

Measuring error is undertaken on a case-by-case basis, as well as through the regular review of processes for reliability. Equipment is rigorously maintained to agreed standards, and ionizing radiation in particular is highly regulated in its use.

All diagnostic units and departments are now expected to create the infrastructure and internal programmes that help them to understand where errors can occur and to take action to reduce or remove these risks. Within the NHS the quality standard for imaging (QSI, formerly known as ISAS) is designed for the purposes of quality improvement. Similarly, for endoscopy, the joint accreditation standards for endoscopy (JAG) define the service standards that cover all aspects of an endoscopy service to ensure safe high-quality diagnosis. The NHS National Safety Standards for Invasive Procedures (NatSSIPs) provide examples and guidance on how to minimize the risk of harm in surgery and other situations where an invasive procedure is undertaken—renal biopsy or chest drain insertion, for example. The combined approach of agreed standards, a formal accreditation system, and regulatory oversight share and develop best practice and inspire confidence that the latter is being adhered to.

Making the patient's diagnostic journey safer

[illegible]

Making the patient's diagnostic journey safer

Before the test

The decision to request the test:

1. Referrer's knowledge, including the evidence base and decision support systems:
   a) Test requesting is designated according to the experience of the referrer (example: only a consultant or a senior staff member can request or authorize tests).
   b) Knowledge and accreditation of the referrer is required (example: Ionizing Radiation (Medical Exposure) Regulations (IR(ME) R) for requesting ionizing radiation).
   c) Easy and required access to decision support/evidence base supporting appropriate tests (examples: I Refer; Image Wisely). If requesting is computerized, such decision support can be a mandatory part of the ordering sequence.
2. Patient information:
   a) Three or more unique identifiers for the patient need to be produced at and on every request.
   b) Relevant history of the patient is required, not just symptoms and signs.
   c) Co-morbidities are described and defined where they add to the risk of the examination (example: renal function when impaired and IV contrast may be used).
3. Referrer–diagnostician communication and relationships:
   a) There needs to be openness of communication and mutual access between referrer and diagnostician.
   b) There needs to be shared responsibility for the patient's outcome and agreement among all that the test is required and as to how and when it should be performed.
4. The feedback and learning system:
   a) regular review of cases together, to learn and share new knowledge or understand the role of the test in the patient's journey (example: multidisciplinary weekly meetings);
   b) regular review and open discussions on errors of omission or commission identified by the department or referring clinicians (example: READ newsletter from the Royal College of Radiologists);
   c) whole departmental review of errors or near misses related to referral or the scheduling of diagnostic examinations.

Delivery of the test

1. Protocols and their adjustment so as to maximize diagnostic accuracy:
   a) A pre-diagnostic test 'imaging strategy' maximizes the value of comprehensive clinical information and the patient's co-morbidities to ensure that contrast use is safe and optimized (example: renal function checks are required to avoid contrast induced nephropathy).

2. Scheduling and prioritization:
   a) The timing of the diagnostic test optimizes the benefit to the patient and his or her outcome and coordinates with referring teams plans (example: agreed time of referral to CT scan in the management of patient with an acute abdomen likely to need a laparotomy).
   b) Access to diagnostics meets current best practice on all occasions (example: the interval between clinical symptom onset and CT/MRI scan for people with a head injury or an acute stroke.)
3. Key process reliability and protocol compliance (including radiation dose and cumulative dose over repeated examinations):
   a) Comprehensive programmes of equipment maintenance and testing ensure that calibrations, dose, and performance are optimized (example: unknown variations in radiation exposure can limit the diagnostic value of an image as well as add to the radiation burden of the patient).
   b) Regular observations and spot audits ensure that key processes for patients are delivered as planned and only varied if there is a specific patient need or diagnostic indication.
4. Team safety culture:
   a) A positive safety culture ensures that staff values, attitudes, competencies, and behaviours are completely focused on preventing and mitigating harm or error.
   b) Communication is founded on mutual trust, shared perceptions of the importance of safety, and the efficacy of preventative measures.
   c) The non-technical skills of team members, for example their situational awareness and safe decision-making, are well developed and continually nurtured ('stop and check' site mark).
   d) Work pressures are acknowledged and dealt with effectively by the whole team in order to reduce risk to patient and staff members.
5. Diagnostic department safety culture and work systems:
   a) 'Red rules' that must always be undertaken are agreed on (example: patient ID checks).
   b) Communication is clear among team members, especially in handover or complex situations where bidirectional clarity is critical.
   c) Speaking up about uncertainties and escalating concerns is expected and respected by everyone.
   d) Routine briefing and debriefing in all interventions and complex situations will enable reflection on possible improvements.
   e) Checklists are always used when required and ownership of this process is shared equally by the whole team.
   f) The regular simulation of emergency events to review room and staff procedures ensures that the team can work optimally under pressure or in an exceptional situation.
   g) National Safety Standards for Invasive Procedures (NATSIPPS) are used as a guide to reducing the risk of never events (room safety/wrong site discipline).

Post-test, reporting, and next steps

1. Interpretation errors:
   a) Reporting of images is undertaken by those trained in the modality and specifics of the test. Appropriate supervision supports those in training.
   b) Various types of reformatting in multiple planes are routinely used to increase the perceptivity of lesions. Automated computer software is used to flag up important information such a micro calcification in breast imaging or nodules in the lung in order to aid detection rates.
   c) The double reporting of complex, specific, or unusual cases, if it does not add delay, will add robustness to a report and may be organized as a routine or as a regular systematic approach for learning.
2. Reporting and transcribing errors:
   a) Reporting environments enable high levels of concentration with limited disturbance, to reduce the risk of errors of commission (interpretation) and omission (failure to see or include findings in report) (example: ensuring optimal lighting for the viewing screens and temperature for the staff).
   b) Reporting templates co-designed by diagnosticians and referrers ensure that key aspects of the study are always included and reduce the accidental omission of normal findings. This also enables the referring clinician to read and respond to reports more easily.
3. Communication between diagnostician and referring clinician or team:
   a) Systems for swiftly and precisely communicating urgent or unexpected and important findings to referring clinicians are in place. This process may be aided by computer automation. Any system in place should be tested regularly for reliability and accuracy.
   b) The onward communication of all reports should be understood by all parties, and if there are changes due to technical or manpower issues all parties should be informed.
4. Affirmation from the referrer that the recommended next steps are understood and are being carried out in line with best practice and optimal time scales:
   a) This is part of the system referred to in 3. Close working relationships and regular multiprofessional clinical team meetings ensure that all parties are clear on the optimal timescales for treatment options or communication with the patient to ensure the best outcome.
   b) Standard approaches are in place for identifying new research or best practice guidelines and for adapting existing systems to match what is now needed.

5. Feedback and a learning system for referrers and diagnosticians on errors, near misses, and collaborative approaches to continuously improve and reduce avoidable harm:

An open learning culture requires all parties to share their interpretations of images and, where there are differences in opinion or judgement, to find a constructive means to resolve them with the patient's best interests at heart (example: develop a regular whole team review meeting where errors of commission and omission and interesting cases are considered).

6. The patient's experience and feedback as a core element of safe design:

The patient's feedback and involvement are used to co-design a safer and more effective care (examples: designing children's services to reduce anxiety included parents' or children's involvement in or advice about decorating the endoscopy or scanner area; approaches to venepuncture to reduce anxiety and improve procedural quality).

Summary box

Safety theories and improvement methods that can be used to enhance diagnostic safety
Human factors analysis (example: work environment, task design)
Process reliability (example: patient ID check and scanning protocols)
Team building and team performance (example: open culture and regular review of near misses and errors of commission and omission)
Standardized communication tools (example: request and report templates)
System resilience (example: well defined and tested process for reporting unexpected and or significant findings)
Technical resilience (example: comprehensive equipment maintenance and repair programme)
Co-production (example: using the patient's experience to reduce the risk of harm or the use of excess radiation or sedation

Further reading

American College of Radiology, Radiological Society of North America, American Society of Radiological Technologists and American Association of Physicists in Medicine. Image Wisely 2021. https://www.imagewisely.org/

Brink JA, Amis ES Jr. Image Wisely: a campaign to increase awareness about adult radiation protection. *Radiology* 257(3) (2010): 601–2. doi:10.1148/radiol.10101335. PMID: 21084410.

NHS England. National Safety Standards for Invasive Procedures (NatSSIPs). 2015 London. https://www.england.nhs.uk/wp-content/uploads/2015/09/natssips-safety-standards.pdf

Royal College of Physicians. Joint Advisory Group on Gastrointestinal Endoscopy (JAG) accreditation standards for endoscopy services. 2021. London. https://www.thejag.org.uk/

Royal College of Radiologists. Standards for learning from Discrepancies meetings. 2014. London. Royal College of Radiologists. https://www.rcr.ac.uk/publication/standards-communication-radiological-reports-and-fail-safe-alert-notification

Royal College of Radiologists. Standards for the communication of radiological reports and fail-safe alert notification. 2016. London. Royal College of Radiologists. https://www.rcr.ac.uk/publication/standards-communication-radiological-reports-and-fail-safe-alert-notification

Royal College of Radiologists. *I Refer*. London: Royal College of Radiologists, 2019. https://www.rcr.ac.uk/clinical-radiology/being-consultant/rcr-referral-guidelines/about-irefer

Chapter 26

Safety in primary care and general practice

Key points

- Adverse events in primary care and general practice are common.
- The care provided in primary care is complex, heterogeneous, and longitudinal. This leads to unique safety challenges.
- Higher-risk aspects of general practice are identified and more specific safety concerns explored.
- Rates of remote consultation have increased significantly owing to COVID 19. Advice for safer remote consulting is included.
- Practical approaches to improving safety in primary care and general practice are presented, including leadership, mitigation and risk control.
- Useful strategies for measuring and learning from safety culture, processes, and events are detailed.

What are the key safety issues in primary care and general practice?

Approximately 90% of all patient encounters in the United Kingdom occur in general practice (over 300 million each year). There is a lack of robust epidemiological data to quantify the current level of safety in primary care accurately. It is estimated that 1%–2% of all consultations involve an adverse event, and it is thought that 11% of all prescriptions contain an error (Health Foundation 2017). It is believed that most errors do not affect patients adversely or cause harm; however, given the enormity of the overall number of patient interactions, it is possible that the total burden of harm is greater in primary than in secondary care.

While much of the science of patient safety originated in secondary care, there is an ever increasing emphasis and recognition of its importance in primary care. In the unique environment of primary care the challenges, measures, and tools associated with providing safe care must be adapted and made suitable to the particular nature of the care provided.

Why is it a challenge to be safe?

General practitioners interact with large numbers of patients in relatively short consultations. Patients are living longer with multiple comorbidities, which involve increasingly complex care. Patient care often involves multiple care providers, spread across both primary and secondary care, with relatively poor levels of integration across care interfaces. In addition to this, general practitioners are expected to provide unparalleled levels of personalized care, responsive to patient values and preferences in a community context.

The number of general practitioners practising single-handedly continues to fall, as care shifts to larger group practices, with resultant impacts on the continuity of care for individual patients. There is also an increasing emphasis on the provision of allied health and multidisciplinary care closer to home for patients. In this context, improving patient safety in primary care is challenging.

How can one be safe?

What is safer care?

The concept of providing safer care in primary care is different from that in secondary care. [illegible]

Focus areas to prevent harm

[illegible] Focus areas for patient safety in primary care are listed in Box 28.1.

Box 28.1 Focus areas for patient safety in primary care

[illegible]

Prescribing and medicines management

[illegible] Adverse drug events are more commonly associated with prescribing the following types of medications:

- Cardiovascular medications
- Non-steroidal anti-inflammatory drugs
- Anticoagulants
- [illegible] medication
- Antimicrobial medications

Diagnosis

General practice [illegible] When managing large volumes of minor problems, it is neither feasible nor good practice to investigate every patient to the level where absolute diagnostic certainty can be achieved. Over-investigation is a recognized cause of patient harm.

How can one be safe?

What is safer care?

The context of providing safer care in primary care is different from that of secondary care. Within primary care there is significant heterogeneity of organizational structures: different working structures, systems, and treatment practices; patient care delivered across a wide variety of different sites (e.g. in a consultation room, in a care home, in the patient's home, over the phone, and now, in the COVID-19 era, increasingly via online video platforms). To enable and achieve safer care, it is essential to recognize this context and dynamic environment. Safer care in general practice encompasses an acceptance of the inherent diversity of primary care provision and the adoption of an applicable safety culture by every primary care professional who provides care to all patients all the time.

Focus areas to prevent harm

The approach to patient safety in primary care is holistic and involves the entire patient journey. Focus areas for patient safety in primary care are listed in Box 26.1.

Box 26.1 Focus areas for patient safety in primary care

- prescribing and medicines management;
- diagnosis, misdiagnosis, and delayed diagnosis;
- communication challenges;
- environmental and human factors;
- variation;
- out of hours;
- remote consultation;
- the essence of time.

Prescribing and medicines management

The rate of medication-related error in general practice is high. Repeat prescribing systems, medication reconciliation across care interfaces, and communication around medication use carry an error rate of up to 50%. Medication monitoring is also particularly challenging in the context of increasing multimorbidity and multiple medications. Adverse drug events are more commonly associated with prescribing the following types of medications:

- cardiovascular medications;
- non-steroidal anti-inflammatory drugs;
- anticoagulants;
- hypoglycaemic medication;
- antimicrobial medications.

Diagnosis

General practitioners (GPs) are expert at managing uncertainty in diagnosis. When managing large volumes of minor problems, it is neither feasible nor good practice to investigate every patient to the level where absolute diagnostic certainty can be achieved. Over investigation is a recognized cause of patient harm.

However, it is also incumbent upon GPs to diagnose and appropriately manage more rare serious conditions within this milieu. The rate of diagnostic error in general practice is estimated to be approximately 4%. Diagnostic error can be attributed to one incident in time, for example to the misinterpretation of a laboratory result, or can unfold over weeks or months, with an accumulation of errors. The most common cause for litigation in primary care is failure or delay in diagnosis, particularly for cancer and myocardial infarction in adults and meningitis in children. Common features contributing to diagnostic difficulty include:

- co-morbid illnesses;
- non-specific presentations;
- atypical presentations of the disease;
- very low prevalence of the condition.

Communication

Modern models of healthcare require patients and their data to cross care boundaries regularly, both between providers in primary care and between providers in primary and secondary care. Communication of essential patient data is often suboptimal. Errors can arise in communicating referral and discharge information, investigation requests and results, and medicines reconciliation. Poor and ineffective communication between primary care and the many other elements of the healthcare and social care system are a major source of error and patient safety incidents (see Box 26.2).

Box 26.2 Examples of inadequate communication

- poor communication between professionals;
- poor communication with patients;
- unclear lines of responsibility;
- reliance on automated systems to prevent error;
- inadequate systems to share information about errors, which hampers analysis of causes and improvement strategies;
- fragmented reporting systems;
- lack of coordination, including with secondary care;
- drug names that look or sound alike.

Environmental and human factors (HFE)

As described in the chapter on human factors, there is a growing recognition of the need to consider the stress, fatigue, increasing workload, and burnout that many clinicians experience. These can all contribute to error and potential harm. To address the problem, one needs to apply HFE principles as follows:

- principles related to physical environment such as practice layout, working postures and materials handling;
- principles related to cognitive behaviours such as doctor–computer interaction, decision-making capability, skill levels, mental workload, work stress, and extent of training;
- principles related to organizational systems such as practice culture, supervision, teamwork, and scheduling.

Variation

There is widespread variation in how different conditions are managed across all healthcare sectors, but especially in primary care, given its heterogeneity. Safer care requires the consistent application of best evidence-based practice where appropriate in the care of each individual patient. This can be achieved through the application of reliability theory. The use of care bundles for chronic illnesses such as chronic obstructive pulmonary disease, diabetes, and hypertension, as well as the use of standardized community antimicrobial prescribing guidelines, can assist in reducing unwanted variation.

Out-of-hours work

Care provided in out-of-hours settings is different in many ways from routine general practice. Many out-of-hours care structures provide nurse-led phone triage services and scheduled appointments at centralized care settings. In most cases, the care provider is not the patient's usual GP, and the consultation is more likely to focus on a single presenting complaint. However, as the treating doctor may not have access to comprehensive health and medication records, previous clinical knowledge of the patient, or the opportunity to provide further follow-up care, the level of error is recognized as being considerably higher, with an estimated error rate of 2% to 6% for all out-of-hours consultations.

Remote consultation

With increasing demand on services and changing patient expectations, general practices are increasingly caring for patients via remote consultation (see Box 26.3). This type of consultation can be synchronous (telephone or video call) or asynchronous (email, text message, or instant messenger).

While currently there is a lack of robust data on specific safety concerns related to consultation through these media, tailoring the appropriate medium of consultation to the clinical concern to ensure diagnostic accuracy and timely, effective management is essential. For example, emailing a photograph of a chronic intermittent rash may be safe and could aid diagnosis, but email would not be a suitable or safe means of assessing a patient with central crushing chest pain.

When using electronic media, it is advisable, where possible, to ensure good quality and a fast and reliable connection, in order to optimize communication and enhance the clinician's sensitivity to illness cues (verbal and non-verbal). It is also important to plan how these types of consultations can be safely accommodated and organized during a busy working day.

The essence of time

In general practice, time is often used as both a diagnostic tool and a treatment for illness. Monitoring the evolution of symptoms and of the disease over time is a key management strategy in primary care and often annuls the need to intervene clinically. The use of time in this way aids GPs by helping patients to avoid over investigation and its potential harms, as well as by reducing overtreatment.

In this sense, time and its use are intrinsically linked to both risk and patient safety. Poor management of the dynamic relationship between time, disease, and patient care can contribute to error and patient harm. Different streams of time in primary care called 'tempos' have been proposed to inform how care can be improved and made safer in this real-world context (see Box 26.4).

Box 26.3 Top tips for remote consultation (telemedicine)

Prepare

Ensure a quiet, well-lit room with access to the patient's medical record, a good internet connection, correct contact or link details, and adequate training on the technology to be used.

Begin

Ensure that communication will be adequately clear (quality of sound and video) and that confidentiality will be maintained depending on where the patient is; and assess early whether remote consultation is appropriate (e.g. in view of factors like language barrier or acuity of the presenting complaint).

Consult

Address the camera rather the patient's picture on the screen to enhance rapport; take an appropriate history; assess objectively what you can; and consider asking the patient to perform any reasonable self-tests or examination.

Conclude

Close by sharing decisions for further assessment, treatment, and care as necessary; use a tool such a 'teach back' (see Person-Centred Safety Chapter 4) to ensure adequate understanding and safety in the agreed treatment plan; and complete medical records, prescriptions, and referrals before moving to the next consultation.

Safety issues to consider

- equipment limitations;
- equity of access and barriers to connection;
- the patient's health literacy;
- diagnostic challenges;
- confidentiality.

In primary care, risk is managed over the course of the evolution of the presenting symptoms or during the patient's journey through the healthcare system. Primary care clinicians constantly balance benefit and risk in relation to time so as to maximize benefit for patients. As time proceeds, risk inevitably accrues.

Box 26.4 The impact of time

Disease Tempo	Is based on average disease evolution time. Error arises when disease or treatment effects do not follow the expected time pattern for a given condition, be they too slow or too fast.
Office Tempo	Relates to the organization of working time (e.g. consultation times, interruptions, non-work commitments). Risk arises when the availability or capability of the GP to provide focused care is compromised, often as a result of competing demands.
Patient Tempo	Considers the perspectives and behaviours of individual patients. Risk can increase if patients minimize their symptoms, do not have the same health priorities as their GP, or fail to arrange follow-up as planned.
System Tempo	Comprises the time spent navigating through the healthcare system outside the GP surgery. Patient safety can be compromised if referral pathways are ineffective, if there are unexpected delays in the system, or if communication across care interfaces is suboptimal.
Doctor Tempo	Refers to how time affects the clinical performance of the doctor. Safety can be compromised if the doctor cannot cognitively synthesize all the available information effectively, if knowledge or expertise is not used in the correct way, or if expected steps in examination are neglected.

What do you need to do to be safe?

Three types of intervention can [illegible]

Leadership for a culture of safety

- [illegible] leadership [illegible] safety [illegible] is essential to being able to [illegible]. [illegible] necessary to prioritize [illegible] training [illegible] patient [illegible] development [illegible] primary care [illegible] safety systems [illegible] would [illegible] require strong leadership.

Mitigation

- Mitigated patient safety [illegible] less frequent and less severe harm to patients. [illegible] can be the clinician, the patient, or a family [illegible] that [illegible] mitigation [illegible] quarter of [illegible] events [illegible] for patient safety improvement.

Risk control

- Proactive management of risk will decrease harm. [illegible] at the level of the individual GP or the system.
- [illegible] prescribing [illegible] individual GP [illegible] that [illegible] particular medication be discussed in [illegible] on a weekly basis [illegible] medications [illegible] and discussing high-risk medications [illegible] and interaction in [illegible] settings.
- [illegible] risk control strategy [illegible] individual GP [illegible] number of patients [illegible] under their care [illegible] time.

What do you need to do to be safe?

Three types of interventions can improve safety in primary care.

Leadership for a culture of safety

- The understanding of patient safety theories and methods is essential to being able to deliver safer care. To achieve such understanding, it is necessary to prioritize these areas in postgraduate training curricula and in continuing professional development. Orienting the educational approach in primary care around a culture of safety, safer systems design, and real-world safety application will require strong leadership.

Mitigation

- Mitigated patient safety events result in less frequent and less severe harm to patients. The mitigator can be the clinician, the patient, or a family member. It is estimated that mitigation ameliorates almost a quarter of all harm events and is an often overlooked tool for patient safety improvement.

Risk control

- Proactive management of risk will decrease harm. Risk control strategies can occur at the level of the individual GP or of the system.
- To take prescribing as an example, an individual GP may control risk by insisting that a particular medication be dispensed in fixed amounts on a weekly basis. At a system level, medication risk control may include restrictions around prescribing and dispensing high-tech medications, some medications requiring a prescription or administration in specialist secondary care settings.
- Other examples of risk control strategies are individual GPs capping the number of patients that they will see in a day or the number of patients under their care at any one time.

How do you measure your safety?

Many of the measures that follow have reported excellent [illegible] to drive improvement.

Measures of culture

- [illegible] practice safety climate survey tool [illegible]
  - The climate tool measures safety [illegible] responses [illegible] summary of the team and can be used to [illegible] differences [illegible] concerns within the practice, as well as comparisons with other practices.
- Safety culture maturity, for example the Manchester Patient Safety Framework (MaPSaF).
  - The MaPSaF makes the concept of patient safety culture accessible and enables teams to reflect upon and explore the safety culture within their organization.

Measures of process

- Safety [illegible] to get [illegible] process [illegible] and [illegible] ([illegible]).
  - The safety checklist is a comprehensive systems-based approach aiming to [illegible] existing [illegible] processes [illegible] system [illegible] general [illegible] environment [illegible] everyday [illegible] routines.
- Prescribing quality indicators, e.g. the [illegible] developed by the British [illegible] (PRISCALLA tool).
  - These tools [illegible] identify situations where patients [illegible] potentially unsafe [illegible] and [illegible] can be [illegible] to [illegible] and [illegible] locally and nationally.
- Medicines reconciliation tool, e.g. the National Institute for Health [illegible] (NIHR [illegible]) [illegible] tool.
  - This identifies [illegible] for [illegible] the quality of [illegible] following discharge of a patient from [illegible].
- Patient safety [illegible] (e.g. the Patient-Reported Experiences and Outcomes of Safety in Primary Care (PREOS-PC)).
  - The [illegible] tool assesses patients' experiences of safety in the general practice.

Measures of safety incidents or events

Always events

- A very [illegible] list of practices or behaviours that [illegible] patients and family experience [illegible] implemented consistently. They should be measurable, [illegible] and feasible as part of routine healthcare delivery.

Trigger tool review (see Chapter [illegible], p. [illegible])

- The trigger tool is a [illegible] structured checklist [illegible] to review a random sample of electronic patient files to identify and learn from previously undetected incidents and potential harm events.

How do you measure your safety?

Many of the measures that follow also represent excellent focal points to drive improvement.

Measures of culture

- General practice safety climate survey tools (e.g. GP-SafeQuest):
  - The climate tool measures safety perceptions among all members of the primary care team and can be used to facilitate reflective discussions on safety concerns within the practice, as well as useful comparisons with other practices.
- Safety culture frameworks, for example the Manchester Patient Safety Framework (MaPSaF):
  - The MaPSaF makes the concept of patient safety more accessible and enables teams to reflect upon and explore the safety culture within their organization.

Measures of process

- Safety checklist for general practice (e.g. the monitoring risk and improving system safety (MoRISS) checklist):
  - The safety checklist is a comprehensive systems-based approach aiming to combine existing checking processes into a single checking system within the general practice environment. Ideally it is undertaken every four months.
- Prescribing safety indicators (e.g. the indicators developed by the *British Journal of General Practice* and the PINCER Audit Tool):
  - These indicators identify scenarios where there is potentially unsafe prescribing. They can be adapted for use in individual practices or expanded with online software to allow benchmarking both locally and nationally.
- Medicines reconciliation tool (e.g. the National Institute for Health Research School for Primary Care Research (NIHR-SPCR) Medicines Reconciliation Tool):
  - The medicines reconciliation tool is an audit tool for assessing the quality of medicines reconciliation following discharge of a patient from secondary to primary care.
- Patient safety questionnaire (e.g. the Patient Reported Experiences and Outcomes of Safety in Primary Care (PREOS-PC):
  - The patient survey tool assesses patient experiences of safety in the general practice.

Measures of safety incidents or events

Always events

- Always events are an indicative list of practices or behaviours that encourage optimal patient and family experience when implemented consistently. They should be measurable, deliverable, and feasible as part of routine healthcare delivery.

Trigger tool review (see Chapters 12, 13, and 30) –

- The trigger tool is a simple and quick checklist for screening a small sample of electronic patient files to identify and learn from previously unrecognized risks and potential harm events.

Significant event analysis (SEA)

- The SEA is a team-based systematic approach to identifying and learning from significant occurrences, both positive and negative, in order to improve quality and safety in general practice. Enhanced SEA incorporates and applies human factors principles to this learning (see Box 26.5).

Box 26.5 Significant event analysis

Definition of a significant event

Any event thought by anyone in the team to be significant in the care of patients or in the conduct of the practice.

- Stage 1: Awareness and prioritization of a significant event
- Stage 2: Information gathering
- Stage 3: The facilitated team-based meeting
- Stage 4: Analysis of the significant event

1. What happened?
2. Why did it happen?
3. What has been learned?
4. What has been changed or actioned?

- Stage 5: Agree on, implement, and monitor change
- Stage 6: Write it up
- Stage 7: Report, share, and review

Enhanced significant event analysis

- Enhanced analysis applies human factors principles to the significant event analysis. This enables care providers and care teams to engage with the process more objectively, through greater appreciation of the individual emotional impacts and wider systems influences on significant events.

Never events

Never events are a list of serious but preventable patient safety incidents used to focus on, and drive, safety improvements in general practice. Examples include prescribing a drug to a patient with an allergy to that drug, failing to send a referral for a patient with a suspected diagnosis of cancer, or prescribing a teratogenic drug to a pregnant patient (see Box 26.6).

Box 26.6 Never events in general practice

1. Prescribing a drug that is recorded as having previously caused a significant adverse reaction.
2. Not discussing or arranging emergency transport for a patient deemed to need emergency admission.
3. A clinician's failure to review an abnormal investigation result received by the practice.
4. A referral for a patient with a suspected diagnosis of cancer is not sent.
5. Prescribing a drug with known teratogenic potential to a pregnant patient (unless the prescription is initiated by a clinical specialist)
6. Systemic oestrogen-only hormone replacement therapy prescribed to a patient with an intact uterus.
7. Prescribing methotrexate daily rather than weekly (unless the prescription is initiated by a specialist for a specific clinical indication).
8. Prescribing aspirin for a patient under 12 years of age (unless recommended by a specialist for a specific clinical indication)
9. Adrenaline (or equivalent) is unavailable when needed for a medical emergency in the practice or on a home visit.
10. Failure to dispose of 'sharps' appropriately, resulting in a needlestick injury.

Summary box

Key tips

- Appreciate the unique challenges in providing safe care in primary care, given its complexity and heterogeneity.
- [illegible]
- [illegible]
- [illegible]

Reference

[illegible]

Further reading

[illegible]

Summary box

Top tips

- Appreciate the unique challenges in providing safe care in primary care, given its complexity and heterogeneity.
- Maintain awareness of, draw attention to, and measure known high-risk aspects of primary care and general practice.
- Recognize the role and relationship that time can have with risks to safety in primary care and general practice.
- Apply the theories and tools presented in this chapter towards creating a culture of safety in primary care and general practice.

Reference

The Health Foundation. Evidence scan: Levels of harm in primary care. The Health Foundation, 2011, November. https://www.health.org.uk/publications/levels-of-harm-in-primary-care.

Further reading

Amalberti, R. and Brami, J. 'Tempos' management in primary care: A key factor for classifying adverse events, and improving quality and safety. *BMJ Quality & Safety* 21.9 (2012): 729–36. doi: 10.1136/bmjqs-2011-048710.

Bowie, P., De Wet, C., and Pringle, M. *Significant Event Analysis: Guidance for Primary Care Teams.* NHS Education for Scotland, 2011. http://www.cpdconnect.nhs.scot/media/1362/sea-guidance-for-primary-care-teams.pdf.

de Wet, C., O'Donnell, C., and Bowie, P. Developing a preliminary 'never event' list for general practice using consensus-building methods. *British Journal of General Practice* 64.620 (2014): e159–e167. doi: 10.3399/bjgp14X677536.

Garfield, S. et al. Quality of medication use in primary care: Mapping the problem, working to a solution: A systematic review of the literature. *BMC Medicine* 7.50 (2009). doi: 10.1186/1741-7015-7-50.

Greenhalgh, T., et al. Planning and Evaluating Remote Consultation Services: A New Conceptual Framework Incorporating Complexity and Practical Ethics. *Frontiers in digital health* 3 726095. (2021), doi:10.3389/fdgth.2021.726095

Healthcare Improvement Scotland. Scottish Patient Safety Programme: Primary Care. https://ihub.scot/improvement-programmes/scottish-patient-safety-programme-spsp/spsp-programmes-of-work/spsp-primary-care/

Royal College of General Practitioners. Patient safety toolkit for general practice. RCGP, 2021. https://www.rcgp.org.uk/clinical-and-research/resources/toolkits/patient-safety.aspx.

Singh, H. et al. Identifying diagnostic errors in primary care using an electronic screening algorithm. *Archives of Internal Medicine* 167.3 (2007): 302–8. doi: 10.1001/archinte.167.3.302.

Vincent, C. and Amalberti, R. *Safer Healthcare: Strategies for the Real World.* Springer Open, 2016. https://link.springer.com/book/10.1007%2F978-3-319-25559-0.

Wallace, E. et al. The epidemiology of malpractice claims in primary care: A systematic review. *BMJ Open* 3 (2013): e002929. doi: 10.1136/bmjopen-2013-002929.

Chapter 27

Safety in the emergency department

Key points

The emergency room offers several safety challenges:

- The environment may not be ideal due to overcrowding.
- Patients have varying degrees of acuity that require rapid assessment.
- The tasks required are varied and the clinical staff needs to have a range of skills to complete these tasks.
- Organization culture is important if one is to have situation awareness.
- People's cognitive biases can lead to diagnostic error.
- Solutions require teamwork and effective communication.

What is the safety issue?

Clinical practice in the emergency department contains the same patient safety risks and challenges as all other areas of medicine. However, there are environmental and organizational factors that are specific to emergency medicine and cause unique problems that require bespoke solutions.

A definition of emergency medicine has been suggested by the International Federation of Emergency Medicine: 'A field of practice based on the knowledge and skills required for the prevention, diagnosis and management of acute and urgent aspects of illness and injury affecting patients of all age groups with a full spectrum of undifferentiated physical and behavioural disorders' (https://www.ifem.cc/about-us).

This definition is relevant because it emphasizes that a core component of emergency medicine is the management of undifferentiated patients. An emergency medicine environment requires staff to understand how to diagnose and treat a range of conditions across a range of ages. The risk of cognitive biases, that is, of unknowingly making incorrect decisions through reliance on heuristics, is high. It is not possible to provide complete management in a short period of time in some cohorts of patients, as to do so would structure processes and resources that would be impossible to deliver in any healthcare system.

Clinicians must work with limited information to make appropriate diagnoses in a timely fashion, and then determine which patients need further investigation and treatment and which ones can be discharged to other environments, including their own residence.

In order to do this with large numbers of patients, there need to be systems of triage (ordering of patients by degree of urgency and acuity), rapid assessment, treatment, resuscitation, and risk stratification. Specific to emergency medicine are four factors that impact on the effectiveness and safety of the department regardless of its location in the world (see Figure 27.1).

Crowding

In order to process patients effectively, it is important for the outflow from the department to be high—that is, when a decision to admit or discharge is made, this should happen swiftly. Many hospitals reach their bed capacity very quickly, and therefore there is nowhere to 'bed' patients from the emergency department (inflow being greater than outflow). Patients who remain in the emergency area take up a physical resource (a bed) and a practical resource (clinical staff must continue to care for them while looking after newly arriving patients as well).

Crowding is consistently related to increased mortality rates, which are multifactorial. Crowding is also related to decision-making within the emergency department, which may cause crowding (repeated unnecessary investigations) or be impacted by it (cognitive fatigue). Ultimately crowding demonstrates that flow through the department is not optimized; and flow is essential to ensure processes are safe.

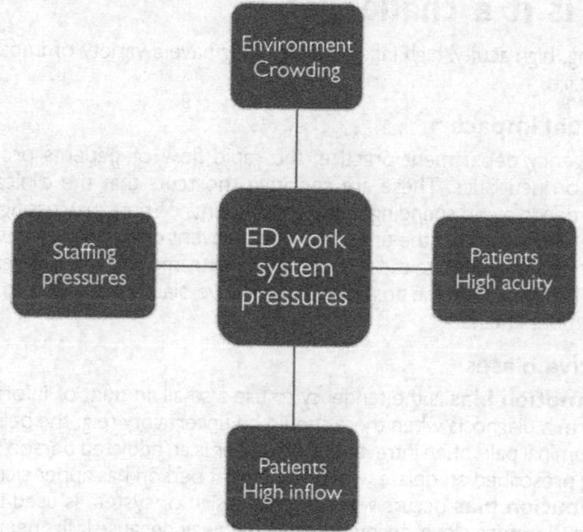

Figure 27.1 Pressures on the emergency department work system.

High acuity

Patients with higher than average acuity may demand increased observation and investigation if they are acutely unwell—with appropriately reversible pathology and therefore greater resource per patient. It is difficult to predict periods of high acuity, but seasonal changes (e.g. a flu epidemic) or mass casualty incidents are common triggers.

High inflow

Attendance per unit time can overwhelm triage and assessment processes, regardless of whether outflow is good. A long time to initial triage can be detrimental, since high-risk patients may not always be visibly unwell but can be at high risk of sudden, unexpected deterioration (e.g. a neonate with a fever).

Staffing

The management of undifferentiated, undiagnosed patients from first principles is very different from the actual experience of in-hospital medicine. Operating at the limit of competence—a situation many staff members assigned to the emergency department will initially find themselves in—places an increased burden on them and requires the presence of a senior decision maker to facilitate the correct patient management. While staffing levels impact all clinical environments in the emergency department, there are also particular dependencies on skilled staff in certain areas. Triage is a particular practice that needs to be performed by a specifically trained staffing group, often according to set protocols and towards the end of the patient's journey in an emergency department. The absence of competent decision makers affects patient flow, and therefore increases crowding.

Why is it a challenge?

Crowding, high acuity, high inflow, and staffing have a variety of impacts on patient care.

Individual impact

In emergency department practice, the rapid flow of patients promotes reliance on heuristics. These are cognitive shortcuts that the clinical staff use in order to avoid spending significant amounts of time processing all the available information all the time; heuristics prevent delays in the delivery of patient care and expedite the flow. They are extremely useful and generally reliable, but introduce the possibility of cognitive biases in the decisions that staff members make.

Cognitive biases

Assumption bias is the tendency to use a small amount of information to confirm a diagnosis when there should be uncertainty (e.g. the belief that the abdominal pain of an intravenous drug user is an addicted person's route to being prescribed an opiate, when in fact that person has appendicitis).

Attribution bias occurs when a specific sign or system is used to confirm, and therefore close, an investigative pathway because it fits neatly with the presenting pattern of the disease that the clinician has in mind. For example, if a person presents with chest pain and the diagnosis is solely considered to be cardiac in origin, without other possibilities considered such as pulmonary embolism. The presence of flow charts and algorithms (thought to improve safety) may have the opposite effect here, encouraging an incorrect patient to be put on the 'correct' pathway.

Diagnostic momentum is also prevalent in patient pathways in the emergency department, especially when the staff are under pressure to see as many patients as possible in a short period of time. The patient with breathing difficulty, chest pain, and a mild elevated temperature is easily placed on a sepsis pathway rather than being worked up properly for the pulmonary embolus he or she actually has.

These cognitive biases increase when internal and external pressures are placed on an emergency department and staff members do not have sufficient time or sufficient access to senior staff to 'sense-check' decisions.

The diversity and complexity of patients and the gruelling shift in patterns to cope with workloads give emergency medicine a higher than average incidence of burnout. Burnout impacts patients' safety through individual disenfranchisement, compassion fatigue, and system resource issues, as members of staff are absent in increasing numbers and rotas struggle to complement.

Finally, unprofessional behaviours are recognized to impact on the quality of care and on patient outcomes, doing moral injury to members of staff. The mixing of specialty groups in emergency departments often causes disputes over the best approach to management with differing attitudes to risk and responsibility. While these issues may be present at any time, during peak demand or when crowding, acuity, and inflow are high, both the emergency department and other hospital staff may display maladaptive behaviours to each other, further decreasing the chance of effective communication.

System factors

Emergency departments have a suite of processes they use to balance the large number of patients who need to be seen by a relatively finite group of staff members. During periods of high acuity or overcrowding, these systems can begin to fail. While escalation policies with defined and measurable end points should be in place for exceptional circumstances, the high-pressure state is increasingly the norm, creating a constant platform for errors to occur. Housing patients in corridors, with significantly long waits until the initial assessment, and managing patients through staff not familiar with their underlying illness both contribute to an increase in mortality when demand exceeds the capacity of the hospital. This creates a patient safety issue at all the levels of potential harm for the individuals involved—patients and providers.

One could mitigate the risk by sharing it throughout the hospital. For example, if the emergency department is housing patients for considerable periods of times (more than 12 hours), all wards in the hospital could take extra patients, even if it meant that their nurse-to-patient ratio is exceeded; in this way the risk would be shared.

How can one be safe?

Several initiatives can be implemented to improve safety and to mitigate the impact of external factors on emergency department flow, over which the department may have little control.

Effective triage and assessment processes

Triage should be a robust process where a small amount of information is used to categorize patients into distinct groups on the basis of how long they can safely wait for until they are seen.

Triage should not be applied if there are sufficient staff members to meet the flow of the patients. Nonetheless, most patients require initial triage and early formal assessment, including initial observations, vital signs, and preliminary details. This assessment process can be used to segment patients so that they are seen by the most appropriate person. This may include a primary care stream for patients who are best managed by general practitioners or family doctors, an injury stream specifically for limb fractures, lacerations, soft tissue injuries, and burns, and a stream for medical issues.

At times of peak demand, when waiting for assessment is prolonged, patients may deteriorate between arrival to the emergency department and assessment. Where pre-hospital treatment has been administered by paramedics, it could normalize previously abnormal observations; then the patient's condition deteriorates as the effect of that treatment wears off (e.g. a febrile, tachycardic patient who has received fluids/antipyretics). Recording the worst observations obtained before hospital onto the observations charts helps to highlight this.

Improved situational awareness using emergency department specific huddles

Safety huddles focus on the general situation in the emergency department, the capacity of the hospital, and the core metrics relevant to patient safety. These metrics include the number of critically ill patients in the resuscitation room, the number of patients awaiting an in-patient bed, the patients deemed to be at high risk of deterioration ('watchers'), and those suitable for discharge but awaiting specific final interventions. The huddle may include only critical staff from different areas of the department who will feed back on focused issues. Improving situational awareness includes the appropriate handover of patients, especially in recognized high-risk areas. The use of full shift systems means that this is an increasingly common occurrence, both within the emergency department and between it and in-patient specialties, and needs to be robust. The use of a SBAR (situation, background, assessment, recommendation) technique or similarly focused communication tools is helpful for ensuring that critical issues are highlighted.

Deployment of specialist practitioners

Emergency medicine was an early adopter of practitioners with focused roles. Advanced care practitioners, often nursing staff that has specific skills in managing illness and injury, are able to expand clinical roles and to provide focused, effective patient care.

Adopting best evidence

Deviation from best practice guidelines is common. The standardization of protocols is important, bearing in mind the risks of cognitive biases. There have been significant improvements in outcomes for specific conditions such as myocardial infarction and stroke by applying set response criteria such as care bundles. A commitment to standardization has led to a supra-regionalization of services whereby patients with certain clinical features are taken only to certain emergency centres. This has proved extremely successful in managing trauma.

Enabling reliability by using a checklist

One of the main problems in an emergency department is ensuring reliable care, that is, ensuring that the processes rehired from registration to triage, assessment, diagnosis, and treatment are followed every time. The emergency department checklist developed in Bristol provides a template that can be adapted by any emergency department (visit www.weahsn.net/ed-checklist). Use of a checklist will standardize care and improve outcomes (see the case studies that follow).

Implementing time-related standards

To ensure that people receive timely care, national standards are often introduced; these limit the amount of time any person spends in an emergency department. Previously 4-hour or 6-hour limits led to significant investment in emergency care and can highlight system issues when the set time is breached. However, this is a blunt tool, as some clinical conditions require a longer workup than others.

Case studies

Examples of emergency medicine-centred innovations

ED Checklist (Bristol)

In order to improve situational awareness in its emergency department, the Bristol Royal Infirmary created a checklist to apply to all patients present there. This checklist ensures that observations have been taken, that any urgent treatments have been delivered, and that specialty teams are aware of the patient. Its introduction led to significant reductions in mortality locally, despite increasing attendances. The challenge is whether this system would be appropriate to roll out in other departments, as this specific approach may not have similar effects in areas with different cultures and working patterns.

West of England Academic health Science Network. Emergency Department Safety Checklist. https://www.weahsn.net/emergency-department-ed-safety-checklist/

Paediatric emergency care

Children and young people have specific health and emotional needs; in particular, they are at risk of harm if exposed to adult patients who may display behaviours not appropriate for children. There are several standards for improving the care of children. They include the use of play specialists, ensuring that children's areas are audio-visually distinct from adult areas, and ensuring the provision of specialist paediatric advice within the department when a threshold of attendances is reached.

Geriatric emergency care

Frail older people are fast emerging as one of the biggest categories of users of emergency care. These people have multiple morbidities and present unique challenges to the traditional 'one person, one problem' approach to managing patients in emergency departments. A frail older person is the personification of a complex system; and 'geriatric syndromes' such as falls, immobility, incontinence, polypharmacy, and other, 'non-specific' presentations are akin to 'emergence' or developing phenomena, as they represent final common pathways in which decompensated frailty tends to present to emergency care. A subsequent systemic inability to deal with complexity makes it common to rely on simplistic approaches for making sense of such presentations and to compartmentalize frailty within typical emergency department pathways. This leads to over-reliance on urine dipstick and much unnecessary testing to strengthen confirmation bias. Poorly studied sensitivity and specificity of many diagnostics in older people leads to both overtreatment and undertreatment.

The 'gold-standard' approach to assessing and managing older people is to do it through 'comprehensive geriatric assessment' (https://doi.org/10.1002/14651858.CD006211.pub3) delivered by multidisciplinary teams. There is little evidence of emergency departments taking on this approach. Stratifying older people in emergency departments through the use of frailty scores allows the delivery of personalized care and reinforces the need for addressing outcomes that matter to the individual. Emergency departments need to develop the right relationships with multidisciplinary teams and to incorporate appropriate processes and resources to deliver person-centred care for frail older people. It is by such means that we can develop safe and high-quality care systems that befit frail older people.

Trauma systems

There is considerable evidence supporting the treatment of patients with significant injuries in departments that are used to dealing with these patients. To ensure that the most appropriately trained staff is available, some emergency departments do not receive such patients, while others become major trauma centres where patients are preferentially taken, even if this means a longer journey. The benefits of this approach are well documented; and there is a similar initiative in stroke and myocardial infarction. In England, the Trauma and Audit Research Network (TARN) is a national organization that collects data on all significant injuries in patients presenting to emergency departments; and TARN has highlighted the importance of specialist and experienced staff being available to improve outcomes.

Summary box

Five key interventions can make a difference in safety in the emergency department

1. Effective triage and assessment processes to ensure rapid recognition of acuity.
2. Improved situational awareness, using emergency department-specific huddles to ensure that everyone knows who is mostly at risk at all times.
3. Deployment of specialist practitioners to meet specific needs of the patients.
4. Adopting best evidence and learning from works.
5. Use of a checklist to improve the reliability of care.
6. Implementing time-related standards so that delays are minimized.

Further reading

Amaniyan, S. et al. Learning from patient safety incidents in the emergency department: A systematic review. *Journal of Emergency Medicine* 58.2 (2020): 234–44. https://doi:10.1016/j.jemermed.2019.11.015.

Ramlakhan, S. et al. The safety of emergency medicine. *Emergency Medicine Journal* 33 (2016): 293–99. http://dx.doi.org/10.1136/emermed-2014-204564.

Chapter 28

Safety in ambulatory care

Key points

- Ambulatory care has been introduced to provide person-centred care in a safe environment and thereby avoid unnecessary admissions to hospital.
- Safety risks include deterioration, lack of adequate facilities and equipment, and lack of robust procedures to ensure safe care.
- The proactive mitigation of risk includes using human factors and reliability theories to design a safe work system and a standardized process of care.
- Good communication is an essential factor in safety in ambulatory care.

What is the safety issue?

The meaning of the term 'ambulatory care' varies in different settings. In this chapter we define ambulatory care units as clinical settings where people who would have historically been admitted to an in-patient bed can be managed as their clinical condition allows. This way of managing such people requires rapid reviews, timely assessments and investigations ideally performed on the same day.

The avoidance of unnecessary admissions will always carry an element of risk, requiring careful management of processes and pathways. These processes must certify that patients are appropriately selected for ambulatory care, as well as managed safely while on the unit.

There are significant gaps in ambulatory safety research, as few studies focus on patient engagement and on accurate diagnosis. Ambulatory care differs substantially from in-patient care, and studies have identified the following points as key safety issues pertinent to ambulatory care (Box 28.1).

Box 28.1 Main safety challenges in ambulatory care

Clinical:
- medication safety and adverse drug events;
- missed or delayed diagnosis;
- treatment delays or lack of preventive services.

Communication and care transition:
- ineffective communication between the patient or the family and the clinical teams;
- the 'communication chain' from patient to GP and the primary care team to speciality referral;
- lack of communication between primary and secondary or tertiary care;
- multiple handoff points on the continuum of care.

Investigations:
- missing laboratory reports, imaging procedures, and consultations;
- separate IT programmes for the unit, the emergency department, and other departments, whose results other teams in the hospital may not be able to access.

Designing a safe unit

The challenge faced when designing for safety is that, despite increasing numbers of patients being managed in ambulatory care settings worldwide, there has been less research and scrutiny into quality and safety in such settings than in high-risk in-patient settings. There may be risks and unintended consequences that are not well recognized. The management of some patients and the assessment of the suitability of patients for ambulatory care may vary among clinicians. Lines of responsibility between multiple clinicians may become blurred. To address this problem, a human factors approach is beneficial when designing the work system, as described in Chapter 11. Careful consideration of the works system and of the agreement of processes is required (see Box 28.2).

Box 28.2 Actions to take in design of the work system in ambulatory care

Organization

- communication to all about the unit and its purpose;
- scope and function of the unit specified;
- limitations: inclusion and exclusion criteria clearly defined;
- safety culture enhanced.

Process

- standard operating procedures agreed and followed;
- referral pathways agreed with all stakeholders;
- management of out-of-hours referrals;
- clear processes for the transfer or redirection of patients who attend, but are not safe to stay in the environment;
- safety net provisions in the event of a deterioration in patients.

People

- engagement and co-design with patients, to manage expectations;
- appropriate skills in staffing.

Tools and technology

- These should be equipped to manage expected clinical conditions.

Tasks

- All staff should be skilled enough to undertake the procedures and the monitoring.

Environment and location

- The environment should be designed to be safe and the people should be friendly.
- A common model is to co-locate with an acute medical unit or an emergency department.

Measurable outcomes

- The unit measures process and outcomes as well as staff and patient satisfaction and experience.

How can one be safe?

Maintaining safety in a constantly developing and evolving service is often difficult and needs to have clear systems and operational policies in place to communicate and document procedures and ensure that the staff can follow these to maintain patient safety. The key areas of safety are patient selection and standardized processes (see Box 28.3).

Box 28.3 Key safety intervention

- Select the right patients.
- Standardize the process.
- Ensure governance and management and measure the outcomes.
- Communicate and engage stakeholders and clinical teams.
- Implement safety huddles.
- Know the safety risks and address them proactively.

Select the right patients

While this action may differ in different organizations, the general principles are available.

- Generally, patients should be mobile or able to sit in a waiting room and should have had an assessment to ensure they are not critically unwell.
- Various tools are in use to assess the suitability of patients for ambulatory care, for example the AMB Score (Ala et al, 2012:420) or the Glasgow Admission Prediction Score (Cameron et al. 2015:174) Many hospitals will use these assessments differently, but a tool or an assessment and screening technique should be chosen by each organization, so that the ambulatory care team and referrers may follow a standardized process.
- Depending on the location and environment of the ambulatory care unit, consideration also needs to be given to particular patient groups and to their suitability for the ambulatory care environment. Examples of suitable patients are those with mental health conditions or who are intoxicated, since the environment may not be appropriate to maintain staff safety in their presence.

Standardize the processes

There are increasing numbers of disease-specific guidelines published by national societies with the intention of helping to identify patients suitable for potential ambulatory management. Here are a few examples:

- the British Thoracic Society guideline published for the initial out-patient management of pulmonary embolis;
- the out-patient management of deep vein thrombosis (DVT);
- uncomplicated pyelonephritis in selected patients;
- the management of cellulitis.

Each pathway should outline clear exclusion and inclusion criteria for patients. There should also be an agreed integrated pathway that details the diagnostic, follow-up arrangements, and the lines of responsibility in each case. For example, the use of OPAT (out-patient parenteral antimicrobial therapy) is well described, with clear specifications for any class, dosing, and duration of antibiotics, microbiologist and pharmacist oversight, and community nursing and primary care support. These pathways should be clear and communicated to all relevant parties.

Ensure governance and measurement

The governance of the ambulatory care unit must have a forum to discuss issues and challenges, to develop standardized operating procedures, and to measure adherence to these procedures and the clinical outcomes. The safety measures could include waiting times for assessment or treatment and the proportion of patients admitted as in-patients from ambulatory care. This would give an overview of the efficiency and safety of the unit. It would assist in highlighting, and thereby reducing, inappropriate referrals and reviews and would ensure that governance is maintained, so as to minimize delays in diagnosis and treatment and monitor any deviance from agreed pathways and standards. The measurement of processes and outcomes is routine.

Communicate and engage stakeholders and clinical teams

It is essential to ensure that the staff in the organization is aware of the operational procedures, referral criteria, and measurements of the ambulatory care service. This will reduce the element of risk and will prevent inappropriate referrals to the unit.

Implement safety huddles

Safety huddles can increase situation awareness on the unit and will allow for safety and flow issues to be addressed proactively. This will lower the complexity of the additional steps in communication in ambulatory care and will define the roles and responsibilities. A brief meeting at the start of a shift, clinical huddles during the shift, and a debriefing session at the end of the shift will improve communication and reduce medical errors.

Summary box

- Ambulatory emergency care comes with its own distinct and specific challenges for managing safety.
- Managing patients on the same day and avoiding unnecessary admissions is always a risk, which should be carefully managed through sensible patient selection and clearly defined pathways and processes. These should highlight roles and responsibilities.
- A clear governance structure and a process of communication and engagement of key stakeholders are also imperative if we want to ensure a smooth running service with minimal risk to staff or patients.
- Given the busy environment of ambulatory care and the heightened potential for communication errors, a 'brief—huddle—debrief' model can reduce harm by increasing situation awareness.

References

Ala, L. et al. Selecting ambulatory emergency care (AEC) patients from the medical emergency intake: The derivation and validation of the Amb score. *Clinical Medicine* 12.5 (2012): 420–6.

Cameron, A. et al. A simple tool to predict admission at the time of triage. *Emergency Medical Journal* 32 (2015): 174–9.

Further reading

Webster, J. S. et al. Understanding quality and safety problems in the ambulatory environment: seeking improvement with promising teamwork tools and strategies. In K. Henriksen et al. (eds), *Advances in Patient Safety: New Direction and Alternative Approaches, vol. 3: Performance Tools.* Rockville, MD: Agency for Healthcare Research and Quality, 2008. http://www.ncbi.nlm.nih.gov.

Chapter 29

Safety in the operating theatre

Key points

- The operating room (theatre) is a complex adaptive system that presents risk for staff and patients.
- The application of reliability, human factors, and resilience theories can assist proactively in decreasing the risk to patients.
- Psychological safety is an essential component of a safe surgical team.
- Non-technical skills (human factors) and social cognitive and personal resource management are important to developing safe care.
- Teamwork, communication, and situation awareness are essential to delivering high-quality patient care.
- Care bundles and checklists can improve safety.
- Designing the environment facilitates safe care.

What is the problem?

- Surgery involves complex and high-risk procedures.
- The potential for error is high and adverse events are common.
- Near misses are more frequent than errors with serious consequences.
- Surgical site infection rates vary between different subspecialties.
- Never events, such as wrong site surgery and retained foreign bodies, occur in surgery because of process errors.

Box 29.1 Case study: The wrong kidney

- A 65-year-old man, otherwise fit, with a painful, non-functioning right kidney was scheduled for a nephrectomy.
- During the consent process the registrar incorrectly indicated the patient for a left nephrectomy.
- The registrar was not in the operating room for the operation.
- In the operating room the consultant checked the scan, but it was inverted.
- A junior nurse and a medical student in the theatre realized that the surgeon was operating on the wrong side but did not speak up.
- After a prolonged stay on intensive care, the patient died.

Why do things go wrong?

The operating room is a highly complex system with multiple interdependent procedures. While some of these processes can be standardized, others are too complex to be made completely reliable. [illegible]

Unfortunately, adverse events can and do still occur, and many of their causes have risks. While it may be impossible to eliminate them entirely, the goal should be to minimize their probability and to learn when errors and harm occur in order to reduce the chance of the same [illegible] happening.

Non-technical skills are important in the delivery of safe surgical care. The non-technical skills that have been identified as contributing to safety and efficiency in the operating room are:

- social: [illegible] communication, teamwork, leadership
- cognitive: [illegible] decision-making and situation awareness
- personal resource skills: [illegible] stress and coping with fatigue.

These skills can be assessed [illegible] (see Chapter [illegible] on human factors), which provides a framework [illegible] the system factors in the organization and work that can affect safety adversely (see Figure 22.1).

In Table 22.1 an analysis of the [illegible] framework [illegible] is demonstrated.

Table 22.1 Application of [illegible] to the operating theatre

[illegible]	Factors [illegible]
Organizational [illegible]	[illegible] [illegible] communication [illegible] [illegible] [illegible]
[illegible] factors	[illegible] [illegible] [illegible] [illegible]
[illegible] factors	[illegible] [illegible] [illegible] [illegible]
[illegible]	[illegible] [illegible] [illegible] [illegible]
[illegible]	[illegible] [illegible] [illegible]

Why do things go wrong?

The operating room is a highly complex system with multiple interdependent processes. While some of these processes can be standardized, others are too complex to be made completely reliable.

Unfortunately not all adverse events can be predicted, as all medical procedures have risks. While it may not be possible to eliminate human error, the goal should be to minimize risk proactively and to learn when errors and harm occur, in order to reduce the chance of the same errors reoccurring.

Non-technical skills are important in the delivery of safe surgical care. The non-technical skills that have been identified as contributing to safety and efficiency in the operating room are:

- social skills of communication, teamwork, leadership;
- cognitive skills of decision-making and situational awareness;
- personal resource skills of managing stress and coping with fatigue.

These skills can be assessed within the SEIPS model described in Chapter 9 on human factors, which provides a framework for examining the system factors in the operating room work that can affect safety adversely (see Figure 29.1).

In Table 29.1 an analysis of the risks in the work system is demonstrated.

Table 29.1. Application of SEIPS 2.0 to the operating room

Work System	Factors Impacting on Safety
Organization/ Team Factors (Culture)	Poorly functioning team: 'we don't get on' Steep hierarchy preventing good communication: in the example, the junior members of staff did not feel they could speak up Checklist becoming a tick box exercise Silo working
Patient Factors	Unknown allergies Unexpected anatomy and disease process Abnormal clotting Poor functional baseline Comorbidities such as heart failure, sepsis, lung disease
Staff Factors	'Simple' mistakes (slips) leading to a never event: in the example, the registrar wrote the wrong side on the consent form New team members (locums) Reduced individual resilience (tiredness, distraction, inexperience)
Environmental Factors	System factors/ergonomics Poor room layout Distraction (talking in theatre, interruptions)
Tools and Equipment	Equipment that is confusing to use Equipment that is not available
Tasks	Tasks beyond the team's capability Complexity of the tasks that require integrated teamwork

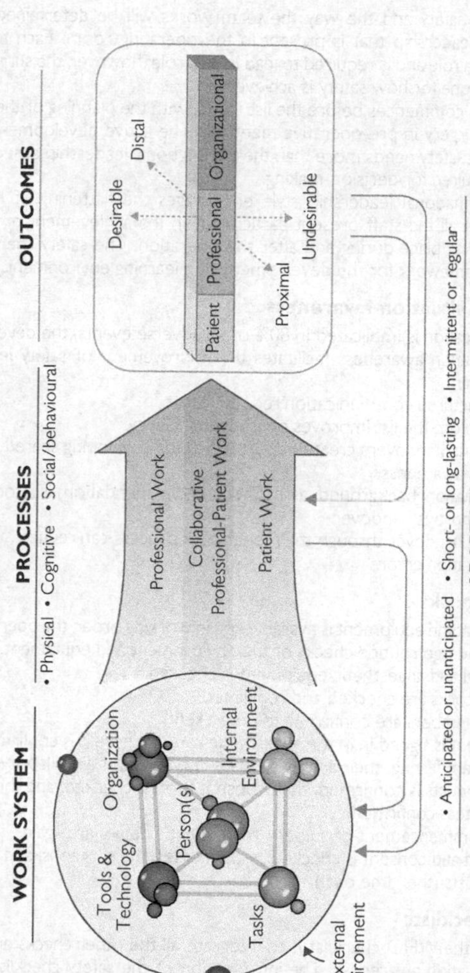

Figure 29.1 SEIPS 2.0 (Reproduced with permission from Holden et al. (2013)).

Interventions to mitigate harm

Leadership

A culture of safety and the way the team works will be determined by the type of leadership that is present in the operating room. Each team member has a role and is required to lead in that role; however, the surgeon may set the tone for how safety is achieved.

Leadership commences before the list starts, with the planning of the list and of the surgery in pre-operative meetings. The active development of psychological safety needs more than the transactional leadership based on the tasks required for decision-making.

A transformational leadership style encourages the flattening of hierarchy, so that all the staff present participates in the achievement of safe care. This takes place during and after the operation. The safety checklist provides a framework for the development of a learning environment.

Improving situation awareness

As communication is implicated in 80% of all adverse events, the development of situation awareness facilitates the improvement of safety in the operating room.

- Clear, structured communication reduces error.
- Briefing before the list improves operative efficiency.
- Briefings and handovers create opportunities for developing shared situational awareness.
- SBAR (situation, background, assessment, recommendation) is a tool that can improve handover.
- Verifying a handover through the repeat-back process can reduce communication error.

Routine checks

To ensure that the equipment is available and in working order, the operating room will undergo routine checks of the environment and equipment.

- All surgical and anaesthetic equipment is checked.
- All drug stocks are checked and confirmed.
- All staff members are confirmed to be present.
- Each patient is signed in in the anaesthetic room, where it is confirmed that they are fasting, their allergy status is confirmed, the availability of blood products is confirmed, their consent form is checked, and the surgical site is confirmed.
- Before commencement of surgery, the patient's details are again confirmed and consent is checked by the nurses, the surgeons, and the anaesthetists (the 'time out').

Safety checklists

The aim of the WHO checklist is to integrate all the other checks and to facilitate situation awareness. The introduction of the safety checklist has had a major impact on the reduction of safety events. A study published in the NEJM in 2009 demonstrated a significant reduction in mortality with a three-stage checklist coupled with team training and briefings. This checklist is a tool that requires attendance and the active participation of every member of the team in the operating room, no matter the seniority. The checklist will identify actions that may need to be taken to improve safety. To be effective, it requires training and a culture of safety.

While there are different versions, the basic steps are the five ones indicated in Table 29.2.

Table 29.2. Five steps to safer surgery

Step	When	Content
Briefing	Before the start of the list, or for each patient if staff changes	• Introduction of team and designation of individual roles • Order of the list; potential breaks • Anticipated issues • Concerns relating to staff/equipment/surgery/anaesthesia
Sign in	Before anaesthetic is administered	• Confirm patient/procedure/consent form • Allergies • Airway issues • Anticipated blood loss • Machine/medication check • Surgical site check
Time out	Before the start of the surgery	• Team member introduction • Verbal confirmation of patient information • Surgical/anaesthetic/nursing issues • Surgical site infection bundle • Thromboprophylaxis • Imaging available
Sign out	Before the staff leaves the OR	• Confirmation of recording of procedure: instruments, swabs, and sharps correct • Specimens correctly labelled • Equipment issues addressed • Postoperative management discussed and handed over
Debriefing	End of the list	• Evaluate list performance • Learn from any incidents that occurred • Remedy problems, eg equipment failure

Adapted from Vickers 2011.

People-related factors

Human beings are the most important defence against error. However, their mistakes significantly contribute to a high proportion of errors. This being so, their individual performance and how the wider team affects them are key to safety. Here are some of the factors that affect performance.

- Tiredness due to the lack of sleep has an effect on human performance. It may result from extended work hours or to home circumstances.

- External stress, for example relationship and financial problems, can impact work performance.
- The safety climate and safety culture of the operating team present in the room will affect how staff members think and behave. Psychological safety is essential: it guarantees that the fallibility of senior staff is acknowledged; it encourages questioning; and staff members are asked to look out for potential safety risks.
  - Performance is higher in supportive environments.
  - The behavior of senior members of the team sets the climate.
- Learning from mistakes is important. However, learning from situations in which things go well (i.e. learning from excellence) creates a more positive conversation.

Team-related factors

The way the team functions is important to effectiveness and safety in the operating theatre. Teams may develop organically; however, safe clinical teams often require planning and training.

In high reliability organizations the development of safe teams is not taken for granted and training is considered mandatory. Such training will include ensuring that senior staff members are able to mentor and coach within the concept of psychological safety, that simulation is routine, and that teams learn together. Skills and assessments are standardized. Methods to improve team performance include:

- assessment of team performance using non-technical skills assessments;
- human factors team training using programmes such as crew resource management (CRM);
- team training such as TeamSTEPPS, which may improve team performance.

Design of the operating room and ergonomics

The design of the operating room uses the principles of human factors and ergonomics to ensure that the layout of the room and the equipment used are optimal for performance and for the safety of all healthcare workers. A tidy and well-designed operating room will enhance a safely operating theatre.

Here are some environmental factors that may challenge safe surgery:

- The physical size of operating rooms can be a limiting factor, as newer equipment is large and takes up space, leaving theatres cramped.
- Increasing amounts of electrical equipment and electrical cables running across floors are a trip hazard for all staff.
- The location of the theatre may be suboptimal and can be isolated. For example, new procedures may result in new venues for interventions: interventional radiology, catheter laboratories, endoscopy suites. When things go wrong, help is far away.
- The availability of computers and screens in the room to display essential imaging during surgery may be limited, or, as an add on, these machines may be in suboptimal positions. For example, the height of video displays when performing laparoscopic operations affects performance and can cause musculoskeletal injury.

- The height of the operating table is also important. Theatre staff members are most comfortable and effective when the elbow joint is bent by 100 to 120 degrees, that is, with the hands slightly below the elbow. If possible, sitting while operating reduces shoulder and neck pain.
- Optimal room temperature and avoidance of distractions will improve performance.

Care bundles for reliability

Care bundles, as described in Chapter 10, bring together evidence-based practice to ensure reliability in care delivery, for the prevention of an undesired outcome. The surgical site infection care bundle is an example of how a multidisciplinary team must work together to prevent the surgical site from getting infected.

There are key elements in the bundle, each of which is the responsibility of a different member of the team (see Table 29.3).

Table 29.3. Surgical site infection prevention

Responsible	Action
Surgeon	**Identification:** person at risk when booking surgery
Ward staff	**No shaving:** in preparation for surgery, to decrease micro spread of bacteria
OR staff	**Hypoglycaemia:** prevention, therefore delay fasting and attend to delays in operating lists
OR staff	**Hypothermia:** prevention
Anaethetist and surgeon	**Antibiotic administration:** in the 30 minutes before knife to skin
Surgeon and surgical team	**Aseptic technique** and use of chlorhexidine at opening and closure of incision

https://pathways.nice.org.uk/pathways/prevention-and-control-of-healthcare-associated-infections#path=view%3A/pathways/prevention-and-control-of-healthcare-associated-infections/preventing-and-treating-surgical-site-infections.xml&content=view-index

The use of statistical control charts has demonstrated that the reliable application of the bundle can decrease infection rates.

How do you measure safety?

The measurement of safety requires a multifaceted approach to the patient's journey, from the moment of the decision for surgery until at least thirty days after surgery (see Table 29.4).

Table 29.4. Measuring safety in the operating room

Type of measure	Type of measures	Measure
Outcome measure	1. Unplanned return for same procedure 2. Surgical Site infection 3. Mortality 4. Incident rates	1. Number or number per surgery performed 2. Days since last; or rate per surgeon, per organization 3. Rate within 30 days of surgery 4. Ratio of minor to major incidents
Process measure	1. Waiting list for surgery 2. Cancelled surgeries 3. Operating room utilization time 4. Waiting time for surgeons 5. Start time of operations 6. Surgical checklist 7. Time antibiotic given	1. This is an indication of the performance of the system 2. Number of cancelled surgeries for non-clinical reasons 3. Ratio of time spent by patients in OR to total OR time available 4. Length of time spent by surgeons waiting prior to the start of scheduled surgeries 5. Percentage of lists that start within 15 minutes of scheduled time 6. An all or nothing measure, completed in full with all staff present. 7. Percentage of antibiotics given in full within 30 minutes of start of surgery
Patient centric	1. Measures of pain 2. Post-operative delirium 3. Starvation time	1. Patient reported pain scores 2. Patient reported delirium rates 3. Waiting time of patient prior to the start of their scheduled or urgent surgeries.
Team measures	Safety climate/ culture Team working	Different ways of assessing both (as in Chapter 4)

Summary box

References

Further reading

Summary box

1. Leaders demonstrating the importance of briefings and checklists.
   - If the lead surgeon conducts the first checklist effectively, this will set the tone for the rest of the day.
2. Involving all staff in the briefing.
3. Creating psychological safety by flattening the hierarchy and encouraging staff to speak up.
4. Team training improves team resilience.
   - This can and should include the team's socializing together.
5. Getting the room ergonomics right.
6. Developing individual resilience.
   - Supporting staff with well-being: During long cases, take a break.
7. Learning from positives and not just from previous mistakes.
8. Using safety culture surveys and learning from the results.

Reference

Holden, R. J. et al. SEIPS 2.0: A human factors framework for studying and improving the work of healthcare professionals and patients. *Ergonomics* 56.11 (2013): 1669–86. https://doi.org/10.1080/00140139.2013.838643.

Vickers, R. Five steps to safer surgery. *Annals of the Royal College of Surgeons of England* 93.7 (2011): 501–3. http://doi:10.1308/147870811X599334.

Further reading

Guidance

NICE. Perioperative care in adults. NG180, August 2020. https://www.nice.org.uk/guidance/ng180/chapter/Recommendations

Incidents

Bosma, E., Veen, E. J., and Roukema, J. A. Incidence, nature and impact of error in surgery. *British Journal of Surgery* 98.11 (2011): 1654–9. http://doi:10.1002/bjs.7594

DiCuccio, M. H. The relationship between patient safety culture and patient outcomes: A systematic review. *Journal of Patient Safety* 11.3 (2015): 135–42. http://doi:10.1097/PTS.0000000000000058.

Hyman, N. Nature, causes and consequences of unintended events in surgical units. *British Journal of Surgery* 97.11 (2010): 1730–40. http://doi:10.1002/bjs.7204.

Human factors

Holden, R. J. et al. SEIPS 2.0: A human factors framework for studying and improving the work of healthcare professionals and patients. *Ergonomics* 56.11 (2013): 1669–86. http://doi:10.1080/00140139.2013.838643.

Leadership

Hu, Y. Y. et al. Surgeons' leadership styles and team behavior in the operating room. *Journal of the American College of Surgeons* 222.1 (2016): 41–51. http://doi:10.1016/j.jamcollsurg.2015.09.013

Stone, J. L. et al. Effective leadership of surgical teams: A mixed methods study of surgeon behaviors and functions. *Annals of Thoracic Surgery* 104.2 (2017): 530–7. http://doi:10.1016/j.athoracsur.2017.01.021.

Checklist

Bethune, R. et al. Use of briefings and debriefings as a tool in improving team work, efficiency, and communication in the operating theatre. *Postgraduate Medical Journal* 87.1027 (2011): 331–4. http://doi:10.1136/pgmj.2009.095802.

Haynes, A. B. et al. A surgical safety checklist to reduce morbidity and mortality in a global population. *New England Journal of Medicine* 360.5 (2009): 491–9. http://doi:10.1056/NEJMsa0810119.

Treadwell, J. R., Lucas, S., and Tsou, A. Y. Surgical checklists: A systematic review of impacts and implementation. *BMJ Quality & Safety* 23 (2014):299–318. http://dx.doi.org/10.1136/bmjqs-2012-001797.

Teams

AHRQ. TeamSTEPPS. n.d. https://www.ahrq.gov/teamstepps/index.html.

Gross, B. et al. Crew resource management training in healthcare: A systematic review of intervention design, training conditions and evaluation. *BMJ Open* 9 (2019): e025247. doi: 10.1136/bmjopen-2018-025247.

Hull, L. and Sevdalis, N. Advances in teaching and assessing nontechnical skills. *Surgical Clinics of North America* 95.4 (2015): 869–84. http://doi:10.1016/j.suc.2015.04.003

Li, N. et al. Systematic review of methods for quantifying teamwork in the operating theatre. *BJS Open* 2.2 (2018): 42–51. http://doi:10.1002/bjs5.40.

Pronovost. P. J. and Freischlag, J. A. Improving teamwork to reduce surgical mortality. *JAMA* 304.15 (2010): 1721–2. http://doi:10.1001/jama.2010.1542.

Sevdalis, N., Hull, L., and Birnbach, D. J. Improving patient safety in the operating theatre and perioperative care: Obstacles, interventions, and priorities for accelerating progress. *British Journal of Anaesthetics* 109 Suppl. 1 (2012): i3–i16. http://doi:10.1093/bja/aes391.

Surgical site infection

Phelan, L. et al. Evaluation of a bundle of care to reduce incisional surgical site infection after gastrointestinal surgery. *Journal of Infection Prevention* 21.2 (2020): 52–9. http://doi:10.1177/1757177419892072.

Williams, V. and Leis, J. A. Applying rigour to the interpretation of surgical site infection rate. *BMJ Quality & Safety* 29 (2020): 446–8. http://dx.doi.org/10.1136/bmjqs-2019-009964.

Measurement

Ilieş, I. et al. Large-scale empirical optimisation of statistical control charts to detect clinically relevant increases in surgical site infection rates. *BMJ Quality & Safety* 29 (2020): 472–81. http://dx.doi.org/10.1136/bmjqs-2018-008976.

Russ, S. et al. Measuring safety and efficiency in the operating room: Development and validation of a metric for evaluating task execution in the operating room. *Journal of the American College of Surgeons* 216.3 (2013): 472–81. http://doi:10.1016/j.jamcollsurg.2012.12.013

Chapter 30

Safety in paediatrics and child health

Key points

- Safety in paediatrics requires a focus on providing highly reliable, effective care and reducing avoidable harm in both lower-income countries, where the emphasis is on neonatal care, and higher-income countries, where hospital care is increasingly complex as a result of preventable harm.
- Safety is a challenge in paediatrics because children present four main differences from adults—namely in development, in dependence, in differential epidemiology, and in demographics.
- Most of the preventable harm is related to medication, deterioration, sepsis, and hospital-acquired infections. Early warning systems, care bundles, and other frontline tools and initiatives outlined here can help to reduce harm and improve situation awareness.
- A multidisciplinary approach to safety—one based on human factors principles and supported by a culture of patient–parent engagement—is crucial.
- The paediatric trigger tool is a useful way to measure harm and identify areas for improvement.
- Multisite collaborative improvement networks are a good starting point for improving paediatric patient safety.

What are the key safety issues in paediatrics?

When one considers paediatric patient safety, one needs to look at it in the context of where the child lives. Globally, according to the World Health Organization, the under-five mortality rate has dropped from 93 deaths per 1,000 live births in 1990 to 38 per 1,000 in 2019. (https://www.who.int/data/gho/data/themes/topics/topic-details/GHO/child-mortality-and-causes-of-death). This is largely due to public health measures that focus on conditions that can be prevented or treated with access to immunization, oral rehydration, and safe water. Now, nearly half of the deaths of children under the age of five worldwide occur during the neonatal period, which makes safe childbirth and effective neonatal care an important safety aim.

In high-income countries, the key safety goals concentrate around reducing preventable deaths and harm in paediatric hospital departments, where care is provided in an increasingly complex environment. The 2007 UK CEMACH report 'Why Children Die' found preventable factors in 26% of reviewed cases. These factors were predominantly related to poor communication and delayed recognition of the condition of the deteriorating child—mainly sepsis. Children are at an increased risk of adverse events from medication.

Safer care means that children receive appropriate, evidence-based care the first time and every time, in the right environment. This includes attention to psychological safety. The focus should be on providing highly reliable care to all children, in the higher- and lower-income countries alike, and on preventing avoidable harm.

Harm can be defined as anything that one would not like to happen to oneself, one's own child, or a member of one's family. (Chapman, 2014:2) This allows us to take a broad view of harm. For example, in the hospital environment, harm ranges from ventilator-acquired pneumonia to multiple failed attempts at cannulation or inadequate psychological support; in the community, it may extend over the poor control of diabetes, failures to identify child protection concerns, or inappropriate equipment for children with neurodisability. Examples of preventable harm are shown in Box 30.1.

Box 30.1 Preventable harm in paediatrics

- medication error (especially dosing errors and administration);
- failure to recognize deterioration;
- failure to recognize sepsis and other life-threatening illness early;
- hospital-acquired infections (e.g. central line infections);
- preventable pain and distress;
- tissue injury from extravasation or pressure ulcer;
- failure to recognize early and manage procedural or surgical complications;
- failure to recognize safeguarding concerns early;
- unnecessary admissions, investigations, procedures, and treatments;
- psychological harm or not providing a positive experience of healthcare

Adapted from Fitzsimons and Vaughan 2015.

Why is it a challenge?

Children have changing physiology as they develop and cannot be treated as 'little' adults. The following differences are key factors that influence safety in paediatrics.

The harm listed here is mostly related to hospital paediatrics, and it is important to recognize that there is relatively little research into the burden of harm that occurs in the home or in community settings. Incidents in primary care are under-reported, and there is a need for improved communication and listening skills when providing healthcare to children. The National Patient Safety Agency has already signalled both a lack of recognition and appropriate management of mental health issues in young people and the lack of an integrated approach to children's risk management—an approach that should incorporate health, education and social care.

Difference in children: the four Ds	Potential impact on safety
Development: Children go through different developmental physiological stages Size Weight Physiology Psychology	Clinicians often do not have knowledge of child development There is a range of equipment needed as a result of growth Vital signs (heart rate, blood pressure) are dependent on the child's age and height Drug dosing is dependent on weight Drug metabolism is dependent on age The margin of error in diagnosis and treatment is smaller than in adults The child's ability to understand and communicate varies
Dependency: Children rely on adults to advocate for them and often cannot speak up for themselves	Difficulty identifying parental concerns or failure to act upon these concerns Poor communication between clinicians, both within teams (handover) and between specialist and community healthcare professionals Poor communication with patients and their parents or carers Lack of focus by clinicians on the child's mental health Listening to the voice of the child if there are safeguarding concerns

Difference in children: the four Ds	Potential impact on safety
Differential epidemiology: Children suffer from different diseases at different ages	Adult-trained health providers often provide care with little knowledge of the disease spectrum and the changing needs of a child There is resultant missed diagnoses and undetected deterioration Paediatric healthcare is often provided in adult-oriented facilities, with lack of training and inappropriate equipment Children with chronic illness and special healthcare needs are at a higher risk of harm in hospital settings Mental health services for children and young people are under resourced or absent Provision and clinician experience of adolescent health are lacking
Demographics: Children are impacted by social determinants of health	Poverty, war, ethnicity, economic crises, and natural disasters impact children Educational settings provide an important access to healthcare and to the identification of safeguarding concerns

How can one be safe?

Safe care in paediatrics relies on integrated care with clinical leadership and a culture of patient–parent engagement, governance, teamwork, and education. Crucial also to creating a culture of safety is knowledge of, and capability for, safety and quality improvement.

A systems approach to safety for children is essential; where possible, the design of the work system should take human factors principles and standardizing processes into account.

Interventions to reduce harm

Four key safety dangers for children in healthcare account for most of the harm experienced by children (see Box 30.2).

Box 30.2 Main safety dangers
- medication harm;
- deterioration;
- sepsis;
- hospital-acquired infections.

Safety initiatives aimed at reducing medication error, improving the recognition of deterioration, recognizing and managing sepsis early on, and reducing hospital-acquired infections (preventable harm 1–4) are outlined below. All initiatives require a multidisciplinary approach, with the engagement of children, young people, and their families and carers. Increasingly, information technology will help to support safety interventions such as decision support rules for e-prescribing drug dosing schedules and order sets (with guideline reminders), or alerts of early warning scores. There are also initiatives to improve communication with children and young people, such as the 'Me First' communication model (visit http://www.mefirst.org.uk/the-model).

Interventions to reduce medication harm (Chapters 20 and 21)

Children are at risk of medication error because drug dosing is weight- or age-dependent and errors in prescribing (including information technology or e-prescribing) are common. There are often errors in the dispensing or administration of drugs and in medicines reconciliation. A multi-disciplinary approach is crucial if we want to reduce the harm caused by medication errors. This requires a focus on the safe prescribing, dispensing, and preparation of medication (both in hospital and in the community) and on medicine administration (Box 30.3).

Strategies to improve recognition of deterioration (Chapter 24)

Children are at risk of deteriorating quickly, and early intervention is crucial. Early warning systems are a means of identifying deterioration to prevent intensive care admission or cardio-respiratory arrest. This is especially important in children, since it is well recognized that children who have died or required intensive care have shown signs of physiological or behavioural disturbance in the period before collapse.

Box 30.3 Interventions to decrease medication harm

- checking of drug prescriptions by a paediatric pharmacist and identification of errors;
- dedicated prescribing desks with paediatric formulary to reduce interruptions;
- use of electronic paediatric drug calculators;
- electronic prescribing, and use of protocols and checklists;
- feedback to prescribers on errors, empowering all members of a multidisciplinary team (MDT) to identify errors;
- guidelines on administration techniques;
- double-checking of drug dose, concentration, and route;
- accurate patient identification;
- engagement of parents and carers in medicine reconciliation;
- use of patient hand-held medication records;
- increase in the reporting and measuring of, and learning from, medication incidents.

(Also see Chapter 21)

Situation awareness is crucial to reducing unrecognized deterioration, and it can be improved through regular multidisciplinary safety huddles (Chapter 8). The aim is to anticipate deterioration and to mitigate it as needed, by continually predicting the clinical course of the child and by taking the views of all involved into account, including those of parents and families (visit www.rcpch.ac.uk/SAFE). Parents and carers are often the first to recognize changes in their child's behaviour and signs of deterioration. The factors that can prevent deterioration are presented in Box 30.4.

Box 30.4 Five important factors that help to prevent deterioration

1. Family concerns should always be taken seriously, even if vital signs are normal.
2. High-risk therapies raise the risk and make the child a potential candidate for deterioration.
3. Presence of an elevated early warning score is a marker, though it is not always present.
4. Special attention needs to be paid if any member of staff senses that the child is 'not right'. The patient is termed to be a "Watcher'—a patient who needs added attention as there is an undefined risk of deterioration.
5. Concerns about communication with the patient, the parent, or the family are discussed (e.g. they speak a different language from yours and your team's).

Source: Brady et al. 2013.

Systems to recognize and manage sepsis early (Chapter 23)

Globally it is estimated that almost 60% of deaths in children under 5 years can be attributed to sepsis. Children still die of sepsis in the hospital environment in developed countries, but early recognition and aggressive management in a time-critical manner can improve the outcome.

Paediatric sepsis is often difficult to recognize and symptoms may mimic other common childhood or neonatal illnesses. Febrile illness is a common presentation to primary care or the emergency department, and the UK NICEs 'Fever in under 5s: Assessment and Initial Management' (visit https://www.nice.org.uk/guidance/ng143) provides a traffic lights system for identifying those at risk of serious illness. Not all children with sepsis will present with fever, and the detection of shock caused by sepsis is more difficult due to the greater ability of children to compensate until the late stages.

The Paediatric Sepsis 6 toolkit offers a system for rapidly identifying children who are at risk of sepsis. The main challenges to an early recognition of sepsis include those of general lack of early recognition (compounded by lack of understanding of children's physiology), plus difficulties of securing vascular access, inability to administer fluids quickly, and a lack of knowledge concerning recommendations, such as initiating vasopressor therapy for fluid resistant shock. A reliable identification system is difficult to achieve because the vital signs (e.g. heart rate) are dependent on the child's age. The diagnosis of severe sepsis relies on the clinical acumen of the healthcare professional and on raising awareness and suspicion of sepsis (visit www.sepsistrust.org/professional-resources/clinical).

Interventions to reduce hospital-acquired infections (Chapter 22)

Hospital acquired infections are no longer considered to be an inevitable consequence of hospital care; but they are preventable and unacceptable, often causing considerable harm to paediatric patients. Such harm includes central line-associated blood-stream infections (CLABSIs), ventilator-acquired pneumonia, surgical site infections, and peripheral line infections. Care bundles are collections of proven interventions required to safely and effectively deliver reliable care for patients who undergo treatments with inherent risks, such as central line insertion.

How do you measure paediatric safety?

The Paediatric Trigger Tool is a structured case note review tool; the review in undertaken by medical and nursing teams on a regular basis, in order to identify unintended harm within the local department. Although trigger tools are designed to identify common causes of harm, they also pick up other causes when broad definitions of harm are used. By understanding the types of harm that occur, the organization may focus its improvement work on areas of greatest impact and monitor improvements over time (see Chapter 12).

The tool measures adverse events with high sensitivity and specificity, through a rapid (maximum 20-minute) structured review of randomly selected case notes. Triggers listed in the tool are identified (e.g. INR > 5), then a closer examination of the notes determines whether an adverse event has occurred (e.g. bleeding). If an adverse event has occurred and harm has resulted, then the category of harm is assigned. The purpose of the review is to identify harm, not to discuss whether it could be prevented.

The use of trigger tools has revealed how frequently harm occurs in the paediatric in-patient hospital setting. Studies have suggested that as many as one in four children experience at least one episode of harm during their hospital stay. The most common cause of harm in hospitalized children has been identified in one study as tissue injury related to intravenous cannulas.

System-wide data are also important: they provide a greater understanding of harm, allowing consensus on the most prevalent adverse events and generating opportunities to learn about infrequent but definite harms (e.g. hyponatraemia caused by 0.18% saline fluid) and to share quality improvement interventions from different sites.

Summary box

The application of the safety theories presented in this book will enable you to provide safe care for children. A good place to start is to explore paediatric collaborative improvement networks that use multisite data to drive safety initiatives—for example the Pediatric International Patient Safety and Quality Community (PIPSQC at www.pipsqc.org), Making It Safer Together (www.mist-collaborative.net), and Solutions for Patient Safety (www.solutionsforpatientsafety.org).

Box 30.5 Key actions one can take to improve paediatric patient safety

All frontline staff in paediatrics, be it in the community or in hospital, can execute the following four actions to improve safety:

1. pay attention to hand hygiene, in order to decrease hospital-acquired infections;
2. ensure that prescribing is accurate and that all medications are really needed and are stopped on time;
3. work within a team to ensure that all have real-time situation awareness;
4. make sure that all records are accurate and have no abbreviations and that communication is simple and effective, especially with handover, which should be standardized.

References

Brady, P. W. et al. Improving situation awareness to reduce unrecognized clinical deterioration and serious safety events. *Pediatrics* 131.1 (2013), e298–e308.

Fitzsimons, J. and Vaughan, D. Top 10 interventions in paediatric patient safety. *Current Treatment Options in Pediatrics* 1 (2015): 275–85. https://doi.org/10.1007/s40746-015-0035-3.

Further reading

Chapman SM, et al. Prevalence and severity of patient harm in a sample of UK-hospitalised children detected by the Paediatric Trigger Tool. *BMJ Open*. 2014 Jul 3;4(7):e005066. doi: 10.1136/bmjopen-2014-005066.

Cheung, R., Roland, D., and Lachman, P. Reclaiming the systems approach to paediatric safety. *Archives of Disease in Childhood* 104.12 (2019): 1130–3. https://doi:10.1136/archdischild-2018-316401.

Kirkendall, E. S. et al. Measuring adverse events and levels of harm in pediatric inpatients with the Global Trigger Tool. *Pediatrics* 130.5 (2012): e1206–e1214.

Mueller, B. U. et al. Principles of pediatric patient safety: Reducing harm due to medical care. *Pediatrics* 143.2 (2019): e20183649.

Stockwell, D. C. et al. A trigger tool to detect harm in pediatric inpatient settings. *Pediatrics* 135 (2015): 1036–42.

Important resources

Example of a paediatric early warning system: https://www.england.nhs.uk/patientsafety/re-act/design/what-works/pews-charts.

Example of a hospital huddle: http://pediatrics.aappublications.org/content/pediatrics/131/1/e298/F1.medium.gif (the Cincinnati Children Hospital Medical Centre safety huddle).

Example of care bundles to reduce CLABSI: http://pediatrics.aappublications.org/content/pediatrics/early/2012/08/28/peds.2012-0295.full.pdf.

[illegible]

[illegible]

References

[illegible]

Further reading

[illegible]

Important resources

[illegible]

Chapter 31

Safety in maternity care

Key points

1. Pregnancy and childbirth are safe and are associated with successful outcomes. However, serious preventable harm still occurs, and systems issues can be contributory.
2. Challenges in the provision of maternity services include the complexity of patients who attend maternity services and the recruitment and retention of highly skilled staff for safe service provision.
3. Frameworks such as the PIER (prevention, identification, escalation and response) framework and standards can be used at the system level to address key issues in maternity care.
4. Independent statutory authorities can promote safety and quality in the provision of maternity services.
5. The development and use of care bundles make it easier for healthcare providers to work closely with women so as to prevent adverse events.
6. Every maternity team should have performance measures in place that can be used for quality improvement.
7. Improvement-led groups known as 'improvement collaboratives' can help maternity and neonatal care providers to improve safety and outcomes by reducing unwarranted variation.

What are the key issues in maternity care?

Optimal maternal health, together with safe, high-quality maternity care in pregnancy and throughout the puerperium, can have a marked effect on the future health of both mother and baby.

For most women and their partners, pregnancy and childbirth are safe and are associated with successful outcomes. However, despite high levels of safety and patient satisfaction with maternity services, serious preventable harm still occurs.

Serious preventable incidents can result in preterm birth, stillbirth, early neonatal death, serious brain injury in term babies, and direct and indirect maternal death. Behind these devastating endpoints are very important systems issues.

What are the challenges in maternity care?

Clinical complexity

The need for maternity services is likely to remain high. Factors such as increasing maternal age, increased rates of medical co-morbidity, and increasing rates of obesity contribute to the complexity of patients who attend maternity services.

Maintaining safe clinical teams

Critical to the delivery of safe, high-quality care is the safe, sustainable, and productive staffing of maternity services. Furthermore, all multidisciplinary team members must have the appropriate skills to deliver this high-quality care. The occurrence of serious preventable harm can undermine confidence in maternity services and can impact on staff morale. The staff needs to be supported to deliver woman-centred care; it should work in highly efficient teams, in well-led organizations that are open, transparent, innovative, and constantly learning to improve their services.

The recruitment and the retention of obstetric, midwifery, maternity support, anaesthetic, and neonatal staff remain ongoing challenges for safe service provision. Increased workloads affect the staff's well-being, and there is a high level of attrition among staff members as a result of poor work–life balance, rota gaps, more out-of-hours working, less supervision, and fewer training experiences. Work to improve organizational culture and focus on workforce planning and intelligence are of paramount importance in the development of a long-term maternity workforce strategy.

What is required for safe maternity care?

Liberati et al. 2020 have developed a framework named For Us (For Unity Safety), which identifies seven key features of safety in maternity units (see Box 31.1). Each feature of the framework is synergistic in nature and each one is necessary, but none is sufficient on its own. This framework can be used at the system level, to address the key issues in maternity care.

Box 31.1 The seven key features of the For Us framework

1. commitment to safety and improvement at all levels, with everyone involved;
2. technical competence, supported by formal training and informal learning;
3. teamwork, cooperation, and positive working relationships;
4. constant reinforcement of safe, ethical, and respectful behaviours;
5. multiple problem-sensing systems, used as basis of action;
6. systems and processes designed for safety and regularly reviewed and optimized;
7. effective coordination and ability to mobilize quickly.

Adapted from Liberati et al. 2020

Standards of care

The Health Information and Quality Authority (HIQA) in Ireland has developed national standards to address the challenges faced in maternity care by using eight central themes. These eight themes are grouped into two central concepts—'safety and quality within a service' and 'services capacity and capability' (Table 31.1)—and form a template for designing a safe service that incorporates the themes in Box 31.1.

Table 31.1. The delivery of safety and quality within a services capacity and capability

Safety and Quality within a Service	Services Capacity and Capability
Person-Centred Care A woman and her baby at the centre of care delivery, which includes access to care and equity and protection of rights	**Leadership, Governance, and Management** Arrangements put in place by a service for clear accountability, decision-making, and risk management that meets its strategic, statutory, and financial obligations
Effective Care and Support How services deliver the best achievable outcomes for women and their babies in the context of that service, reflecting the best available evidence and information	**Workforce** Planning, recruiting, managing, and organizing a workforce with the necessary skills and competencies
Safe Care and Support How services avoid, prevent, and minimize harm to women and their babies	**Use of Resources** Using resources effectively and efficiently in order to deliver best possible outcomes for women and their babies
Better Health and Well-Being Working in partnership to improve health and well-being for mother and baby.	**Use of Information** Actively using information as a resource for planning, delivering, monitoring, managing, and improving care

Adapted from Health Information and Quality Authority 2016.

Drivers of safe care

The delivery of a high quality safe service for women is imperative. Quality standards are levers for the improvement of patient care.

The Better Births framework was published in 2016 with the overarching aim of making care safer and more personalised. This initiative is built around the PIER framework for women in personalised care, [illegible] a number of tools and processes designed to support women and empower them to make decisions about their care, including continuity of carer and support in planning. The Maternity Transformation Programme seeks to deliver the vision set out by the Better Births initiative by bringing together a wide range of organizations to lead and deliver across ten workstreams (Figure 11.1).

Figure 11.1 Ten workstreams to achieve the Better Births vision.

Strategies for safety

To deliver outcomes in the Better Births vision, the government set out ambitions for safer maternity care—The National Maternity Safety Strategy: Progress and Next steps ([illegible]). It commits to halving key maternal and neonatal outcomes by the end of 2025—the rates of stillbirths, neonatal and maternal deaths and brain injuries that occur during or soon after birth. Another goal is to reduce the rate of preterm births from 8% to 6% in England and Wales over the same period.

Drivers of safe care

The delivery of a high-quality safe service for women is imperative.

Quality standards are levers for the improvement of patient care.

The Better Births framework was published in 2016 with the twin aim of making care safer and more personalized. This initiative is built around the PIER framework. Improvements in personalized care are based on a number of tools and processes designed to support women and empower them to make decisions about their care, including continuity of carer and support planning. The Maternity Transformation Programme seeks to achieve the vision set out by the Better Births initiative by bringing together a wide range of organizations to lead and deliver across ten work streams (Figure 31.1).

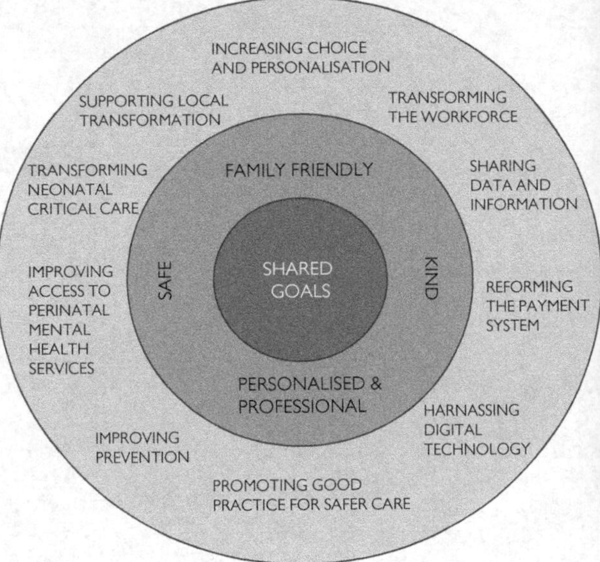

Figure 31.1 Ten work streams to achieve the Better Births vision.

Strategies for safety

To deliver outcomes in the Better Birth work steams, a national strategy for safer maternity care—The National Maternity Safety Strategy: Progress and Next Steps (visit https://www.gov.uk/government/publications/safer-maternity-care-progress-and-next-steps)—was developed; and it highlights key maternal and neonatal outcomes, with the aim of halving, by 2025, the rates of stillbirths, neonatal and maternal deaths and brain injuries that currently occur during or soon after birth. Another aim is to reduce the rate of preterm births from 8% to 6% in England and Wales during the same period.

Several steps are required to achieve the outcomes. The main steps are system-wide learning, enhanced training, and incentives for quality improvement.

An example of the potential of system-wide learning is shown in Box 31.2, which highlights seven actions derived from recurrent themes from previous investigations, reports, and publications.

Box 31.2 Immediate and essential actions to improve care and safety in maternity services: Seven themes

- enhanced safety and the culture of safety;
- listening to women and families;
- staff training and working together;
- improving the management of complex pregnancies;
- better proactive risk assessment throughout pregnancy;
- improved monitoring of foetal well-being;
- informed consent at all stages of the process.

Adapted from Ockenden Report 2020

These actions correlate with the action plan for the safer maternity care programme, which focuses on five key drivers of the delivery of safer maternity care (Box 31.3).

Box 31.3 Five key drivers of safer maternity care

Leadership	Developing leaders at every level
Learning	Identifying and sharing best practice Learning from investigations
Teams	Prioritizing and investing in the skills of the workforce and promoting team working
Data	Improved data collection and linkages between maternity and other data sets to enable benchmarking
Innovation	Creating space for accelerating improvement at local levels

Adapted from Department of Health 2017

The achievement of these-high level aims requires improvement at the front line through the core values of person- and family-centred integrated care of a safe and accessible nature. In this system both the mother and the neonate are looked after by skilled multiprofessional teams.

Clinical standards in maternity care

The Royal College of Obstetricians and Gynaecologists (RCOG) has recommended key standards for maternity care (Table 31.2).

Table 31.2. Summary of RCOG standards for maternity care

	Key Standards
Pre-pregnancy services	Key public health messages should be promoted (e.g. regarding diet, exercise, smoking) Pre-pregnancy counselling should be provided for women with complex medical needs
Antenatal Care	Should be accessible to women at the right time and from the appropriate provider
Vulnerable Women	Local and regional perinatal mental health strategies should be in place Multidisciplinary care for alcohol and substance misuse should be in place Multiagency partnerships for women who are at risk of, or experience, domestic abuse should be in place
Medical Complexity	Access to specialized care with a multidisciplinary team should be secured Each case to be reviewed by a senior obstetrician before discharge, with a clear plan for the postnatal period
Inpatient Care	Coordinated care should be underpinned by clear, accurate information exchange between healthcare professionals
Elective Birth	Options for birth should be discussed, including pros and cons of different modes of delivery, with available written information
Intrapartum Management	Choice of birth setting and transfer of care, if required Clinical leadership, accountability and governance Learning and improving by audit and review Staffing, training, and communication across the MDT
Postnatal Care	Smooth transition between birthing unit and ongoing care in the community Monitoring and reporting of postnatal readmission rates Breastfeeding support
Foetal Medicine	All women whose foetus has a suspected or confirmed disorder should have timely access to patient-focused high-quality evidence-based care
Perinatal Loss	Implement strategies to prevent perinatal loss Offer care and support when perinatal loss occurs Learn lessons from perinatal loss Communicate when perinatal loss occurs

Adapted from Royal College of Obstetricians and Gynaecologists 2016.

How do you improve safety?

[illegible] safety methodology.

System-wide drivers: Independent statutory authorities

An independent statutory authority can be used to promote safety and quality in the provision of maternity services for the benefit of the health and welfare of women and their babies. The HIQA in Ireland and the Care Quality Commission (CQC) are examples. These authorities can be responsible for setting standards, monitoring services, and undertaking health technology assessment and health information (Table [illegible]).

Table [illegible]

Setting standards for [illegible]	[illegible]
Monitoring services	[illegible]
Health technology assessment	[illegible]
Health information	[illegible]

[illegible]

Improvement at the front line

Measurement for safety

Every maternity team needs to have several measures that demonstrate performance so that improvement can take place.

Examples of measures are given in box [illegible].

[illegible] measures and then develop an improvement programme.

Care bundles in maternity care

The development and use of care bundles (see Chapter [illegible]) in maternity care [illegible] greater focus on surveillance and makes it easy for healthcare providers to work closely with women in preventing adverse events. An example of a care bundle is the Saving Babies' Lives (SBLCB) care bundle, which brings together five elements of care that are recognized as evidence-based and [illegible] good practice [illegible].

How do you improve safety?

To implement the standards, one needs to apply improvement and patient safety methodology.

System-wide drivers: Independent statutory authorities

An independent statutory authority can be used to promote safety and quality in the provision of maternity services for the benefit of the health and welfare of women and their babies. The HIQA in Ireland and the Care Quality Commission (CQC) are examples. These authorities can be responsible for setting standards, monitoring services, and using health technology assessment and health information (Table 31.3).

Table 31.3. The role of an independent statutory authority in maternity care

Setting standards for maternity care	Developing person-centred standards and guidance on the basis of evidence and international best practice
Monitoring services	Monitoring standards and compliance against most of the national standards assessed during this monitoring programme
Health technology assessment	Evaluating the clinical and financial effectiveness of health programmes, policies, medicines, medical equipment, diagnostic, and surgical techniques, health promotion and protection activities, and providing advice to enable the best use of resources and the best outcomes for people who use our health service
Health information	Advising on the efficient and secure collection and sharing of health information, setting standards, evaluating information resources, and publishing information on the delivery and performance of maternity services

Adapted from Health Information and Quality Authority 2020

Improvement at the front line

Measurement for safety

Every maternity team needs to have several measures that demonstrate performance, so that improvement can take place.

Examples of measures are given in Box 31.4.

Out of these measures one can develop an improvement programme.

Care bundles in maternity care

The development and use of care bundles (see Chapter 9) in maternity care places greater focus on surveillance and makes it easy for healthcare providers to work closely with women in preventing adverse events. An example of a care bundle is the 'Saving Babies' Lives' (SBLCB) care bundle, which brings together five elements of care that are recognized as evidence-based and as best practice (Box 31.5).

Box 31.4 Measures in maternity

Outcome measures

Obstetric events:

- eclampsia
- uterine rupture
- peripartum hysterectomy
- pulmonary embolism

Perinatal events:

- stillbirth
- perinatal mortality
- hypoxic ischaemic encephalopathy
- admission to NICU
- low birth weight

Process measures

- Delivery metrics
    - Induction
    - Instrumental delivery
    - Caesarean section
- Number of clinical incidents

Adapted from Health Information and Quality Authority 2020

Box 31.5 'Saving Babies' Lives' care bundle

- reduced smoking in pregnancy;
- risk assessment, prevention and surveillance for foetal growth restriction;
- raising awareness of reduced foetal movement;
- effective foetal monitoring during labour;
- reduction of preterm births.

Adapted from NHS England 2019.

Improvement collaboratives

Improvement-led collaboratives can help maternity and neonatal care providers to improve safety and outcomes by reducing unwarranted variation.

An example is the Maternity and Neonatal Safety Improvement Programme (MatNeoSIP; see Box 31.6). Driver diagrams and change packages have been developed that can be used as part of a systematic approach designed to improve maternity and neonatal services. The programme identified five drivers underpinned by a strong focus on safety culture, systems and processes, engaging with staff members, women, and families, and learning from error and excellence.

Box 31.6 Five driver and change packages (MatNeoSIP)

- improving the proportion of smoke-free pregnancy;
- optimization and stabilization of the preterm infant;
- detection and management of diabetes in pregnancy;
- detection and management of neonatal hypoglycaemia;
- early recognition and management of deterioration of mother or baby.

Adapted from NHS England and NHS Improvement 2016

In Scotland, the Maternity and Children Quality Improvement Collaborative (MCQIC) brings together maternity, neonatal, and paediatric care communities, promoting the use of improvement methodologies among frontline staff in order to improve the quality of care and build global capacity and capability through support visits, online educational sessions, and networking events.

Summary box

- Important identifiable systems issues are responsible for many serious but preventable incidents. These incidents can result in preterm birth, stillbirth, early neonatal death, serious brain injury in term babies, and direct and indirect maternal death.
- Although there are significant challenges to the provision of safe, high-quality maternity care, for example challenges related to clinical complexity and the maintenance of safe clinical teams, there are several standards and frameworks in place to guide healthcare providers.
- Additionally, safety bundles and improvement collaboratives are useful tools that can be used at an institutional level to improve safety and outcomes by reducing unwarranted variation.

References

Health Education England. *Maternity Workforce Strategy: Transforming the Maternity Workforce*. March 2019. https://www.hee.nhs.uk/sites/default/files/document/MWS_Report_Web.pdf.

Health Information and Quality Authority. *National Standards for Safer Better Maternity Services*. 2016. https://www.hiqa.ie/sites/default/files/2017-02/national-standards-maternity-services.pdf.

Health Information and Quality Authority. *Overview Report of HIQA's Monitoring Programme against the National Standards for Safer Better Maternity Services, with a Focus on Obstetric Emergencies*. 2020. https://www.hiqa.ie/sites/default/files/2020-02/Maternity-Overview-Report.pdf.

Liberati, E. G. et al. Seven features of safety in maternity units: A framework based on multisite ethnography and stakeholder consultation. *BMJ Quality & Safety* 30.4 (2020): 444–56. doi: 10.1136/bmjqs-2020-010988.

NHS England and NHS Improvement. Maternity and neonatal safety improvement programme. NHS, December 2016. https://improvement.nhs.uk/resources/maternal-and-neonatal-safety-collaborative.

Ockenden Report: Emerging findings and recommendations from the independent review of maternity services at the Shrewsbury and Telford Hospital NHS Trust. 2020. https://assets.publishing.service.gov.uk/government/uploads/system/uploads/attachment_data/file/943011/Independent_review_of_maternity_services_at_Shrewsbury_and_Telford_Hospital_NHS_Trust.pdf.

Royal College of Obstetricians and Gynaecologists. *Providing Quality Care for Women: Obstetrics and Gynaecology Workforce*. 2016. https://www.rcog.org.uk/globalassets/documents/guidelines/working-party-reports/ogworkforce.pdf.

Further reading

Department of Health. *Safer Maternity Care: The National Maternity Safety Strategy: Progress and Next Steps*. Department of Health, 2017. https://assets.publishing.service.gov.uk/government/uploads/system/uploads/attachment_data/file/662969/Safer_maternity_care_-_progress_and_next_steps.pdf

Healthcare Inspectorate Wales. National Review Maternity Services, Phase One. 2020. https://hiw.org.uk/sites/default/files/2020-11/20201118HIWNationalReviewofMaternityServicesEN_0.pdf.

Kirkup, B. *The Report of the Morecambe Bay Investigation*. 2015. https://assets.publishing.service.gov.uk/government/uploads/system/uploads/attachment_data/file/408480/47487_MBI_Accessible_v0.1.pdf

National Maternity Review. BETTER BIRTHS. 2016. https://www.england.nhs.uk/wp-content/uploads/2016/02/national-maternity-review-report.pdf?PDFPATHWAY=PDF.

National Quality Board. *Safe, Sustainable and Productive Staffing: An Improvement Resource for Maternity Services*. 2018. https://improvement.nhs.uk/documents/1353/Safe_Staffing_Maternity_final_2.pdf.

NHS England. *Saving Babies' Lives Version Two: A care bundle for reducing perinatal mortality*. 2019. https://www.england.nhs.uk/wp-content/uploads/2019/07/saving-babies-lives-care-bundle-version-two-v5.pdf.

Royal College of Obstetricians and Gynaecologists. *Each Baby Counts*. 2015. https://www.rcog.org.uk/globalassets/documents/guidelines/research--audit/each-baby-counts-2015-full-report.pdf.

Scottish Government. The best start: A five-year forward plan for maternity and neonatal care in Scotland. 27 January 2017. https://www.gov.scot/publications/best-start-five-year-forward-plan-maternity-neonatal-care-scotland/pages/3.

Scottish Patient Safety Programme. Maternity and children quality improvement collaborative. n.d. https://ihub.scot/improvement-programmes/scottish-patient-safety-programme-spsp/maternity-and-children-quality-improvement-collaborative-mcqic.

Welsh Government. Maternity care in Wales: A five-year vision for the future, 2019–2024. https://gov.wales/sites/default/files/publications/2019-06/maternity-care-in-wales-a-five-year-vision-for-the-future-2019-2024.pdf.

Chapter 32

Safety issues in mental health

Key points

People with mental health conditions are at a specific risk of harm when in healthcare.

The main areas of concern are:

- self-harm, including suicide;
- delayed diagnosis and misdiagnosis;
- medication harm.

These risks are amplified in health facilities that do not have the skills to meet the needs of individuals with mental health problems.

What are the key issues in mental health?

- When it comes to mental health, general hospitals report the most frequent harmful events and safety incidents of all healthcare facilities.
- They are followed by psychiatric hospitals and mental health units.
- Self-harm is the most frequently reported safety incident in mental health.

Why is it a challenge to be safe?

Understanding what is meant by harm

[illegible]

[illegible]

Diagnosing common health issues is complex

[illegible]

Balancing patient autonomy against safety

[illegible]

[illegible]

Why is it a challenge to be safe?

Understanding what is meant by harm

There is a lack of consensus on what is meant by 'harm' in mental health. Most indicators are based on the physical symptoms or outcomes of the patient, to the neglect of psychological and emotional aspects. Box 32.1 highlights the different harm indicators identified in a recent Delphi study.

Box 32.1 Harm indicators

Type of harm in mental health, identified from roundtable discussions

Diagnostic errors
Non-drug treatment errors
Medication errors
Errors related to coercive measures
Errors related to the management of aggression against self and others
Errors in treatment of suicidal patients
Communication errors
Errors in interfaces of care
Structural errors

Adapted from Mascherek and Schwappach 2016.

Diagnosing mental health issues in people

Unlike in physical health, in mental health diagnosis is based on clinical symptomology rather than on physical tests. The misdiagnosis of patients presenting difficulties is common in general settings. For example, a study exploring GPs' ability to identify depression found that they were correct in 47.3% of cases (Mitchell, Vaze, and Rao 2009). This can lead to situations where no treatment is received or the wrong treatment is dispensed, causing unnecessary side effects. Additionally, for mental health conditions such as bipolar disorder, there is often a long delay between symptom onset and treatment.

Balancing patient autonomy against safety

Clinicians treating individuals with a mental health difficulty have to balance risk, the patient's preferences, and their own capacity. This may even be more challenging for young people who are doubly challenged, both through their age and by having a mental health difficulty. Coercive measures may have to be used in some situations to protect or benefit a person, overriding his or her expressed wishes. This can be at odds with patient-centred care and shared decision-making.

Coercive measures include forced administration of medication, confinement or isolation, and restraint. The use of coercive measures results in patients staying longer in hospital. While there is a general move to lower the frequency of coercive measures, there is evidence that the use of restraint has risen in high-secure settings for people with learning disabilities, high-dependency rehabilitation wards, medium and high-security mental health wards, and children and young people's non-forensic services (Care Quality Commission 2017).

Patients' absconding is a further consideration when considering risk and patient autonomy. Patients with mental health difficulties who abscond are more likely to commit suicide or self-harm, neglect themselves, and miss medication, which interrupts treatment.

Stigma and discrimination

Some mental health difficulties are seen to be not as 'valid' as others. This creates a hierarchy in which some patients are not deemed as deserving of care. Personality disorders fall under this umbrella. The result can be that clinicians do not take patients' concerns seriously, which can impact on treatment.

Clinicians' lack of cultural competence can impact care. Clinicians are more likely to misdiagnose certain groups. For example, Black Asian and Minority Ethnic (BAME) individuals are also more likely to be misdiagnosed with schizophrenia than white individuals (Gara et al. 2019).

Harm from talking therapies

When it comes to talking therapies, there is even less understanding of how harm is caused. Dimidjian and Hollon (2010) attribute this phenomenon to the following causes:

- Therapists have difficulties predicting treatment; examining side effects may even be harder, as they may attribute them to patient behaviour.
- The nature of the therapeutic relationship and of the harm caused through treatment means there could be legal consequences for the therapist.
- Untangling adverse events from negative events in a patient's life is difficult.
- Discerning positive and negative effects is challenging, owing to their subjective nature.
- Given the lack of procedural guidelines, it is difficult to separate therapeutic dosage from the therapist's behaviour.

Medication knowledge and errors

The safe prescription and administration of medication designed to treat or manage mental health difficulties is underpinned by various factors, including:

- the clinician's knowledge of drug interactions and polyphamacy;.
- the clinician's knowledge of how to administer and manage higher-risk medications (e.g. clozapine);
- the patient's knowledge of the medications he or she is taking.

A recent systematic review of medication errors in psychiatric hospitals found that medication errors ranged from 10.6 to 15.5 per 1,000 patient days, while adverse drug events ranged from 10.0 to 42.00 per 100 patient days. As for adverse drug events, between 13% and 17.3% were found to be preventable (Alshehri et al. 2017).

How do you measure safety in mental health?

- Like definitions of harm, metrics tend to be based on physical characteristics. These can be calculated at different levels, depending on their purpose or on the need: for example, hospital level, ward level, bed numbers, number of admissions, and bed occupancy.
- Internationally, there is a push towards zero suicides on wards and in the community. Zero Suicide outlines organizations that collect data for the numbers of patients who are screened for suicide risk. For those who are deemed high risk, Zero Suicide recommends that metrics should be collected and recorded on the following themes: whether a risk assessment was carried out; whether there was a developed safety plan; whether lethal means counselling was offered and undertaken. Additionally, the organizations in question should check whether there were missed appointments for those with a suicide care plan and whether there was contact within 24 hours after acute care transition for those who had been hospitalized or who had attended emergency services.
- For measures to consider in mental health, see Box 32.2.

Box 32.2 Measures to consider in mental health

The UK five-year forward plan outlines the need for evidence-based pathways and pillars of quality, one aspect of which is safety. Specific safety metrics for suicide prevention include:

- age-standardized mortality rate from suicide per 100,000 individuals;
- age-standardized admissions to hospital for self-harm per 100,000 individuals;
- percentage of people on the Care Programme Approach followed up within seven days of an in-patient's discharge.

In Scotland the following metrics have been used:

- unscheduled care presentations where self-harm is a presenting feature;
- percentage of people prescribed lithium who experienced toxicity in the past 12 months.

- For mental health professionals delivering psychological interventions, a checklist has been developed to capture side effects and adverse treatment reactions: the UE-ATR checklist. This list covers the following domains: symptomology, the well-being of the patient, the therapeutic relationship, the patient's social and family networks, and changes in the patient's circumstances and situations.

Factors that affect safety

Developing safe care in mental health means targeting factors across the following levels: patient, provider, organization, and physical environment (Brickell et al. 2009). Table 32.2 outlines some of the different areas that should be considered at each level:

Table 32.2. Factors affecting patient safety

Factor	Consideration
Patient factors	Impact of diagnosis: it can affect communication
	Self-stigma can affect whether patients seek help and communicate in case harm has been caused
	Co-morbidity combined with substance misuse can lead to aggression
Provider factors	Limited time and high workloads lead to low or poor interaction with patients and harm is missed
	There can be poor communication between staff, other providers of care, and patients' families
Organizational factors	Low retention of staff can cause new procedures not to be embedded
	The embedding and revisiting of safety training programmes can be affected
Physical environment	There can be inadequate resources to minimize aggression, boredom, or impulsive behaviour
	Mixed-sex wards can make patients feel vulnerable
	Fittings can increase the risk of injury or death

Adapted from Brickell et al. 2009.

How can one be safe and what is safer mental healthcare?

Clinicians, services, and organizations can employ the following methods to deliver safer care in mental health (see Emanuel et al. 2013):

1) delivery of high quality personalized care;
2) education, training, and reviews of safety indicators;
3) creation of safer physical environments;
4) creation of open and honest environments.

Delivery of higher-quality personalized care

- Recovery-oriented care: recognising the patient as an expert in the lived experience of his or her illness and a collaborator in his or her own recovery. This prompts shared decision-making and removes the hierarchical imbalance that lies at the heart of paternalistic care.
- Trauma informed care: approaching care from the perspective that a patient may well have experienced trauma and that that patient's understanding of it shapes his or her experience. Care and treatment, when not managed properly, can result in re-traumatization.
- Culturally responsive care: taking into account the patient's background, religion, and culture. Where appropriate, both the patient and others (e.g. family, spiritual leader) are included and asked to collaborate on drawing up a care and treatment plan that respects their values and beliefs.

Education, training, and reviews of safety indicators

- Training should be organized around the models of care described so far.
- Education should focus on how harm is defined and training should explain what harm and safety indicators need to be captured and recorded.
- Training and education should be refreshed periodically.

Creation of safer physical environments

- Make sure environments are adequately staffed.
- Co-design wards and care environments with patients and families, so as to make them accessible, usable, and stimulating.
- Have single-sex spaces for men and women, so they both feel safe from sexual advances and assault.
- Remove or, where not possible, limit furniture, fittings, and items that could be used for self-injury and harm. For example, installing two-way doors limits the possibility that patients block entrances with furniture in order to self-harm.

Creation of open and honest environments

When a safety incident occurs, have robust procedures in place, for example:

- a review committee made up of a diverse range of individuals, with clinical, administration, information management, legal, and ethical expertise;
- a process for incident management and review in steps:
  - debriefing the team after the safety incident occurred;
  - recording the incident with the healthcare provider;
  - reviewing the incident with a focus on improving processes rather than blaming clinicians or other individuals. Findings and recommendations should be fed back to all members of staff and those involved in the incident and any improvements implemented using QI methodology;
- acknowledging that all individuals have a role to play in monitoring safe care in mental health. This task includes engaging the patient and the family in discussions—as well as the wider team, which sits outside the patient's immediate care or treatment plan. Huddles may be used on wards to help achieve this task.

Examples of developing safer care

Mental health practitioners as well as clinicians in a general hospital can undertake improvement projects to benefit the safety of their patients. The two case studies in Box 32.2 and Box 32.3 show an application of the theories presented in the book, with a focus on the patient's specific needs.

Box 32.2 Case 1: The Zero Suicide initiative

With evidence of increasing suicide rates in the USA, the Henry Ford Health System set out to transform the healthcare system and to commit to zero suicides (Coffey 2006). After mapping out the patient's journey, it made key changes across three areas: partnership with the patients; making sure they were active partners in treatment; and measuring satisfaction.

Clinical care

A protocol was developed for assessing patient risk and for steps to be undertaken at each level of risk.

- Access – improved patient access via drop-in group medication appointments, same-day access appointments, and e-mail 'visits'.

Communication

- Information flow – information systems were updated to allow confidential information to flow better, and a secure website was developed for patients and family members.

Research comparing mortality data suggested a statistically significant decrease of 75%.

Box 32.3 Case 2: Reducing prone (face down) restraint on wards (adapted from 2gether NHS Foundation Trust 2017)

There is increasing debate around the use of prone restraint, which can prove harmful to both patients and staff. As a result, the 2gether NHS Foundation Trust attempted to reduce the amount of prone restraint within its wards.

Study and learn

First an internal review was undertaken, where findings showed that 2/3 of tranquilizations involved prone restraint, by comparison with 1/3 supine (face up) restraint.

Change, test, and introduce new process

After this, the trust's guidelines were updated to reflect that tranquilization can be given in the quadriceps area during supine restraint. This was supplemented with training on supine restraint for all new staff and retraining on supine restraint for all existing staff.

Findings showed the use of supine restraint increased: 2/3 of all incidents in February 2017 were of the supine kind.

Summary box

Safety in mental health can be challenging. However, if one applies the principles of patient safety and the specific requirements of mental health, one can achieve safety. In general hospitals this can be difficult, and the approach described here can make a difference to the safety of this vulnerable group of patients.

Deliver high quality personalized care. This should draw on the principles of:

- recovery-oriented care;
- trauma-informed care;
- culturally responsive care.

Understand what safety metrics should be captured and how these are recorded.

Training and education on safety indicators should be refreshed periodically.

On inpatient wards or wards where patients may be staying, create environments in day rooms that are stimulating and engaging. Minimize fittings and fixtures, which could be used for self-harm and injury.

References

Alshehri, G. H., Keers, R. N., and Ashcroft, D. M. Frequency and nature of medication errors and adverse drug events in mental health hospitals: a systematic review. *Drug Safety* 40.10 (2017): 871–86.

Brickell, T. A. et al. *Patient Safety in Mental Health*. Edmonton: Canadian Patient Safety Institute and Ontario Hospital Association, 2009.

Care Quality Commission. The state of care in mental health services 2014 to 2017. Newcastle, 2017. https://www.cqc.org.uk/sites/default/files/20170720_stateofmh_report.pdf.

Coffey, C. E. Pursuing perfect depression care. Psychiatric Services 57.10 (2006): 1524–6

Dimidjian, S. and Hollon, S. D. How would we know if psychotherapy were harmful? *American Psychologist* 65.1 (2010): 21–33.

Emanuel, L. L. et al. (eds). *The Patient Safety Education Program, Canada: Module 13: Mental Health Care*. Ontario: PSEP-Canada, 2013.

Gara, M. A., et al. A naturalistic study of racial disparities in diagnoses at an outpatient behavioral health clinic. *Psychiatric Services* 70.2 (2019): 130–4.

Mascherek, A. C. and Schwappach, D. L. Patient safety priorities in mental healthcare in Switzerland: A modified Delphi study. *BMJ Open* 6.8 (2016): e011494.

Mitchell, A. J., Vaze, A., and Rao, S. Clinical diagnosis of depression in primary care: A meta-analysis. *Lancet* 374.9690 (2009): 609–19.

2gether NHS Foundation Trust. Improving patient safety by reducing prone restraint, through better use of data, targeted training and other improvement initiatives. NHS Improvement Report, June 2017.

Patient safety in critical care

Key points

- Patients in intensive care are at risk of several specific safety risks, owing to the complexity of the care processes.
- Safety must be planned and risk proactively managed.
- The application of human factors and reliability theory can mitigate the risk and decrease harm.
- A culture of safety with teamwork, good communication, and situation awareness will facilitate safe care.

Key safety issues in critical care

As healthcare professionals, we strive to provide safe, effective, and person-centred healthcare, because a failure to do so can cause our patients temporary or permanent harm, and even death. Critical care provides life-saving interventions for patients who are at their most vulnerable and, as such, is often associated with significant risks of adverse events.

The focus of this chapter is on safety. In this respect, some of the key issues related to critical care are:

1. ventilator-associated pneumonia (VAP);
2. central line-associated bloodstream infections (CLABSI);
3. other intensive care-acquired infections (e.g. methicillin-resistant *Staphylococcus aureus* (MRSA) and *Clostridium difficile*);
4. complications associated with critical illness and invasive interventions (e.g. stress ulcer and venous thromboembolism prophylaxis);
5. equipment-related errors;
6. medication-related errors;
7. handover and communication;
8. reintubation rate.

These are just a few examples of safety-related issues in critical care and by no means form an exhaustive list. Later in this chapter we will discuss in greater detail some of the issues mentioned here.

Why is it a challenge to be safe?

Modern critical care arose from the poliomyelitis epidemic in the 1950s; patient safety within critical care has been considered a challenge around the globe since its inception. If one analyses the work system using the Systems Engineering Initiative for Patient Safety (SEIPS) model (see Chapter 9), one can see that critical care patients are at an increased risk of harm, as in shown in Table 33.1.

Table 33.1. Examples of risk factors in the critical care work system

Work System	Risk Factors
Environment	ICU is a very complex and demanding environment owing to the severity of disease and patient vulnerability.
Tools and Technology	Patients are exposed to a high number of invasive procedures and procedures attached to multiple devices and infusions.
Tasks	The tasks to be competed are complex and prone to error.
People: Patients	*Patients* • are often either sedated and or incapacitated through medication or disease (e.g. delirium) and, as a result, are unable to fully participate in decisions about their own care; • are usually on multiple drugs (polypharmacy), which increases the risks of medication errors, interactions, side effects, higher sensitivity, and drug accumulation; • are more likely to experience complications related to their treatment or procedures (e.g. acute kidney injury), and these complications may or may not be preventable.
Organization	Multidisciplinary team involvement increases the risk of non-technical errors as well as the risk of communication errors.
People: Staff	Staff members can experience fatigue, which can cause slips and lapses.
Processes	The process or standard operating procedures and guidelines are not always standardized or are not always followed.

Some of these factors are in the very nature that defines critical care, hence there is very little that we can do about it. However, if we focus on the principles of a safe system then we can Prevent, Detect and Mitigate these risks by improving the working environment and making critical care a safer place for both patients and staff.

Types of preventable harms in critical care

Ventilator-associated pneumonia

Ventilator-associated pneumonia (VAP) is the most common nosocomial infection in the critical care unit and accounts for a large proportion of the antibiotics delivered. It is defined as a type of pneumonia that develops in hospital 48 hours or more after the patient was on mechanical ventilation. It is associated with increased lengths of stay, costs, morbidity, and mortality.

Several strategies have been found to reduce the incidence of VAP. When combined to create a care bundle of evidence-based interventions, the output and benefits of the bundle are greater than the sum of individual parts. Using a bundle approach to improve ventilator care processes and reduce ventilator-associated pneumonia has subsequently led to significant improvement in reducing the incidence of VAP.

VAP bundle

1. Avoid invasive ventilation.
2. Sedation is to be reviewed and, if appropriate, stopped each day.
3. All patients will be assessed for weaning and extubation every day.
4. Avoid the supine position and aim to have the patient at least 30° head up.
5. Daily oral care with toothbrushing.
6. Use subglottic secretion drainage in patients who are likely to be ventilated for more than 48 hours.

Central line-associated blood stream infections

A central line-associated bloodstream infection (CLABSI) occurs when organisms (usually bacteria) enter the bloodstream via a central venous catheter, causing serious infection and bacteraemia. CLABSI is defined as a laboratory-confirmed bloodstream infection not related to an infection at another site that develops while a central line is in situ or within 48 hours of a central line's being in place. This is the costliest of all healthcare-acquired infections and is thought to be preventable if central lines are inserted using strict aseptic technique, with proper surveillance and a maintenance strategy for daily use.

CLABSI bundle

- hand washing;
- full-barrier precautions during the insertion of the central line;
- cleaning the skin with chlorhexidine;
- avoiding the femoral site if possible;
- removing unnecessary catheters.

This central line care bundle was used in 103 intensive care units (ICUs) in Michigan and demonstrated decreased infection rates by up to 66% following implementation.

Pressure ulcers

Pressure ulcers can cause significant morbidity for patients and their families. They are a real problem for the NHS, costing between £1.4 billion and £2.1 billion annually, or 4% of the NHS budget. Critical care patients are at increased risk of pressure ulcers, mainly because of their increased vulnerability (hypotension/sedation) and immobility. Pressure ulcers are defined as localised injuries to the skin or to the underlying tissues, usually over bony prominences; they are due to pressure, or to pressure in combination with shear.

Hospital-acquired pressure ulcers are mostly preventable occurrences. Many interventions have been taken to minimize the risk; these include improving staff education and knowledge of pressure ulcer prevention, guidelines and policies with evidence-based practices, and risk assessment of all patients within six hours of admission. Critical care patients are at risk of both device-related (e.g. endotracheal tube ties) and non-device-related pressure sores. The SKIN bundle is an evidence-based checklist designed to assist the staff in implementing pressure ulcer prevention strategies.

Pressure ulcer bundle

S. SKIN: assess and manage;
S. SURFACE: keep surface dry; relieve pressure (mattresses)
K. KEEP MOVING/TURNING to ensure decreased pressure;
I. INCONTINENCE management to prevent skin irritation and integrity;
N. NUTRITION and HYDRATION to maintain skin viability and promote wound healing

Medication errors

Critical care patients are at higher risk of medication errors and harm: the risk is around 2–3 times greater than for non-critically ill patients and has a probability of mortality that is approximately 2.5 times higher when the error happens. This is due to the complexity of the patients' drug regimens and to the stressful environment. They are often on heavier medication than non-critically ill patients, and this can result in drug interactions and altered pharmacokinetics owing to organ failure. Critical care patients are also more likely to develop drug-induced events such as acute kidney injury and coagulopathies. Unsuccessful medication reconciliation and interruptions during medication preparation and administration can also increase the chance of errors.

Over the years there have been many interventions intended to make it easy to do the right thing and more difficult to do the wrong thing, all in an attempt to improve medication safety. These interventions are listed in Box 33.1:

Box 33.1 Interventions to decrease medication error and harm

- standardizing intravenous drug concentrations;
- preventing the preparation of medication in the critical care area with pre-prepared products readily available;
- implementation of technology that aims to eliminate human error, including:
  - robots for filling and dispensing medications;
  - computerized prescriber order entry;
  - clinical decision support;
  - bar code medication administration;
  - advanced infusion pumps;
- promoting and encouraging a culture of patient safety;
- comprehensive surveillance programme involving:
  - adverse drug event (ADE) monitoring and reporting;
  - ADE detection;
  - management;
  - documentation;
  - evaluation; and
  - developing preventative strategies and programmes.

How can one be safe in a critical care environment?

How can one be safe in a critical care environment?

1. reducing harm from deterioration;
2. reducing harm in critical care;
3. reducing harm in perioperative care;
4. reducing harm from high risk medications.

In recent years, patient safety has been at the forefront of patient care. There has been a huge drive to improve the quality of care as well as the patient's safety, with national campaigns such as the Scottish Patient Safety Programme and the Patient Safety First Campaign in NHS England. There are four common interventions associated with these campaigns:

The first two interventions involve critical care directly, and the last two interventions have direct impact on both critical care and its patients.

As healthcare professionals of the modern era, we are familiar with care bundles, processes, and checklists that exist to improve patient safety. For example, the World Health Organisation (WHO)'s safer surgical checklist prevents never events from happening and improve surgical outcomes.

The situation is no different in critical care. Critical care driver diagrams and improvement plans are composed of numerous standardized care bundles related to daily practice and frequent tasks in the ICU that, when carried out together, can improve a patient's outcome. Some examples are:

1. the ventilator-associated pneumonia bundle;
2. the central line insertion bundle;
3. the central line maintenance bundle;
4. the peripheral venous catheter bundle; and
5. the sepsis care bundle.

In addition to the care bundles, we also use various checklists in critical care, in order to prevent the error of omission, which is usually noticed because of slips and lapses. Here are some examples of the checklists used:

1. multidisciplinary ward rounds with daily goal checklists: these are meant to ensure, as a matter of daily routine, the consideration of interventions such as stress ulcer prophylaxis, VTE prophylaxis, medicine reconciliation, sedation interruption, and spontaneous breathing trials, as well as the consideration of therapeutic targets such as blood gas parameters and weaning plans;
2. rapid sequence induction intubation checklists;
3. routine interventions for patients admitted with out-of-hospital cardiac arrest or major trauma;
4. transfer checklist for both intra- and inter-hospital transfer;
5. death checklist, to ensure that all the relevant paperwork has been done and the relevant parties have been informed.

All-or-none compliance with the individual elements of the checklist and care bundles is as important as the bundle itself, as this has been proven to improve the effectiveness of the checklist. As a result, it is the implementation of the bundle that affects patient outcome.

In general, there are five knowledge systems that have been identified to support improvement:

1. Generalizable scientific evidence: bundle developed by an existing network of clinicians with interest in the subject and based on best evidence.
2. Awareness of the context: knowing what works best in that department, for example the education of staff may work best in one unit, while using a prompt as part of the daily goals to execute the bundle may work better in another unit.
3. The development and application of systems for a valid and reliable measurement of both processes and outcomes. Collecting and analysing measures for improvement and displaying the data visually in the clinical area has been proven to be a powerful tool in engaging the staff in the improvement process.
4. Plans for change that adapt generalizable evidence to local context: it is important to learn what works and what does not work locally if you want to make sequential changes.
5. Execution of planned changes: this requires having the right leader to promote the safety culture in the critical care unit.

In addition to continued improvement projects, the adverse events reporting system has been used in all areas of healthcare, including critical care. This has prompted the identification of problems and has stimulated a process of conducting root cause analysis, which will lead to learning from error and system change. Moreover, we can use technology to our advantage: for instance we can use electronic health records to prompt interventions, and electronic prescribing to minimize medication errors.

Communication

Finally, poor communication among the critical care team members has been shown to be a contributing factor to errors and adverse events. This can be communication during handover, during ward activities, or during an emergency. Some of the interventions to improve communication that have also been shown to improve patient safety are listed in Box 33.2.

The transport of patients

The safe transportation of critically ill patients, either intra-hospital, for example to radiology for a CT scan, or inter-hospital, for example to a specialist referral centre, can be a safety issue, as maintaining stability in a critically unwell patient is very challenging.

If one implements the human factors SEIPS approach to the work system, one can proactively mitigate the risk of an unfamiliar environment, equipment, and lack of immediately available help. Specific transport bags or trolleys with all-eventuality equipment available are recommended, and these must be checked daily, to ensure that the contents are complete and correct.

Box 33.2 Interventions to improve communication

1. Standardized written handovers are used as prompts, to ensure that all the relevant information is communicated to the receiving team.
2. Safety briefs every morning ensure that all the important safety issues are known to the wider multidisciplinary team.
3. Daily goals written clearly, either on paper or electronically, during the ward round ensure that medical staff plans are communicated and accessible to the nursing staff.
4. Structured SBAR referrals and handovers take place among doctors when reviewing patients without critical care settings.
5. 'Check back' is a simple technique designed to ensure that the information conveyed by the sender is understood by the recipient as intended. Example: Doctor: 'Give 2 mg morphine IV bolus.' Nurse: '2mg morphine IV bolus.' Doctor: 'That is correct.'
6. 'Call out' is a strategy for communicating important information to all team members simultaneously during emergent situations. Example: 'Airway status? Airway clear. Breath sounds? Breath sounds reduced on left side. Trachea? Trachea deviated to the right. BP? BP is 70/30.' 'Call out' helps the team to anticipate the next steps and directs responsibility to a specific individual for carrying out the task.
7. It is important to develop tools for team-training and assess communication and teamwork in critical care (e.g. high-fidelity simulation).

How do we measure safety in ICU?

Measurement is central to a team's ability to monitor and improve care. It is an integral part of both clinical audit and quality improvement, and there is no standard scale for measuring safety. [illegible] identified a approach [illegible] evidence of reduced numbers of incidences of harm to the patient; hence, to measure any improvement in safety, we would need to measure the decrease in the numbers of patients harmed before and after the implementation of an intervention. There are various quality indicators in the critical care unit that are used to measure safety. Therefore, we need to be able to have a data collection process to ensure reliable quality data collection, and we also need frequent analysis of the data to determine whether any changes lead to improvements.

As such, it is important that we adequately measure the following:

- Structure: [illegible] indication [illegible] national comparative audit, such as the Intensive Care National Audit & Research Centre (ICNARC) or the Scottish Intensive Care Society Audit Group is an example.
- Process measures: Are the different steps in the process (e.g. completion of checklists) performing as planned?
- Outcome measures: How is the system performing? What are the results (e.g. has the VAP rate or infection rate decreased?)
- Balancing measures: Looking at the system from a different perspective. Are changes [illegible]

Reporting [illegible] (e.g. [illegible]) [illegible] process [illegible] the [illegible] patients [illegible]

Some examples of quality indicators from published literature in critical care are:

1. the [illegible] rates
2. readmission to critical care within 48 hours of discharge
3. out-of-hours discharges
4. delayed discharges
5. the incidence of ventilator-associated pneumonia
6. the incidence of central line-associated bloodstream infections
7. the incidence of intensive care unit-acquired infections (e.g. MRSA, vancomycin-resistant enterococci, and *Clostridium difficile*)
8. the incidence of pressure ulcers
9. the incidence of medication errors
10. the incidence of critical incidents.

How do we measure safety in ICU?

Measurement is central to a team's ability to monitor and improve care. It is an integral part of both clinical audit and quality improvement; and there is no standard scale for measuring safety. Patient safety can be defined as evidence of reduced harm or of absence of harm to the patients; hence, to measure any improvement in safety, we would need to measure the reduction in the numbers of patients harmed before and after the implementation of an intervention. There are various quality indicators in the critical care unit that are used to measure safety. Therefore we need to be able to have a data collection process that can enable quality data collection; and we also need frequent analysis of the data to determine whether any change is an improvement.

As such, it is important that we monitor key measures of:

- Structure: Participation in a national comparative audit such as the Intensive Care National Audit & Research Centre (ICNARC) or the Scottish Intensive Care Society Audit Group is an example.
- Process measures: Are the different steps in the process (e.g. bundle or checklist compliance) performing as planned?
- Outcome measures: How is the system performing? What is the result? (Examples: the VAP rate or the standardized mortality ratio.)
- Balancing measures: Look at the system from a different perspective. Are there any unanticipated consequences? (Examples: MRSA, VRE, *Clostridium difficile*.)

Running frequent PDSA (plan, do, study, act) cycles and producing statistical process control charts and run charts can help to measure the improvement in patient safety after interventions.

Some examples of quality indicators of patient safety in critical care are:

1. the reintubation rate;
2. readmission to critical care unit within 48 hours of discharge;
3. out-of-hours discharges;
4. delayed discharges;
5. the incidence of ventilator-associated pneumonia;
6. the incidence of central line-associated bloodstream infections;
7. the incidence of intensive care unit-acquired methicillin-resistant Staphylococcus aureus, vancomycin-resistant enterococci, and Clostridium difficile;
8. the incidence of pressure ulcers;
9. the incidence of medication errors;
10. the incidence of critical incidents.

What do we need to do to be safer?

There are many things that we can do, as healthcare professionals, to influence safety in the critical care environment. Here are some examples:

1. Adhere to a strict infection control policy such as the five moments of handwashing, wearing appropriate attire, and using personal protective equipment when in contact with patients.
2. Report any critical incidence, significant events and near misses using the incidence reporting system.
3. Keep up to date with developments in education and evidence-based medicine that will help with the implementation of bundles and guidelines.
4. Participate in exercises designed to improve communications as a team.
5. Ensure compliance and adherence to existing guidelines and care bundles for patient safety.
6. Remember that the patient is at the centre of our care and we can start to improve patient safety with one doctor, one nurse, one patient at a time.

Summary box

In summary, in this chapter we have discussed some of the key issues of patient safety in critical care, the harms we can prevent, and what we can do about them as healthcare professionals. Ensuring patient safety in a high-risk environment such as the critical care unit can sometimes feel like an uphill battle, and one that we may get burnout from. However, when critical care is practised responsibly, with little or no patient safety incidents, it can also contribute to joy at work.

Words like 'safety', or even 'harm', can lose their impact because we use them so often. However, thanks to growing awareness of patient safety issues and different approaches designed to improve critical care (e.g. care bundles and quality improvement projects), over the years we have seen progress: critical care units across the country have achieved a sizeable reduction in the rates of ICU-acquired and device-related infections such as CLABSI and VAP.

At the end of the day, as healthcare professionals, we all share the same dedication to making care better for our patients and their families, and this will serve as a motivation to continue searching for new and better ways to improve patient safety.

Further reading

Chrusch, C. A., Martin, C. M., and The Quality Improvement in Critical Care Project. Quality improvement in critical care: Selection and development of quality indicators. *Canadian Respiratory Journal* 2016 (2016). https://doi.org/10.1155/2016/2516765.

Daniel, M. et al. Details behind the dots: How different intensive care units used common and contrasting methods to prevent ventilator associated pneumonia. *BMJ Quality Improvement Reports* 4.1 (2015). doi: 10.1136/bmjquality.u207660.w3069.

Peden, C. J., and Rooney, K. D. The science of improvement as it relates to quality and safety in the ICU. *Journal of the Intensive Care Society* 10.4 (2009): 260–5.

Pronovost, P. et al. An intervention to decrease catheter-related bloodstream infections in the ICU. *New England Journal of Medicine* 355 (2006): 2725–32.

Resar, R. et al. Using a bundle approach to improve ventilator care processes and reduce ventilator-associated pneumonia. *Joint Commission Journal on Quality and Patient Safety* 31.5 (2012): 243–8.

Rooney, K. *Humanizing Health Care: The Language of Patient Safety*. Institute for Healthcare Improvement, 2016.

Scottish Intensive Care Society Audit Group. *VAP Prevention Bundle Guidance for Implementation*. NHS National Services Scotland, 2012.

Sundaram, R., and Rooney, K. D. Reliable critical care: Making it easy to do the right thing. *British Journal of Anaesthesia* 115.2 (2015), 161–3.

Tayyib, N. and Coyer, F. Effectiveness of pressure ulcer prevention strategies for adult patients in intensive care units: A systematic review. *Worldviews on Evidence-Based Nursing*, 13.6 (2016) 432–44.

Welters, I. D. et al. Major sources of critical incidents in intensive care. *Critical Care*, 15 (2011) https://doi.org/10.1186/cc10474.

Chapter 34

Safety in patients with frailty and complex long-term conditions

Key points

- Frailty is more common in older adults and is characterized by a reduced ability to respond to physiologic stressors.
- Frail and older adults are more likely to have multiple chronic conditions and are at increased risk of developing complications associated with mortality and poor clinical outcomes. These include:
  - delirium;
  - polypharmacy;
  - falls;
  - pressure injuries;
  - infection.
- The application of care bundles can prevent many of these safety risks.
- The COVID-19 pandemic highlighted the increased susceptibility to infection in older adults and the association between frailty and outcomes from serious illness.

The safety challenges with frailty

As society has grown older, the demographic of these attending healthcare facilities has changed across care settings. An ageing population presents unique safety challenges. Any of the potential harms can have a devastating effect on the individual and carry a high cost for the individual and the family, for healthcare facilities, and for the wider society.

This chapter reviews how we can optimize the safety of persons who are at risk for:

- delirium;
- polypharmacy;
- falls;
- pressure injuries;
- infection.

These are five key factors commonly associated with frail older adults. In each of the cases presented here the application of reliability theory will be introduced to ensure that the right care is provided.

Each of these risks may have increased with the impact of the COVID-19 pandemic. Older adults are more likely to present with atypical forms of COVID-19, including delirium and falls.

Preventing and managing delirium

What is the safety issue?

[illegible]

Why is it a challenge?

[illegible]

[illegible]

Preventing and managing delirium

What is the safety issue?

Delirium is an acute change in attention, awareness, and thinking, which usually fluctuates.

Frail older patients are most likely to experience delirium.

It can occur in the community or in hospital, but is most common in hospitalized patients. The highest prevalence of delirium is in the intensive care unit (ICU). Delirium is also common after anaesthesia and surgery, when it has an incidence rate of 20%–30%

Delirium is associated with a higher risk of adverse outcomes, including mortality, discharge to nursing homes rather than home, and persistent cognitive impairment.

Why is it a challenge?

Delirium can be challenging to detect and diagnose unless regular screening takes place. It is also difficult to treat, no effective pharmacological therapies being available to date. There is no evidence that anti-psychotic medications shorten the duration of delirium or lengthen the hospital stay.

As a result, delirium prevention measures and early recognition are of the utmost importance. However, delirium is often under-recognized.

How can one be safe?

Delirium can be prevented by optimizing all the requirements for normal cognitive function. These include optimal hydration, nutrition, sleep, pain control, and avoidance or early detection of acute medical events.

There are several risk factors that either predispose a patient to delirium or precipitate the condition. Recognizing risk factors for delirium is important (Box 34.1). Clinical suspicion should be particularly high in the post-operative setting.

Box 34.1 Risk factors for delirium

Predisposing factors

- older age;
- male sex;
- sensory impairment (hearing, vision);
- cognitive impairment;
- depression;
- alcohol excess.

Precipitating factors

- medications (hypnotics, anticholinergics)
- surgery and or anaesthesia;
- acute illness (infection, stroke, myocardial infarction);
- pain;
- laboratory abnormalities (glucose, electrolytes, thyroid, anaemia);
- withdrawal states (alcohol, drugs).

There are several validated tools available for screening for delirium at the bedside. These include the Confusion Assessment Method (CAM), the Nursing Delirium Screening Scale, and the 4AT.

The American Geriatrics Society, the National Institute for Clinical Excellence, and the Scottish Intercollegiate Guidelines Network have all published guidelines on the prevention and management of delirium.

The prevention of delirium requires reliable delivery of seven key interventions, as indicated in Box 34.2.

Box 34.2 Delirium prevention care bundle

1. Identify risk factors.
2. Ensure that the patient has access to glasses, hearing aids, and dentures.
3. Control the pain.
4. Maintain regular mobilization.
5. Maintain adequate hydration and nutrition.
6. Perform medication reviews and identify potentially inappropriate medications.
7. Care for the patient in a quiet environment and avoid changes.

The management of delirium requires early diagnosis and active interventions, as indicated in Box 34.3.

Box 34.3 Delirium management

1. Train interdisciplinary team members on delirium recognition, prevention, and management.
2. Identify and treat delirium triggers, including postoperative complications.
3. Manage pain proactively.
4. Communicate the diagnosis to patients and caregivers.
5. Perform regular re-orientation.
6. Promote a normal sleep–wake cycle.
7. Avoid physical restraints.
8. Avoid constipation.
9. Aim to treat agitation non-pharmacologically, if possible.

The key intervention is awareness, assessment, and prevention and, if delirium does occur, proactive management.

Polypharmacy and medication safety

What is the safety issue?

Appropriate prescribing for frail older adults is an important safety issue, as this population is more likely to have adverse drug events. The WHO Medication Without Harm initiative has identified polypharmacy as a major risk and aims to reduce harm related to medications by 50% over five years globally.

Why is it a challenge?

Frail older adults are more likely to have multiple chronic conditions and require appropriate therapy. However, they are also more likely to experience polypharmacy. Adverse drug events are also more common, owing to changes in pharmacokinetics and pharmacodynamics that occur as part of the ageing process. These changes include altered distribution of fat soluble and protein-bound medications, decreased renal glomerular filtration rate, and decreased hepatic clearance.

How can one be safe?

A review of medications should be performed for all patients annually, or more frequently if a change in clinical condition arises (Box 34.4).

Box 34.4 Tips for performing a safe medication review

Performing a safe medication review in patients with frailty

- Ask the patient to bring all the medications, including over-the-counter drugs, herbal preparations, homeopathic medications, and nutritional supplements.
- Ask the patient or the caregiver to explain the former's medications and how they are taken.
- Enquire about adherence, difficult administration, and side effects.
- Review the refill history with the patient's pharmacy.
- Observe the patient using complex medications (e.g. inhalers, insulin).

There are two main tools that have been validated to assist in performing a medication review. The Beers criteria and STOPP/START tool are effective at identifying potentially inappropriate medications.

The polypharmacy programme in Scotland suggests seven steps to achieve a person-centred approach to preventing and limiting polypharmacy (see Box 34.5).

Care must be taken to prescribe new medications safely, particularly high-risk ones such as anticoagulation and insulin. Initiation of a medication in a frail older adult must be justified according to need (see the seven steps) and with additional information, as indicated in Box 34.6.

How do you measure medication safety?

Medication safety in frail older adults is measured by:

- adherence to the prescribing checklist;
- decreasing the level of polypharmacy;
- reporting of medication errors;
- reporting of side effects;
- reporting of adverse events.

Box 34.5 Seven-step appropriate polypharmacy bundle

Step 1: What matters to the patient?
Review diagnoses and identify therapeutic objectives.
Step 2: Need
Review the need for *essential* drugs (stop only on expert advice).
Step 3: Need
Review the need for *unnecessary* drugs; consider stopping them or reducing the dose (deprescribe).
Step 4: Effectiveness
Find out whether therapeutic objectives are being met and whether therapy should be added or intensified.
Step 5: Safety
Identify safety risks for the patient.
Identify adverse effects.
Step 6: Cost-effectiveness of the medication determined
Step 7: Patient centredness
Are the outcomes of the review clear?
Do the changes reflect the patient's preferences?
Agree and communicate plan.

Box 34.6 Questions to consider at the initiation of a new medication

- What is the indication? Is the diagnosis clear?
- Is there a safer or more effective alternative medication?
- Is the patient likely to receive benefit when the goals of care and life expectancy are considered?
- Is there a non-pharmacological treatment option for this problem?
- Can the patient adhere to this medication (route and frequency administration, number of pills, monitoring)?
- Could this patient's problem be a side effect of an already prescribed medication?
- What adverse drug events may occur?
- Is the medication being initiated at the lowest possible dose and frequency?
- Has the dose been adjusted on the basis of the patient's creatinine clearance?
- Have I explained all of the above to the patient and to the caregiver?

Preventing and managing falls

What is the safety issue?

Falls can result in serious injury. After a fall, an older adult may be less mobile and is at higher risk for decline in mobility and overall functional status. Injuries sustained after a fall can result in death, particularly if the person was on the floor for a prolonged period after the event or if a fracture occurs.

Why is it a challenge?

Falls do not usually have a single aetiology but are more often multifactorial in origin and require a risk factor assessment to prevent further events.

Older adults are also more likely to have complex neurological conditions, which are associated with increased falls risk. Parkinson's disease and stroke are associated with impairment of gait, which may be difficult to treat.

How can one be safe?

After a single fall, all older adults should undergo an assessment of their balance and gait. A second fall should prompt an interdisciplinary fall assessment.

A home safety evaluation should be conducted. This includes assessing floor coverings, obstacles, lighting, and bathroom safety.

Careful history taking and examination for risk factors for falls should be performed (Box 34.7).

Box 34.7 Risk factors for falls

- history of previous falls/fear of falling;
- inappropriate footwear;
- suboptimal foot care;
- impaired vision and hearing;
- syncope;
- orthostatic hypotension;
- high-risk medications (e.g. benzodiazepines, anticholinergics)
- cognitive impairment;
- gait disorder/musculoskeletal pathologies;
- incontinence;
- environmental hazards.

Gait should be assessed by observing the patient walking, but also by performing a validated balance assessment such as the Timed Get Up and Go test (normal range less than 12 seconds), a 30-second chair stand test or a 4-stage balance test.

There are several scales available to assess a patient's risk for falls while in hospital. The Morse Fall Scale is a widely used and validated tool.

After assessment, a safe mobility plan should be implemented while the patient is in hospital. Falls prevention strategies need to be individualized to reflect the patient's specific risk factors and care needs (Box 34.8).

Box 34.8 Safe mobility care bundle

1. Assess for the presence or absence of delirium.
2. Provide an individualized safe mobility plan.
3. Educate patients and caregivers on falls risk factors.
4. Place the call bell within the patient's sight and reach.
5. Avoid the use of bed or chair alarms.
6. Prepare a continence or toileting care plan.
7. Arrange for an appropriate mobility aid to be within reach.
8. Ensure that adaptive devices for vision and hearing are within reach.
9. Provide appropriate footwear.
10. Assess for medications that increase the risk of falls.
11. Assess for potential syncope and orthostatic hypotension.

How do you measure falls?

Falls can be measured by:

- the number of days since last fall, using a safety cross;
- incidence or frequency of falls, calculated per number of bed days or per number of patients which is more person centred.

Preventing and managing pressure injuries

What is the safety issue?

Pressure injuries are a type of chronic wound characterized by localized damage to the skin and underlying soft tissue over a bony prominence; they can be related to a device. They are associated with increased mortality, longer hospital stay, and higher rates of hospital readmission after discharge.

Why is it a challenge?

Pressure injuries are a challenge because they can be difficult to treat and there is no robust evidence base regarding treatment options.

Prevention is imperative and requires input from all members of the interdisciplinary team.

How can one be safe?

All members of the interdisciplinary team should be trained in assessing risk factors for pressure injuries and prevention strategies.

The SSKIN bundle summarizes the interventions to be undertaken (see Box 34.9).

Box 34.9 The SSKIN care bundle

- SKIN: assess and manage;
- SURFACE: keep surface dry;
- KEEP MOVING to ensure decreased pressure;
- INCONTINENCE management to prevent skin irritation;
- NUTRITION & HYDRATION to maintain skin viability.

All frail older adults should be assessed for the risk for pressure injuries (Box 34.10). A validated risk stratification tool such as the Waterlow score or the Braden or Norton scale can be used.

Box 34.10 Risk factors for pressure injury

- immobility;
- malnutrition;
- older age;
- increased skin moisture (incontinence, sweating);
- medical devices in contact with the skin;
- dementia.

Patient-specific preventive measures should be implemented on the basis of patients' risk factors (Box 34.11).

Specific measures to prevent pressure points are provided in Box 34.12.

Box 34.11 Some prevention measures

- Educate the interdisciplinary team on pressure injury risk factors.
- Implement the SSKIN bundle.
- Don't allow excessive skin moisture.
- Monitor device-related pressure on skin (e.g. urethral catheters).
- Assess and optimize nutritional status.

Box 34.12 Pressure injury prevention measures PRESSURE

Person-centred care planning

Risk assessment on a daily basis, looking at each pressure point (BESTSHOT)

B – buttocks (ischial tuberosities)
E – elbows/ears
S – sacrum (bottom)
T – trochanters (hips)
S – spine/ shoulders
H – heels
O – occipital area (back of the head)
T – toe

Equipment needs to include specialized pressure-relieving cushions for seating and pressure-relieving mattresses

Skin and continence assessment to decease excessive moisture

Skin care

Undertake nutritional screening and optimize

Repositioning on a regular scheduled basis

Evaluate effectiveness of the prevention daily

Visit https://www.nice.org.uk/guidance/cg179/chapter/1-recommendations#management-adults

https://www.hse.ie/eng/about/who/qid/nationalsafetyprogrammes/pressureulcerszero/pressure-ulcers-a-practical-guide-for-review-helen-meagher-050220-cork.pdf

https://www.nationalwoundcarestrategy.net

Management of skin care

If a pressure injury occurs, it should be immediately staged, measured, documented, and, if required, reported to the appropriate reporting body. Pressure injury staging as devised by the National Pressure Ulcer Advisory Board is detailed in Box 34.13.

Box 34.13 Pressure injury stages

Stage 1. Non-blanching redness. Skin intact.

Stage 2. Partial thickness skin loss. No slough or bruising.

Stage 3. Full thickness skin and soft tissue loss. Bone, tendon, or muscle not visible.

Stage 4. Full thickness skin and soft tissue loss. Bone, tendon, or muscle visible

Unstageable. Full thickness soft tissue loss. Base of ulcer obscured by slough or eschar.

Source: https://healthservice.hse.ie/filelibrary/onmsd/hse-national-wound-management-guidelines-2018.pdf

Management of pressure ulcers

- The key management is prevention and detection at stages 1 and 2.
- Proactive relieving of pressure, assisted by appropriate equipment where needed, is essential.
- If a pressure ulcer does occur, it is regarded to be a failure in care.

How do you measure your safety?

The incidence of pressure injuries is a measure of quality both in acute hospitals and in long-term care settings.

In an improvement programme the number of pressure ulcers per day is recorded on a safety cross.

The aim is to increase the number of days between occurrences of a pressure ulcer.

The grade of the pressure ulcer is also measured, and any ulcer over grade 3 could be considered a never event.

Preventing and managing infection

What is the safety issue?

[illegible]

Why is it a challenge?

[illegible]

How can one be safe?

[illegible]

Preventing and managing infection

What is the safety issue?

Frail older adults are more susceptible to infections. They are also more likely to develop opportunistic infections. This is due to age-related changes in the innate and adaptive immune system.

Such changes are known as immunosenescence. The COVID-19 pandemic has demonstrated the susceptibility of the older adult population to infection. Frailty is also associated with mortality following COVID-19 infection, particularly in older adults who reside in nursing home settings.

Why is it a challenge?

Accurate diagnosis and recognition of infection is a challenge.

Frail older adults may have a blunted or absent rise in temperature in response to infection. Rise in white blood cell count may not be present.

The clinical presentation of infection in this population may be atypical; symptoms such as delirium or change in behaviour are more likely to occur.

The diagnosis of infection can be challenging in this patient group. A positive blood culture result does not always confirm active infection. This is particularly so in the case of tract infections (UTIs) where bacteriuria may be present in the absence of symptoms and active infection.

Another challenge is the appropriate use of antibiotics. Frequent use of antibiotics in this population increases the development of drug-resistant pathogens and pseudomembranous colitis.

How can one be safe?

Given that frail older adults are at higher risk for infection and are more likely to receive antibiotic therapy, close adherence to local antimicrobial guidelines is imperative to treating infections appropriately and minimizing antimicrobial resistance.

Indwelling devices such as peripheral venous and urethral catheters must be avoided and, if inserted, removed as soon as possible. This is important for preventing device-related infections and for reducing the incidence of healthcare-acquired infections.

Prophylaxis against infections is often considered for frail older adults. This is particularly the case for urinary tract infections. There is currently no evidence to support the use of prophylactic antibiotics. There is also no evidence for the use of cranberry juice or related products for the prevention of UTIs.

Certain infections, which are more prevalent in frail older adults, can be prevented through immunization (e.g. influenza, pneumococcal disease, and now COVID-19).

Pneumonia in frail older adults carries a higher risk of mortality and is more likely to be caused by gram-positive and gram-negative organisms. Aspiration pneumonia caused by anaerobic organisms is also more common due to the increased prevalence of dysphagia. This should be considered when devising a management plan.

Box 34.14 summarizes important safety issues regarding infections in frail older adults.

Box 34.14 Infections in frail older adults

- Immunizations should be offered as per the local vaccination schedule.
- Fever may be absent, or the elevation in temperature may be blunted.
- White blood cell count may not rise.
- Avoid treating asymptomatic bacteriuria, unless clear symptoms of urinary tract infection are present.
- Adjust the dose and frequency of antibiotics on the basis of creatinine clearance.
- Check for drug interactions when commencing antibiotics.
- Delirium assessment should include an investigation for possible infection.
- Consider aspiration pneumonia in patients with dysphagia.

Summary box

Frail and older adults are at higher risk of safety events. These can all be prevented by following safety principles:

- identification of the risk by pre-assessment;
- preventive measures to decrease the risk;
- constant monitoring to assess changes in risk;
- co-production of preventive measures with individuals and their carers;
- implementation of early interventions when a risk is identified.

Process and outcomes measurement is essential for assessing success in care.

Further reading

Delirium

Bauernfreund, Y. et al. TIME to think about delirium: Improving detection and management on the acute medical unit. *BMJ Open Quality* 7 (2018): e000200. https://doi:10.1136/bmjoq-2017-000200.

Inouye, S. K. et al. Clarifying confusion: The confusion assessment method: A new method for detection of delirium. *Annals of Internal Medicine* 113.12 (1990): 941–8. https://doi:10.7326/0003-4819-113-12-941.

NICE. Delirium: Prevention, diagnosis and management: Clinical guideline (CG 103). 2010. https://www.nice.org.uk/guidance/cg103.

Delirium tests

Gaudreau, J. D. et al. Fast, systematic, and continuous delirium assessment in hospitalized patients: the nursing delirium screening scale. *Journal of Pain Symptom Management* 29.4 (2005): 368–75. https://doi:10.1016/j.jpainsymman.2004.07.009.

Husser, E. K. et al. Implementing a rapid, two-step delirium screening protocol in acute care: Barriers and facilitators. *Journal of the American Geriatrics Society* 69.5 (2021): 1349–56. https://doi:10.1111/jgs.17026

Polypharmacy

American Geriatrics Society. Updated AGS Beers Criteria® for potentially inappropriate medication use in older Adults. *Journal of the American Geriatrics Society* 67.4 (2019): 674–94. https://doi:10.1111/jgs.15767.

Mair, A., Wilson, M., and Dreischulte, T. The polypharmacy programme in Scotland: Realistic prescribing. *Prescriber* 30.8 (2019): 10–16. https://doi.org/10.1002/psb.1779

NHS Scotland. *Polypharmacy Guidance*. Scottish Government, 2018. https://www.therapeutics.scot nhs.uk/wp-content/uploads/2018/04/Polypharmacy-Guidance-2018.pdf.

O'Mahony, D. STOPP/START criteria for potentially inappropriate medications/potential prescribing omissions in older people: Origin and progress. Expert Review of Clinical Pharmacology 13.1 (2020): 15–22. https://doi:10.1080/17512433.2020.1697676.

World Health Organization. *Medication Safety in Polypharmacy: Technical Report*. Geneva, 2019 (WHO/UHC/SDS/2019.11). Licence: CC BY-NC-SA 3.0 IGO. https://apps.who.int/iris/handle/10665/325454.

Falls

Ganz, D. A. and Latham, N. K. Prevention of falls in community-dwelling older adults. New England Journal of Medicine 382.8 (2020): 734–43. https://doi.org/10.1056/nejmcp1903252.

Morse, J. M., Morse, R. M., and Tylko, S. J. Development of a scale to identify the fall-prone patient *Canadian Journal on Aging* 8.4 (1989): 366–77. https://doi.org/10.1017/S0714980800008576.

NICE. Falls in older people: Assessing risk and prevention: Clinical guideline (CG161). 12 June 2013 https://www.nice.org.uk/guidance/cg161.

Royal College of Physicians. FallSafe resources: Original. 13 August 2015. https://www.rcplondon ac.uk/guidelines-policy/fallsafe-resources-original

Pressure ulcers

NICE. Pressure ulcers: Prevention and management: Clinical guideline (CG179). 23 April 2014. https://pathways.nice.org.uk/pathways/pressure-ulcers.

Websites:

HSE Ireland: https://www.hse.ie/eng/about/who/qid/nationalsafetyprogrammes/pressureulcerszero.

NHS Scotland: http://www.healthcareimprovementscotland.org/our_work/standards_and_guidelines/stnds/pressure_ulcer_standards.aspx.

Infections

AGS. Choosing wisely. 2017. https://www.choosingwisely.org/wp-content/uploads/2018/02/Antibiotics-For-Urinary-Tract-Infections-In-Older-People-AGS.pdf.

British Geriatrics Society. COVID-19: Managing COVID-19 pandemic in care homes for older people. 2020. https://www.bgs.org.uk/resources/covid-19-managing-the-covid-19-pandemic-in-care-homes.

Lithander, F. E. et al. COVID-19 in older people: A rapid clinical review. *Age and Ageing* 49.4 (2020): 501–15. https://doi:10.1093/ageing/afaa093.

Chapter 35

Safety in a multidisciplinary team

Key points

- Chronic care requires the integration of different specialties.
- Clinical teams need to come together to coordinate care.
- A multidisciplinary team can increase shared understanding, develop shared goals and decrease the potential for safety events.
- The team will require a change in culture and mutual respect for all members.

What is the safety issue?

In Chapter 6 the development of safe clinical teams was discussed. In clinical care, the complex ways in which services are designed and the increasing number of comorbidities in people with chronic conditions require working across clinical teams.

Healthcare is delivered in many different scenarios, from community and primary care to secondary or tertiary care. This involves many stakeholders from different layers of the treatment pyramid. Within a hospital, clinical teams often work in silos and the patient is seen as a disease entity rather than as a person with multiple problems that require integration. The lack of integrated care can result in safety and quality challenges.

From the perspective of the person receiving care, the main issues are:

- lack of coordinated care;
- exclusion from decision-making;
- communication issues;
- lack of medicine reconciliation;
- delays in treatment;
- confusing and conflicting messages.

From a safety perspective, given the development of chronic illnesses of increasing complexity, the traditional mode of care delivery by a single clinician can be a safety issue. Multidisciplinary teams (MDTs) aim to integrate care, putting the patient and the family at the centre of all decision-making.

The MDT aims to develop shared understanding in order to achieve desired outcomes. Benefits of MDT include improved experience and improved outcomes. Despite this, care remains uncoordinated and the implementation of integrated care remains a challenge. Box 35.1 shows some of the evidence-based benefits of MDT care that have been found in the care of people with chronic conditions and cancer.

Box 35.1 Benefits of MDTs

- They improve clinical outcomes.
- They improve patient satisfaction and experience.
- They improve employee satisfaction.
- They improve staff performance.
- They improve staff retention.
- They decrease the incidence of adverse events.
- They lower the cost of healthcare.

Why is it a challenge?

Despite widespread acknowledgement of the value of person-centred thinking in healthcare, there is still a marked hierarchy in this field, with doctors at the top of the pyramid. This can prevent staff from collaborating, both within a team and across teams, and fosters silo thinking, which has a negative impact on healthcare. Often there still seems to be an emphasis on individual behaviour, as clinicians and team members act as individuals rather than as integrated members of a team with a shared understanding of the care process.

The development of a successful MDT will need to overcome several barriers. Each one needs to be addressed, as they all can impact safety.

Barriers to effective MDTs

- traditional ways of working;
- professional rivalries;
- tribalism and history of silo working;
- different locations;
- use of different languages;
- cultural differences;
- separate documentation;
- lack of awareness and appreciation of the roles and responsibilities of others;
- time constraints.

Who should be in the multidisciplinary team?

Core MDTs usually consist of team leaders and members who are direct care providers, such as nurses, dentists, pharmacists, doctors, allied professionals, and case managers.

A team established to take care of a person with cancer would make a good example. There are numerous specialities involved there, from the primary care team, the hospital physician, and the surgeon to the radiotherapist and the oncologists. They may work in different departments and hospitals. Once they are engaged in the care of the patient, they form the core team. However, without a formal MDT process they may act in silos.

Team members with vastly differing education, experience, backgrounds (both personal and professional) and skills may complement one another well. Yet, whether they deliver chronic care in the community or run a cardiac arrest in the intensive care unit, it is crucial that healthcare providers cooperate, function as effective MDTs, and avoid harmful behaviours such as the silo or halo effect, where individuals may be blamed for failures of the team.

How can one be safe?

Just as building a safe clinical team requires respect for all members and psychological safety, when one brings the MDT together, this is extended across a whole patient journey. The approach to the complexity of care is to have a view of the entire care pathway and of all that is required in order to provide safe care. The Systems Engineering Initiative for Patient Safety SEIPS 3.0 (Figure 35.1) offers a human factors approach to the SEIPS 2.0 model discussed in Chapter 9.

The model enlarges the clinical team, encompassing all the care providers needed for reaching desired outcomes across the entire patient journey. It includes management-level decisions, which define the conditions under which patients are treated. It also includes non-medical areas such as the purchase, supply, and design of services and personnel administration.

To ensure safe care in an effective MDT, a few steps are required.

Build the case and will for the team

The MDT will not simply happen. The case for the team must be made and planned, with clear roles, responsibilities, aims and objectives, and measurable outcomes. Each clinician or provider of support in management or administration, in various other sectors apart from healthcare, needs to be considered. A coordinator for the MDT is essential. The process must be planned and tested—and it should start small.

Include patients and families

It is essential that patients and their families are an integral and equal part of the MDT. Codesign of services and coproduction of health and healthcare are essential for successful outcomes.

Facilitate effective communication

Communication is a key element of effective MDTs. Communication loops that are non-directed, open, or with delayed closure are susceptible to information loss. This can have consequences in chronic care as well as in critical care environments, for instance in the operating room or in resuscitation. Closed loop communication ensures that all have the same understanding and that this understanding is acknowledged through 'read back', for example.

Implement in-patient multidisciplinary rounds

Rounding with all the professionals improves the safety, quality, and experience of care. They can create a culture of collaboration and improvement. The aim is to deal proactively with issues and to develop situation awareness. This can decrease the length of stays, lower the number of central line days, and improve the coordination of care. By pooling expertise, different disciplines can transfer knowledge, set care priorities, establish targets, coordinate patient care, and determine and plan for patient disposition (Box 35.2).

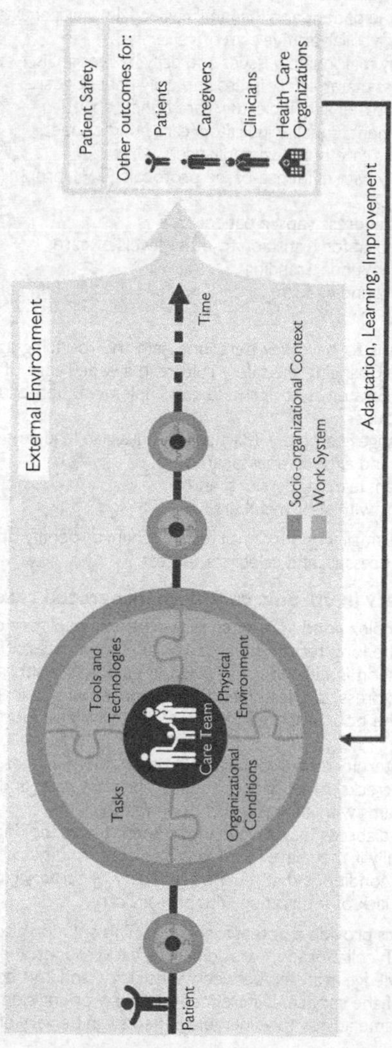

Figure 35.1 SEIPS 2.0 (Reproduced with permission from Holden et al. (2013).

Box 35.2 Key aspects of multidisciplinary rounds

1. They include all those who are involved in the care of patients.
2. They treat the patient and the family as equal participants.
3. They define a collaborative plan of care.
4. They identify major safety issues and daily patient goals.
5. They address major safety issues and daily patient goals.
6. They develop a quality indicator/care bundle sheet.
7. They implement a quality indicator/care bundle sheet.
8. They address care bundle compliance.
9. They comply with evidence-based protocols (DVT prophylaxis, and vaccination).
10. Identify and address gaps in patient care
11. Identify the plan for transition to other levels of care
12. Develop team understanding
13. Implement rounding form

The challenge is to have key personnel join the rounding against competing priorities. Changing the safety culture in a wide range of specialities can be difficult. Strategies to facilitate the implementation of multidisciplinary rounds include:

- identifying change champions (particularly physician leaders);
- defining roles and expectations clearly;
- holding frequent learning sessions; and
- communicating with staff members.

It is best to start small, conduct small tests of change, identify opportunities to streamline processes, and celebrate success.

Maintain safety in chronic care with integrated care

People with complex conditions often require multidisciplinary care in both the short and the long term. The process can sometimes be fragmented and communication is difficult if delivered in different healthcare settings. Patients have expressed dissatisfaction with the varying management approaches and the poorly shared care between clinicians. Here are a few examples:

- Antenatal maternity care. Prospective mothers may feel that they 'fall between the cracks' of obstetrics, medical, primary care, and other healthcare teams with suboptimal communication.
- Patients with diabetes may have many different teams looking after them, especially if they have more than one comorbidity.
- Patients with conditions that require secondary or tertiary care often experience a lack of integration with primary care.

Combined clinics provide a potential solution. This solution also limits hospital visits. MDT collaboration with different backgrounds and viewpoints facilitates knowledge transfer between specialities and can contribute to the evolution of the service. Different specialities working side by side and delivering the same advice to vulnerable patients can be very effective.

Summary box

- [illegible]
- [illegible]
- [illegible]
- [illegible]
- [illegible]

Reference

[illegible]

Further reading

[illegible]

Summary box

- Chronic care is challenging because of increasing comorbidities.
- Silo working presents safety challenges that can be addressed by MDTs.
- Successful MDTs are based on a culture of respect and inclusiveness, where everyone's view is valued.
- Careful planning and coordination are required.
- MDT bedside rounding has benefits for both staff and patients.

Reference

Carayon, P. et al. SEIPS 3.0: Human-centered design of the patient journey for patient safety. *Applied Ergonomics* 84 (2020). doi:10.1016/j.apergo.2019.103033.

Further reading

Clinical Excellence Commission, New South Wales. Multidisciplinary team rounds. NSW 2019. https://www.cec.health.nsw.gov.au/improve-quality/Safety-Fundamentals-for-Teams/multidisciplinary-team-rounds.

Emmel, B. and Golden, J. Multidisciplinary Rounds: Not MORE work, but THE work. Institute for Healthcare Improvement 2019. http://www.ihi.org/resources/Pages/ImprovementStories/MultidisciplinaryRoundsNotMOREWorkbutTHEWork.aspx.

Epstein, N. E. Multidisciplinary in-hospital teams improve patient outcomes: A review. *Surgical Neurology International* 5, Suppl. 7 (2014): S295–303.

Weller, J., Boyd, M., and Cumin, D. Teams, tribes and patient safety: Overcoming barriers to effective teamwork in healthcare. *Postgraduate Medical Journal* 90.1061 (2014): 149–54. doi: 10.1136/postgradmedj-2012-131168.

Safety in the laboratory

Key points

- Up to 95% of the clinical pathways rely on patients having access to pathology services.
- 500 million biochemistry and 130 million haematology tests are carried out per year by the NHS.
- 300,000 tests are performed every working day.
- 50 million reports are sent from labs to GPs every year.
- 2 million units of donated blood are transfused every year.
- 40% of the tests ordered are unnecessary.

Disciplines involved in laboratory medicine and examples of tests performed

There are a variety of subspecialties in laboratory medicine that offer a vast array of tests. Knowledge of the type of test offered, of how to choose the correct test and how to interpret and integrate the result correctly into patient care, is fundamental to patient safety and patient-related outcomes.

The list given here is not intended as a complete record of either specialities or tests; these are just examples of the most common tests.

Haematology	FBC White cell differential PTT, INR, APTT, D-dimers Fibrinogen Pregnancy testing Malaria screens
Blood transfusion	ABO & Rh D Grouping and Antibody Screening Antibody identification Crossmatching blood Direct antiglobulin test Phenotyping
Clinical chemistry	Urea and electrolytes (Na, K, Cl, Urea, Creatinine) Liver function tests (albumin, bilirubin, alkaline phosphatase, GGT, ALT, AST, total protein) Ca, PO4, Mg Amylase Lipids (T. Chol, Tg, HDL Chol, LDL Chol) Glucose Uric acid
Immunology	Anti-nuclear antibody (ANA) Anti-smooth muscle antibody Anti-mitochondrial ANA Anti-dsDNA ANCA Rheumatoid factor (RF) C3, C4 Anti-CCP antibody Coeliac disease: Anti-tTG Anti-EMA
Microbiology and Virology	Culture and sensitivity testing Blood cultures Viral PCR (e.g. respiratory swabs)/viral serology MRSA screening PCR

Histopathology	Fine needle aspiration cytology Fluid cytology Biopsies Staging of cancer resections Interoperative assessment Immunohistochemistry Molecular testing

Laboratory processes

By comparison with other specialities, laboratory medicine is a low-risk speciality if processes for safety are in place; but it is delivered in a pressurized environment, with a vast array of different testing methodologies, complex technology, and variation in input.

Error reduction in the laboratory

- Safety is often viewed through the prism of error and error reduction.
- Laboratory error has been defined by the ISO Technical Report 22367 as a defect occurring at any part of the laboratory cycle, from ordering tests to reporting, interpreting, and reacting to results.

Laboratory testing process

The testing process is illustrated in Figure 36.1. It has the following characteristics:

- It is a complex process.
- It has multiple separate steps.
- Numerous individuals are involved in it.

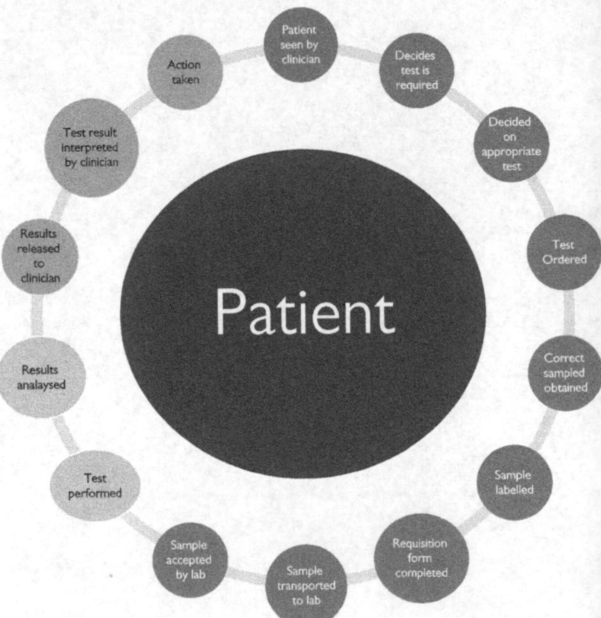

Figure 36.1 Laboratory testing cycle.

- Each step is vulnerable to error and is a potential threat to patient safety.
- For the purposes of analysing patient safety issues, these different processes can be divided into three phases: pre-analytical, analytical, and post analytical.
- The division into these categories does not attempt to suggest that one phase affects patients more than another. The potential consequences are the same in all three.

Errors in laboratory medicine

Pre-analytical error

- Up to 75% of all testing errors occur in the pre-analytical phase
- This phase is the one most prone to error, as it involves the most steps and the most people.
- The phase is also fragmented; the first part of the phase is performed outside of the laboratory, while the second part is performed inside the laboratory
- The pre-analytical phase sees a mixture of non-laboratory staff and laboratory staff that handles the specimen between the time of order and the time of delivery to the laboratory.
- Common causes of error in this phase are displayed in Box 36.1.

Box 36.1 Common causes of pre-analytical error

- inappropriate tests ordered;
- tests ordered on the incorrect patient;
- improper sample collection;
- transport delays;
- illegible handwriting on requisition slips;
- incorrect container used;
- lack of clinical details.

Although these areas are beyond the jurisdiction of the clinical laboratory itself, the credibility of the lab is at stake because of these errors. The laboratories must bear the burden of the inconsistencies or incorrect reporting that can ensue from these preanalytical errors.

Analytical error

The analytical phase of laboratory testing involves the preparation of the sample in the laboratory, testing, interpretation, and verification of the result by a pathologist. Analytical errors in this phase are estimated at 7%–13% (for examples, see Box 36.2).

Box 36.2 Errors that may occur at the analytic phase of testing

- sample mix up;
- incorrect processing prior to analysis;
- equipment malfunctions or failure in test processes;
- incorrect calibration or lack of maintenance;
- interpretation error.

Post-analytical error

The interpretation of the test is complete and, once verified, the results are released to the requesting clinician for their interpretation. Patient safety may impact from errors or omissions in the report provided by the laboratory (see Box 36.3):

Box 36.3 Post analytic errors

- incomplete reports;
- incorrect patient details;
- long turnaround times;
- failure to notify critical values;
- report not read;
- misapplication or misinterpretation of an accurate report by a clinician.

Error reduction

Error reduction in the pre-analytical phase

- As already outlined, the total testing system is a complex and fragmented process.
- Error prevention requires a multidisciplinary approach, led by the laboratory.
- This includes the prevention of errors at the pre-analytical phase (see Box 36.4), which accounts for much of the error rate.
- Laboratory medicine must take ownership of this issue and not dismiss it as coming from an extraneous source, out of the lab's control.

Box 36.4 Prevention of pre-analytical errors

- clear written policies and procedures;
- education and training;
- automation and information technology;
- monitoring of quality indicators;
- interdepartmental cooperation.

A key component of education should be to ensure that the correct test is carried out on the correct patient at the correct time and correctly.

Error reduction in the analytical phase

Error reduction is achieved through the following methods:

- EQA participation;
- continual professional development;
- consultation with colleagues;
- multidisciplinary meetings;
- case reviews;
- competency assessement;
- calibration of measuring systems;
- internal controls;
- SOPS.

Error reduction in the post-analytical phase

Error reduction is achieved through the following methods:

- synoptic reporting;
- consistent format;
- automatic alerts for critical values;
- electronic system to track report acknowledgment.

Critical values

- Critical values are test results that may indicate a pathophysiological state that could be life-threatening or of immediate clinical significance.
- All laboratories should have systems in place to both identify and communicate critical values.
- Having an appropriate system in place to cover the communication of results is an explicit requirement of ISO 15189 from 2012.
- While the importance of critical values is universally accepted, the scope of critical values is not well defined.
- The Royal College of Pathologists offers suggested tests and triggers, but recommends that critical values should be defined according to local clinical needs and circumstances (Croal 2017).

Communication of critical values

When rapid communication of a laboratory test result is indicated, the information on the list in Box 36.5 should be provided to the clinical team.

Box 36.5 Key information for communication of critical values

- the patient's name, date of birth, and unique identifier;
- critical or unexpected test results, with units, along with any reference range, if relevant or requested;
- the date and time of the request;
- the name of the requesting clinician;
- any relevant clinical history that may be available, or any relevant past laboratory test results;
- contact address for the patient and any telephone number, if known (this may be more relevant for primary care locations).

This information should ideally be transmitted electronically, with read receipts if available, to avoid verbal transcription errors. Any unnecessary verbal transmission of results should be avoided if access to electronic means is possible.

Hence an electronic means of recording when results are urgently communicated should be in place; and it should also record the name of the person to whom the result is communicated, the name of the laboratory person communicating the result, and the date and time of the communication.

External quality assessment

The accuracy of laboratory results is vital to providing a safe, high-quality service. One method of ensuring a high-quality service is participation in an external quality assessment (EQA) scheme (for benefits, see Box 36.6). (WHO, 2009)

- EQA allows for an objective measurement of a laboratory's testing performance using an external agency or facility.
- EQA is an essential part of the lab's quality management system.
- It provides information that allows laboratories to assess and monitor the quality status of internal procedures and processes, the suitability of the diagnostic systems, and the accountability and competence of the staff.
- It gives assurance to the laboratories themselves, to their users, and to the public that their work is of an appropriate quality, is reliable, and is in line with the work of their peers nationally.
- EQA participation is usually required for accreditation.

Types of EQA methods

1. Proficiency testing—the external provider sends unknown samples for testing to a set of laboratories, and the results of all laboratories are analysed, compared, and reported to the laboratories.
2. Rechecking or retesting—slides that have been read are rechecked by a reference laboratory; samples that have been analysed are retested, allowing for inter-laboratory comparison.
3. On-site evaluation—usually done when it is difficult to conduct traditional proficiency testing or to use the rechecking/retesting method.

Box 36.6 Benefits of EQA

Allows for comparison of performance and results between different laboratories.
Identifies systematic problems associated with kits or operations.
Offers objective evidence of the quality of testing.
Indicates areas that need improvement.
Highlights where training is required.

EQA performance problems

A poor performance on EQA requires investigation. The problems may lie anywhere along the path of workflow. Possible sources of error include:

In the pre-analytical phase

- The sample may have been compromised during preparation, shipping, or after receipt in the laboratory through improper storage or handling.
- There may have been incorrect labelling or processing.

In the analytical phase

- There may have been issues with reagents, instruments, the methodology, calibrations, and calculations.
- The competence of staff members will need to be considered and evaluated.
- Analytical problems should be investigated to determine whether error is random or systemic.

In the post-analytical phase

- Confusing report format.
- Incorrect interpretation of results.
- Clerical or transcription errors (Croal 2017; Plebani 2006).

Policies, feedback, and risk assessment

One can apply the Juran trilogy (planning, control, improvement) to the development of policies that are an essential part of any laboratory.

Planning

A laboratory must have standard operating procedures (SOP) and policies on the quality required. Quality manuals need to be developed and regularly updated. All aspects of the laboratory service should be covered under standard operating procedures. User manuals should be available online for consultation.

Control

Laboratory quality requires strict measurement over all parts of the process, as well as on the outcomes. Regular user surveys and assessments of complaints with real-time feedback allow laboratories to identify areas that require improvement. Failure to evolve puts patients potentially at risk by either offering the wrong test or the not offering the right test at the right time. The risk management system should assess:

- errors, near misses and non-conformances;
- trends in incidents.

Improvement

A non-conformance management programme should involve corrective and preventive action. A safe laboratory will have a continuous improvement programme is in place that involves all members of staff (see Box 36.7). This programme will aim at taking both corrective and preventive action to maintain the standards, in line with corporate and accreditation requirements.

Box 36.7 Case study: Learning from errors

When errors occur and either patient harm occurs or there is a near miss it is important to investigate, establish causation through root cause analysis, and find methods to reduce the risk. One such programme, established after a high-profile misdiagnosis, is the Irish Histopathology National Quality Improvement Programme. It was the first in the world to report publicly national metrics on the quality of its histopathology system.

Evidence-based targets were established, so that participating laboratories can track their performance and identify areas of strength and weakness. The Histopathology Improvement programme also provides documentary evidence where extra resourcing may be required.

Examples of possible targets are the percentage of cases reviewed at MDT meetings; the percentage of reports reviewed by a second consultant; and the timeliness of reports.

In addition to giving the public an evidence-based assurance of the quality of diagnostic services, the programme also allows for improved communication between participating laboratories, as those that perform well are encouraged to share their best practice approach with other laboratories, which results in improved standards overall.

Safety beyond the laboratory

Laboratory staff members have several roles outside the strict confines of the lab. These roles play an active and essential part in maintaining patient safety. They include haemovigilance, antimicrobial stewardship, multidisciplinary meetings, research, and forming ethics committees and patient safety advisor groups.

Haemo-vigilance

Haemovigilance is defined by EC Directive 2002/98/EC as 'organised surveillance procedures relating to serious adverse or unexpected events or reactions in donors or recipients and the epidemiological follow up of donors'.

- There were 21 transfusion related deaths, 112 patients suffered major morbidity and there were 1671 near misses in the UK in 2017 ('Annual SHOT report 2017', 2018).
- Errors account for 85.5% of all reported incidents ('Annual SHOT report 2017', 2018).

Role of the haemo-vigilance officer

- Promotes the appropriate use of blood, blood products and blood alternatives.
- Provides and organizes education and training for the staff.
- Facilitates the traceability of blood and blood products.
- Monitors adverse reactions, near misses, and non-compliance.
- Identifies and investigates all adverse reactions to transfusion.
- Educates patients or clients and their families.

Antimicrobial stewardship

- Antimicrobial resistance, which renders bacterial infections resistant to standard treatment, is a growing concern globally.
- Antimicrobial resistance increases the cost of healthcare through lengthier stays in hospital and the need for more medical intervention.
- Microbiology laboratories and clinical microbiologists should play a central role in securing the provision of these services leading the development and provision of an antimicrobial stewardship programme. (See Chapter 23, Sepsis and Antimicrobial Stewardship)

Summary box

- The role of the laboratory is to support the clinical staff in the diagnosis and treatment of clinical conditions.
- Laboratories need to have safe processes in order to protect the staff in the laboratory; they also need to provide error-free results in a timely manner, for both clinicians and patients.
- Errors can take place during three phases: pre-analytical, analytical, and post-analytical.
- The application of safety theory to processes in the laboratory will assist by ensuring reliability and safety at all the stages.
- The laboratory has an important role to play in haemo-vigilance and antimicrobial stewardship.

References

Annual SHOT report 2017. SHOT: Serious Hazards of Transfusion. 12 July 2018. https://www.shotuk.org/2017-annual-shot-report-published-12-july-2018.

Croal, B. *The Communication of Critical and Unexpected Pathology Results*. London: Royal College of Pathologists, 2017.

Plebani, P J. Errors in clinical laboratories or errors in laboratory medicine? *Clinical Chemistry and Laboratory Medicine* 44.6 (2006): 750–9.

World Health Organisation. Overview of external quality assessment (EQA) WHO Laboratory Quality Management System Training Toolkit: Strengthening health security by implementing the international health regulations. 2009. Content Sheet 10. https://www.who.int/publications/m/item/overview-of-external-quality-assessment-eqa

Further reading

Badrick, T. et al. External quality assessment beyond the analytical phase: An Australian perspective. *Biochemia Medica* 27.1 (2017): 73–80.

Bonini, P. et al. Errors in laboratory medicine. *Journal of Clinical Chemistry* 53 (2007):1338–42.

Hammerling, J. A. A review of medical errors in laboratory diagnostics and where we are today. *Laboratory Medicine* 43.2 (2012): 41–4.

Lippi, G. and Guidi, G. C. Risk management in the preanalytical phase of laboratory testing. *Clinical Chemistry* 45 (2007): 720–7.

Lippi, G. and Plebani, M. The importance of incident reporting in laboratory diagnostics. *Scandinavian Journal of Clinical and Laboratory Investigation* 69.8 (2009): 811–14.

Medical Laboratories. *Reduction of Error through Risk Management and Continual Improvement*. Online Browsing Platform, 2009. https://www.iso.org/obp/ui/#iso:std:iso:ts:22367:ed-1:v1:en.

National Pathology Programme. *Digital First: Clinical Transformation through Pathology Innovation*. 2004. https://www.england.nhs.uk/wp-content/uploads/2014/02/pathol-dig-first.pdf.

Sandhu, P. K. et al. Effectiveness of laboratory practices to reduce specimen labeling errors at the time of specimen collection in healthcare settings: A laboratory medicine best practices (LMBP) systematic review. *Journal of Applied Laboratory Medicine* 2 (2017): 244–58.

Tang, D. et al. Patient safety issues in pathology: From mislabeled specimens to interpretation errors. *Vignettes in Patient Safety* 3 (2018): 141–59. https://www.intechopen.com. doi:10.5772/intechopen.79634.

Chapter 37

Patient safety in a pandemic

Key points

This chapter addresses patient safety issues and approaches during a pandemic. It explores a system-wide approach, focusing on the following areas:

- public health measures in the community, in work environments, and in clinical pathways for patients and healthcare workers (the suggested actions are derived from Tartaglia 2020 and are based on experiences summarized by clinical risk managers);
- key human factors messages to assist in high-pressured environments;
- a compilation of 'milestones' and indicators for patient safety in a pandemic.

What is the safety issue?

A pandemic is an infrequent event. Health systems need to be prepared for the eventuality of a pandemic. This state of preparedness must be a constant, whether it be in terms of national plans, local interventions, or the application of public health measures. Pandemics are VUCA events: volatile, uncertain, complex, and ambiguous. They present challenges to the health system and society; moreover, they constantly change and renew these challenges.

To be successful in responding to a VUCA event, healthcare systems need to:

- place people first in all decision-making—and by 'people' we mean both citizens at large and healthcare providers more specifically;
- be creative in how they manage operations and work across boundaries and sectors;
- ensure that there is strong teamwork and clear communication.

All this requires a special kind of leadership: compassionate, reflective, and possessed of humility. In this chapter we provide key learning from the COVID-19 pandemic.

Why is it a challenge?

A pandemic is defined as an epidemic that stretches over a very wide area, runs across national boundaries, and affects a very large number of people. In a pandemic it is a challenge to maintain patient safety, that is, to ensure the absence of preventable harm to patients. To declare an infection outbreak to be a pandemic, the infection in question needs to be caused by an emerging pathogen to which the general population, including healthcare workers, is largely susceptible. Depending on infectivity and virulence, a pandemic can cause multiple individuals to be simultaneously affected, generating a massive influx of patients. This can result in hospital overcrowding and staff overload on the one hand, staff shortage caused by illness on the other.

There may be limited but evolving knowledge of the pathogen, its transmission, clinical manifestations, diagnostic work-up, and treatment. This can increase uncertainty and make the field even more slippery for healthcare operators and management.

Given the exceptional characteristics of a pandemic, appropriate preparation and situational awareness can be deficient. For example, the Influenza and COVID-19 pandemics, with their characteristics of diffusion and severity, revealed the unequivocal need for personal protective equipment (PPE).

What is known to work? What is the theoretical basis?

Judging from the experience of pandemics over the past twenty years, the following measures appear to work (Box 37.1):

Box 37.1 What works in pandemics

- Prevent the impact of reduced institutional resilience and address low situational awareness and slow reaction to the danger of the pandemic.
- Apply systems and multidisciplinary approaches to develop solutions.
- Apply human factors and ergonomics theories as a framework.
- Adapt and standardize clinical pathways to have reliable care.
- Implement public health initiatives of testing and contact tracing.
- Work with the public to co-produce solutions.

How can one be safe?

An adequate approach to patient safety in such a context can only be systematic and have a logical approach. It will look at three aspects:

1. the safety of public health measures (the target community);
2. the safety of work systems using human factors and ergonomics;
3. clinical pathways (target patients and operators).

Above all, as the pandemic involves more countries, the root cause of any adverse event is the delayed recognition, and therefore the delayed declaration, initially of an epidemic, then of a pandemic at the international level.

Public health measures

Public health measures (PHMs) include individual protective measures for the target community.

People

- hand hygiene;
- face masks;
- respiratory etiquette.

Environmental

- surface and object cleaning;
- travel restrictions such as border closure, tourist restrictions, entry and exit screening at airports and ports;
- social distancing with an aim to reduce crowded spaces, for example by ensuring that employees can work from home wherever possible:
  - In many countries during the COVID-19 outbreak, this led governments to declare that certain occupations have 'keyworker status', which allowed professionals in these categories to continue work: delivery drivers, refuse workers, teachers for children of keyworkers, supermarket employees, police officers, pharmacists, and other healthcare professionals, and so on. Non-essential activities may be closed, for example, cafes and nightclubs;
- contact tracing, self-isolation of exposed persons, and quarantine of those infected:
  - the length of time suggested for quarantine and self-isolation will depend on the estimated period of infectivity of the pathogen.

These measures are aimed to delay and reduce the size of the peak (see Figure 37.1) and to slow down transmission, so that the impact of the pandemic is mitigated and hospitals are not oversaturated.

Cultural, socioeconomic, and political factors can affect or delay the application of PHMs— with serious preventable harm to the community, lack of integration between health and political authorities, inadequacy of national emergency task force (ETF), and delayed or omitted decisions.

Safety of the work systems

The application of the SEIPS model for healthcare work systems includes any clinical area, either in the hospital or in the community. Safety in the work system is based on:

a. team and organizational culture and communication;
b. environment safety;
c. the tasks required for achieving outcomes and the availability of an appropriate skill mix of staff;

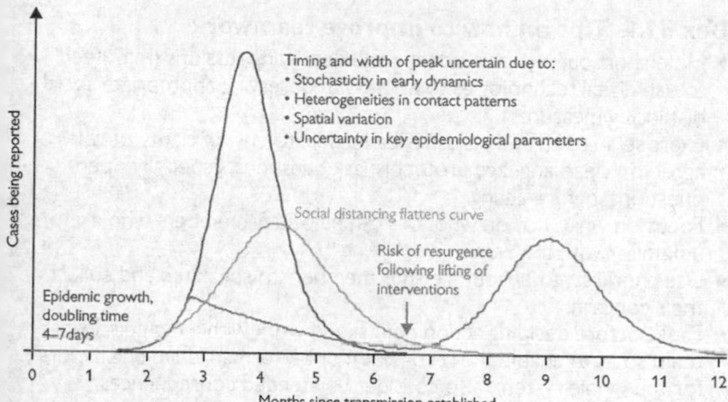

Figure 37.1 Flattening the curve.

Source: Anderson et al. 2020. Reproduced with permission of Elsevier

d. equipment for patient care and for protecting the staff;
e. the people involved, namely the staff and the patients.

Team and organizational culture and communication

A human factors approach can provide value in high-pressure environments. These factors address non-technical skills in order to enhance teamwork and open communication (see Box 37.2).

Attention to culture and communication is essential if we want to ensure effective teamwork. Clinical risk management units can play an important role in this setting through the following activities and operations:

- activation of the local emergency task force (ETF) through a clear chain of command, roles, and responsibilities;
- reliable information-sharing tools and a proactive approach to communication;
- dissemination of clear real-time information to frontline workers;
- maintenance of reporting and learning systems, with rapid reporting tools; and
- collection and dissemination of good practice.

Environmental safety

Safer care in a safer environment involves the following measures:

- Early and appropriate instructions for environment disinfection (detergents, contact time, frequency) to cleaners and domestic staff will prevent in-hospital or clinic transmission. Germicide deficiency can be avoided through galenic preparations.
- A dedicated hospital or clinical area for infected patients is better than a separation between clean and dirty pathways within the same clinical area.
- Screening patients will identify suspected cases on admission to healthcare services, including among those admitted for other reasons (e.g. surgery, coronary angioplasty, labour and delivery).

Box 37.2 Tips on how to improve teamwork

- Hold short but inclusive briefing and debriefing sessions (may need to use digital technologies to assist with observing appropriate social distancing measures)
- Exercise an open and inclusive leadership, to ensure clarity of roles; agree on clear language protocols; ask questions, especially open questions, before acting.
- Focus on what, not on who: this can help staff members who are unfamiliar with the work.
- Use checklists to encourage staff members to speak up; and collect their concerns.
- Pause before deciding action points, and work with a multidisciplinary team so as to enable the recognition of performance-limiting factors for the whole system; also consider unintended consequences.

- Reduction or suspension of non-urgent hospital admissions, routine outpatient clinic appointments and routine surgical procedures is recommended.
- Limit access and implement mandatory precautions for visitors (e.g. surgical masks, two-meter distance between seats in waiting rooms). Restricted numbers of visitors and limited visiting hours will reduce transmission. Healthcare facilities may be asked to limit visits, and a change of clothes for visitors may be required in highly infectious pandemics.

Tasks required and the appropriate skill mix

The following actions are required:

- Staff rotas may need to be revised for frontline workers in order to ensure that sufficient personnel is available to meet demand, especially out of hours.
- Planning should be made for potential sick leave, in case healthcare staff members or their families become infected and need to self-isolate.
- An assessment of tasks and skills is required to manage patients.
- Education plans with simulation training and refresher courses should be developed.
- There should be provision of simulation training and support for the use of medical and protective devices (e.g. for the use of CPAP/NIV machines and how to set them up, especially if special adaptations such as extra filters or alternative masks are required to reduce transmission).
- Human factor principles can be applied to ensure appropriate donning (putting on) and doffing (taking off) of Personal Protective Equipment (PPE)
- Healthcare personnel from other specialties may be called upon to cover work in the pandemic units.

Apply reliability principles of standardization of tasks to ensure effective care (e.g. hand-hygiene; SEPSIS bundle; bundle for the prevention of ventilator-associated pneumonia or central venous catheter infections).

Equipment for patient care and for protecting the staff

Biosafety precautions tailored to the transmission route of the responsible pathogen are essential for staff protection.

- Assessment of the PPE is required, as per infectivity of the pathogen.
- Address supply chains to prevent PPE shortages.
- Consider possible reusable models, or extended use as well as policies for a limited reuse of PPE.
- Identify priority areas.
- Store PPE in a secure facility.

Equipment for treating patients must be available and well functioning in care areas. Examples are stock for pathology labs, gas analysers, pulse oximeters, mechanical ventilators, suction and intravenous pumps, oxygen therapy.

Clinical pathways and processes

The identification of high-risk steps in the diagnosis and treatment of infection, in care transition (hospital discharge), and in special settings or with categories of patients (e.g. surgical, obstetrics, paediatrics, oncology, or immunosuppressed patients) is fundamental to developing reliable clinical pathways and to reducing preventable harm.

Key issues to be addressed for a safe diagnosis and treatment include:

- availability of diagnostic tests, reliability and timeliness of diagnostic processes;
- clear and updated criteria for diagnostic testing, correct methods of performing the test (standardization and quality validation), and appropriate training for the staff;
- awareness of clinical and laboratory red flags and uncommon presentations;
- criteria for severity stratification to assist safe discharge or in-hospital allocation ('clean', non-infected ward vs pathogen-positive 'dirty' ward);
- parameters to monitor patients, with potential need to modify early warning systems and to set clear criteria for an escalation of care;
- clear guidance and hospital policy on drug–drug and drug–disease interactions or on other treatment precautions;
- clear and structured information at discharge, with recommendations for follow-up and social or working life restrictions (is the patient cured or only clinically cured? does the patient need home isolation? what precautions must be observed in case of isolation, next appointments, etc.).

Specific clinical considerations

Obstetrics

In pregnant women, the safety practice is focused on preventing contagion both for the mother (reduction of prenatal care, screening of cases, isolation of infected pregnant women) and for the newborn (mother–infant separation, use of biosafety precautions, or breast pump for breastfeeding). The use of experimental drugs may need special consideration, as well as the decision in favour of pre-term delivery or caesarean section.

Paediatrics

In children there may be differences in clinical presentation, and therefore different management protocols.

Oncology

In patients with cancer and in other immunocompromised patients, the focus is on the safety of the required procedures. Postponement of antineoplastic treatment should be evaluated on a case-by-case basis; immune suppressants must not be suspended, but dose increases should be postponed; a route of administration suitable for home treatment should be considered; steroids can be continued cautiously. It is key to prevent infection with the pandemic-inducing pathogen, therefore individual protective measures must be rigorously applied; visitors in therapy rooms or hospital wards should be limited. These high-risk patients, in whom an infection with the pathogen could prove fatal, are advised to observe longer periods of self-isolation; for example, in the UK, the preliminary 'shielding' during the COVID-19 pandemic lasted 12 weeks.

Surgery

In special settings such as surgery (or morgue/autopsy), particular attention must be paid to environment and operator safety, so as to avoid infection spreading. Bearing in mind that a pandemic is often due to a new and unknown pathogen, autopsy investigation assumes great importance: it helps us to understand the pathophysiology better and to address future treatment.

Most elective, non-cancer, and 'non-urgent' operations may need to be postponed in order to prevent transmission and to increase ICU capacity and availability of equipment.

'Cold sites' may need to be considered; for example, in cases where elective procedures are cancelled, specialist centres can act as cold sites for the admission and management of trauma patients, covering a wider catchment area, to free up local hospital ITU capacity. Any trauma patients who would normally present to the local hospitals could be diverted to such sites. This also allows for specialist skills to be grouped into key sites.

Radiology

There may be increased demand for diagnostic imaging during a pandemic, or for complications that arise from an advanced disease; for example, a CT pulmonary angiogram (CTPA) can exclude pulmonary embolism in COVID-19-positive patients. Develop guidelines and pathways that may guide clinicians, paying consideration to the appropriate transfer of infected patients and to the cleaning time of equipment such as CT scanners between investigations.

General practice and out-patients

Given the isolation precautions, many routine medical out-patient appointments may need to be postponed or cancelled. This will be specialty-dependent. Many specialties such as dermatology and psychiatry have adapted to the use telephone or video calls with patients whenever possible.

Telemedicine may replace face-to-face consultation; and the risks of delayed or missed diagnosis, the communication challenges, and the complications related to confidentiality and person-centred care are a challenge

Emergency room and ambulatory care

Routine ambulatory care would be expected to fall, given the reduction in general, 'non-pandemic-related' attendance to the emergency room (ER) in the early stages. There would also be fewer referrals, given the limited access to hospitals. However, caution needs to be exercised and public health warnings need to be made that patients who require emergency care should still seek medical assistance.

Emergency areas will need to adapt the environment so as to separate those who present with risk of infection on screening from those who do not present with symptoms.

Community care homes and palliative care

Special attention needs to be paid to the prevention of transmission in care homes, as per the PHM principles. This includes safe discharge and the risk of transmission to community facilities.

There must be equal and timely access to appropriate PPE and diagnostics.

What do you need to do to be safe?

The milestones of patient safety in a pandemic include the following rules and principles (Box 37.3):

Box 37.3 Key actions to take be safe in a pandemic

Organisation
- preparedness for the possibility of a pandemic;
- policies that can adapt to changing circumstances;
- simulation of the response needed;
- early recognition and declaration of an epidemic or pandemic;
- development and use of a reporting and learning system (quick, informal reporting tools);
- facilitation of effective teamwork and communication;
- enhanced flexibility and resilience;
- promotion of situation awareness.

Tools and technology
- staff protection with dedicated equipment (PPE);
- provision of resources (people and devices) to care for these patients.

Environment
- implementation of safe environments with separation between the uninfected and the infected.

Tasks and processes
- proactive approach to problems;
- implementation of lean and clear policies;
- safety practices targeted to high-risk steps of clinical pathways, patients, and settings.

How do you measure your safety in a pandemic?

How do you measure your safety in a pandemic?

Measurement is essential to understanding how the system is performing. The following divisions are meant to focus on different areas, each one of which has a safety dimension.

Outcome measures for infected individuals

1. hospitalization rate of infected people (indirect outcome measure of out-of-hospital healthcare);
2. in-hospital mortality rate of hospitalized patients;
3. percentage of patients admitted to ICU;
4. survival rates.

The pandemic will have an impact on the delivery of healthcare to the wider population. These are some of the measures to be considered.

Outcome measures for uninfected individuals

1. percentage of non-infected hospitalized patients who acquired an infection during their hospital stay;
2. in-hospital mortality rate of patients not infected and hospitalized for other conditions such as acute myocardial infarction, stroke, or chronic obstructive pulmonary disease (COPD);
3. percentage of the population vaccinated;
4. community data on other common severe conditions (e.g. heart attacks, strokes, trauma, COPD) to ascertain the impact on people who cannot receive care.

The stress and mental well-being of healthcare workers, as well as their risk of infection, are key factors to keep under observation.

Outcome measures for healthcare workers' well-being

1. staff members' infection rate;
2. staff members' mortality rate;
3. staff members' well-being;
4. illness and sickness rates;
5. mental well-being of staff and patients.

These measures indicate activity and how the system is working.

Process measures include:

1. percentage of infected patients admitted to ICU;
2. percentage of infected patients with comorbidities;
3. percentage of staff with and without correct equipment;
4. number of tests performed on hospital staff;
5. number of patients not treated to the appropriate level of care;
6. percentage of the staff trained to use equipment.

Summary box

The best interventions

Plan:

- multidisciplinary task force;

Manage infected individuals or those potentially infected with the pathogen

- triage of patients outside the ER, to differentiate infected and non infected clinical pathways from the beginning;
- early identification of infection in care homes;

Prevent:

- contact tracing and testing campaigns, to identify cases;
- epidemiological studies on the population to include periodic monitoring of the epidemic's evolution;
- vaccination of the population;

Protect healthcare workers:

- provision of PPE in all facilities, especially in community nursing homes and geriatric wards where there are frail elderly patients.

References

Anderson, R. M. et al. How will country-based mitigation measures influence the course of the COVID 19 epidemic? *Lancet* I 395.10228 (2020): 931–40.

Tartaglia, R., Patient safety recommendations for COVID-19 epidemic outbreak. *Global Clinical Engineering Journal* 2.3 (2020). doi: 10.31354/globalce.v2i.94.

Further reading

Clinical Human Factors Group. Key human factors messages when under pressure. ghfg, 30 March 2020. https://chfg.org/key-human-factors-messages-to-support-the-nhs.

Donaldson, L. et al. *Textbook of Clinical Risk Management and Patient Safety*. Springer, 2021.

Holden, R. J. et al. SEIPS 2.0: A human factors framework for studying and improving the work of healthcare professionals and patients. *Ergonomics* 56.11 (2013): 1669–86. https//doi:10.1080/00140139.2013.838643.

La Regina, M. et al. Responding to COVID-19: The experience from Italy and recommendations for management and prevention. *International Journal for Quality in Health Care* 33.1 (2021). https://doi.org/10.1093/intqhc/mzaa057.

Nembhard, I. M., Burns, L. R., and Shortell, S. M. Responding to Covid-19: Lessons from management research. NEJM Catalyst, 17 April 2020. https://catalyst.nejm.org/doi/full/10.1056/CAT.20.0111.

Pandit, M. Critical factors for successful management of VUCA times. *BMJ Leader* 5.2 (2020). doi: 10.1136/leader-2020-000305.

Porta, M. *A Dictionary of Epidemiology*. 6th ed. Oxford: Oxford University Press, 2014.

Seghieri, C. et al. Looking for the right balance between human and economic costs during COVID-19 outbreak. *International Journal for Quality in Health Care* 33.1 (2021). doi: 10.1093/intqhv/mzaa155.

Tartaglia, R. et al. COVID-19 pandemic: International survey of management strategies. *International Journal for Quality in Health Care* 33.1 (2021). doi: 10.1093/intqhc/mzaa139.

WHO. Non-pharmaceutical public health measures for mitigating the risk and impact of epidemic and pandemic influenza. WHO 2019. License: CC BY-NC-SA 3.0 IGO. https://apps.who.int/iris/handle/10665/329439.

WHO. Patient safety. WHO 2021. https://www.who.int/patientsafety/en.

Safety improvement tools

This chapter contains a list of practically useful safety improvement tools applicable in almost all clinical settings. Many of these tools are referenced and demonstrated in other chapters. Tools and resources that are more specific to areas of care or patient groups are contained within those chapters.

Websites with a safety and improvement focus

International

World Health Organization
https://www.who.int/teams/integrated-health-services/patient-safety

OECD
https://www.oecd.org/health/patient-safety.htm

EU Patient Safety
https://www.oecd.org/health/patient-safety.htm

England

Patient Safety Learning
https://www.patientsafetylearning.org/

NHS England Patient Safety Programme
https://www.england.nhs.uk/patient-safety/patient-safety-improvement-programmes/

Northern Ireland

Safety and quality standards
https://www.health-ni.gov.uk/topics/safety-and-quality-standards

Scotland

NHS Scotland Improvement Hub
https://ihub.scot/improvement-resources/

Wales

Patient Safety Wales
https://du.nhs.wales/patient-safety-wales/

Ireland

National Quality and Patient Safety Directorate
https://www.hse.ie/eng/about/who/nqpsd/

USA

Institute for Healthcare Improvement
http://www.ihi.org/
Patient Safety Movement Foundation
https://patientsafetymovement.org

Australia

Clinical Excellence Commission NSW
https://www.cec.health.nsw.gov.au/

Canada

Health Excellence Canada
https://www.healthcareexcellence.ca/

BC Patient Safety and Quality Council
https://bcpsqc.ca/

Improvement and measurement tools

Improvement and measurement tools be obtained from these websites:

NHS England Improvement Tools
https://www.england.nhs.uk/sustainableimprovement/qsir-programme/qsir-tools/

NHS Fundamentals
https://www.england.nhs.uk/sustainableimprovement/improvement-fundamentals/

NHS Horizons
https://horizonsnhs.com/

East London NHS Foundation Trust QI
https://qi.elft.nhs.uk/resources/

Sheffield Microsystems
https://www.sheffieldmca.org.uk/improving-microsystems

NHS Scotland Improvement Tools
https://learn.nes.nhs.scot/741/quality-improvement-zone

Point of Care Foundation
https://www.pointofcarefoundation.org.uk/

HSE Quality toolkit
https://www.hse.ie/eng/about/who/nqpsd/qps-education/quality-improvement-toolkit.html

Patient perspective

International Alliance of Patients' Organizations (IAPO)
https://www.iapo.org.uk/

Patient stories provide a different perspective to the safety and quality of health care and are a valuable source of information.
https://www.patientstories.org.uk/

NHS England Framework for involving patients in patient safety.
https://www.england.nhs.uk/publication/framework-for-involving-patients- in-patient-safety/

Index

Notes Tables, figures, and boxes are indicated by *t*, *f*, and *b* following the page number

D

N

Q

R

Y

Z